Fat and Cholesterol Don't Cause Heart Attacks and Statins Are Not the Solution

A Tribute to Uffe Ravnskov, MD, PhD
and his Establishment of THINCS,
The International Network
of Cholesterol Skeptics

Paul J. Rosch, MD, FACP, Editor

Published by Columbus Publishing Ltd 2016
www.columbuspublishing.co.uk

ISBN 978-1-907797-53-8
ver 20160903

Cover design by Andy Harcombe

Typesetting by Raffaele Bolelli Gallevi

Brand and product names are trademarks or registered trademarks of their respective owners

The information provided in this book should not be construed as personal medical advice or instruction. No action should be taken based solely on the contents of this book.

Readers should consult appropriate health professionals on any matter relating to their health and well-being.

The information and opinions provided here are believed to be accurate and sound and are based on the best judgments of the authors, but readers who fail to consult appropriate health authorities assume the risk of any injuries. Neither the authors nor the publisher can be held responsible or liable for any loss or claim arising from the use, or misuse, of the content of this book.

COLUMBUS PUBLISHING

Acknowledgements

I would like to thank all the authors for their patience and prompt cooperation in finalizing this tribute to Uffe Ravnskov. Special thanks to Andy Harcombe for facilitating its speedy publication and for his expertise and advice during every stage of this process. I am also grateful for Donna Telyczka's assistance with research and administrative assignments.

Paul J. Rosch, MD, Editor

About The Editor

Paul J. Rosch, MA, MD, FACP is Clinical Professor of Medicine and Psychiatry at New York Medical College, Chairman of the Board of The American Institute of Stress and Honorary Vice President of the International Stress Management Association. He did his internship and residency at Johns Hopkins, and has a Workers Compensation subspecialty rating in cardiology, endocrinology and metabolism. In 1993, he began devoting a series of sessions on the fallacies of the lipid and diet-heart hypotheses at the annual Montreux International Congress on Stress that featured leading authorities from all over the world. This was long before the advent of THINCS and he was unaware of Uffe Ravnskov's contributions at the time.

Dr. Rosch is a Fellow and Life Member of The American College of Physicians, and has served as President of the New York State Society of Internal Medicine, President of the Pavlovian Society and Expert Consultant on Stress to the United States Centers for Disease Control. He has been the recipient of numerous honors here and abroad, including the Outstanding Physician's Award of the New York State Medical Society, the Innovation Award of The International Society for the Study of Subtle Energies and Energy Medicine, and The I.M. Sechenov Memorial Medal from The Russian Academy of Medical Sciences.

Contents

Chapter One

Preface: Why And How This Book Was Written

Paul J. Rosch, MD

What Causes Heart Attacks?

If you ask anyone "What causes heart attacks", the vast majority, including physicians, would undoubtedly blame high cholesterol from eating too much fat, or include this along with unavoidable influences like heredity and stress. That's not surprising, since this dietary fat ⇨ elevated cholesterol ⇨ heart attacks scenario has been repeated over and over so many times for the past 70 years, that it has become accepted as gospel. As William James, the father of American psychology noted. *"There's nothing so absurd that if you repeat it often enough, people will believe it."*

But there was apparently nothing absurd about this. It was easy to visualize how fatty foods could elevate blood cholesterol, which was then deposited in arteries where they reduced and ultimately blocked the flow of blood. Animal studies seemed to support this sequence of events and large scale epidemiologic studies in different countries purportedly showed a close correlation between fat consumption and deaths from heart disease, and in some instances, with cholesterol levels. Proponents of this "Diet-Heart" or lipid hypothesis included eminent researchers and physicians who received the Nobel Prize, Lasker and other Awards for their contributions to this theory.

As a result, reducing fat intake, especially saturated fat, has been U.S. policy for the past 35 years. These official guidelines are the basis for determining the foods that will be used in the military, government cafeterias, schools, food assistance programs, industry food formulations, and restaurant recipes, as well as recommendations made by nutritionists and dieticians. And since they were also endorsed by leading authorities and prestigious organizations such as the American Heart Association and the American College of Cardiology, it was assumed that restricting fats would provide cardioprotective and other health benefits. The advent of statins, which allegedly prevented heart disease by lowering cholesterol, appeared to prove the validity of the lipid hypothesis, and statins quickly became the best selling prescription drugs ever.

How Could We Have Been So Wrong For So Long?

The above erroneous beliefs began 100 years ago based on studies showing that feeding rabbits purified cholesterol obtained from egg yolks for two or three months produced lipid laden lesions rich in cholesterol in the aorta and other arteries. However, since rabbits are herbivorous, cholesterol is a foreign substance and blood levels were 4-5 times higher than those seen in humans. More importantly, these results could not be replicated in rodents or carnivorous animals so they were not relevant to humans. In addition, there was little clinical interest in any of the above, since prior to 1920, less than 10% of all U.S. deaths were due to heart disease.

That changed dramatically in the 1950s, when this had escalated to over 30% as an epidemic of heart attacks in middle-aged men was sweeping the U.S. This was also attributed to increased intake of fatty foods by Ancel Keys, after whom the K-rations used by US troops in World War II had been named. He demonstrated an almost straight line relationship between death rates from coronary disease to fatty food consumption in six countries, with Japan having the least and US the most. This was confirmed in his subsequent much larger Seven Countries study that showed heart attack and stroke death rates were also directly related to serum cholesterol levels and that saturated fats were the main culprit.

The problem was that although Keys had data on 22 countries, he cherry picked the seven that best supported his theory. When all the countries were included, there was no fatty diet-heart disease link, and **had he selected Israel, Sweden, Germany and France, he would have concluded that the more saturated fat consumed, the lower the incidence of coronary heart disease.**

Nevertheless, Keys was featured on the cover of the January 13, 1961 issue of *Time magazine*, was referred to in the media as "Mr. Cholesterol", and triumphantly proclaimed, "***No other variable in the mode of life beside the fat calories in the diet is known which shows such a constant relationship to the mortality rate from coronary or degenerative heart disease***".

The tremendous publicity given to his conclusions stimulated numerous attempts to reduce coronary disease by low fat diets. The Anti-Coronary Club Project launched in 1957 compared two groups of middle-aged New York businessmen. One group followed a "Prudent Diet" with corn oil and margarine instead of butter, cold cereal rather than eggs, and chicken and fish instead of beef. A control group ate eggs for breakfast and meat three times per day. The results published a decade later revealed that cholesterol levels of those on the Prudent Diet were slightly lower than the control group eating eggs and meat but there were eight deaths from heart disease compared to none in the high fat control group. In a final effort to prove his point, Keys fed middle-aged men a very high cholesterol diet but found that their blood cholesterol was no different than a control group who consumed less than half as much. Twenty years later, he was forced to admit, "*There's no connection whatsoever between cholesterol in food and cholesterol in blood. And we've known that all along. **Cholesterol in the diet doesn't matter at all unless you happen to be a chicken or a rabbit**.*"

The Framingham Study has had more of an impact on coronary heart disease research than any other epidemiological project. It was initiated by the NIH in 1950 to validate the lipid hypothesis by following 28,000 residents of Framingham, a small manufacturing town near Boston. It allegedly provided the first "solid evidence" that those with high cholesterols were at greater risk for heart attacks and that smoking and hypertension were also "risk factors" that had an additive effect. George Mann was involved early on to develop a nutritional survey to evaluate the effect of diet on cholesterol. An extensive analysis of the results completed by 1960 was never published, possibly because it found that participants had widely varying cholesterol levels and that "*something explains this inter individual variation, **but it is not diet**.*"

William Kannel, Director of the Framingham Study from 1966 to 1979, never referred to this, but told the press that the Framingham results essentially proved that cholesterol was a powerful predictor of heart disease, and coined the term "risk factor". However, 30 years later the researchers found that "**For each 1% mg. drop in cholesterol there was an 11% increase in coronary and total mortality.**"

Although the study showed that a drop in cholesterol was associated with increased coronary deaths, it was cited as supporting the cholesterol-coronary link! What the public read in the joint AHA-NIH 1990 publication, *The Cholesterol Facts*, was, "**The results of the Framingham study indicate that a 1% reduction in cholesterol corresponds to a 2% reduction in CHD risk**", and these words were followed by a reference to the Framingham-paper with the opposite result. It also stated, "The most important overall finding is the emergence of the total cholesterol as a risk factor of CHD in the elderly". No data was presented to support this erroneous claim, since men over 47 with low cholesterol actually had mortality rates greater than those with elevated levels. The real truth about diet and cholesterol finally emerged in a 1992 editorial by William Castelli, who had replaced Kannel as Framingham Director in 1979, as follows:

> *Most of what we know about the effects of diet factors, particularly the saturation of fat and cholesterol on serum lipid parameters, derives from metabolic ward-type studies. Alas, such findings, within a cohort studied over time have been disappointing, indeed the findings have been contradictory. For example, in* **Framingham, Mass, the more saturated fat one ate, the more cholesterol one ate, the more calories one ate, the lower the person's serum cholesterol.**

In a subsequent article Castelli stated that **nearly 75 percent of heart attacks were in people with normal cholesterol levels**. As indicated in the next chapter, a very recent study by Uffe Ravnskov co-authored by 15 physicians and scientists, many of whom have contributed to this book, demonstrated that senior citizens with high LDL-C live the longest.

The Tecumseh Community Health Study followed 2,000 men and women for two decades in an attempt to demonstrate that cholesterol levels were influenced by fat consumption in the previous 24 to 48 hrs. Based on data that included the composition of over 2.700 foods, it concluded that blood cholesterol and triglyceride levels were unrelated to the quality, quantity, or proportions of fat, carbohydrate, or protein consumed. **Those who ate the least amount of saturated fat had the highest blood cholesterol levels**.

The World Health Organization's MONICA epidemiologic project was undoubtedly the largest study ever designed to explore the relationship between risk factors and cardiovascular disease. It began in 1971 as a collaborative effort involving 32 centers in 21 countries that monitored approximately 10 million men and women aged 25-64 for ten years. It thoroughly discredited the saturated fat–heart disease hypothesis. **All the countries in the top eight for fat consumption had lower death rates for heart disease than all of the eight countries that consumed the least fat**.

Such epidemiologic studies cannot disprove the fatty diet –heart disease hypothesis, nor can they prove it, as illustrated by Keys Seven Countries Study. They can only demonstrate whether there is a statistically significant association between the two, which is quite different. The only way to prove cause-effect relationships is a randomized clinical trial comparing the effect of restricting fat with a control group that followed their regular diet. As noted previously, the Prudent Diet study failed to show any such benefits, but it was limited to a relatively small number of middle aged men and there was little monitoring of what they actually ate. What was required were large scale interventional trials, and these have also failed.

The MRFIT (Multiple Risk Factor Intervention Trial) was the largest and most intensive effort to prove the links between diet, cholesterol and heart disease based on Framingham risk factors. Researchers carefully screened over 350,000 men at high risk for heart disease because they had elevated cholesterol, hypertension and smoked cigarettes. From this group, 12,866 healthy men aged 35 to 57 with no history or evidence of heart disease were enrolled in the study and randomly assigned to either an intervention group that received treatment for all risk factors or a control group that received usual care. A 1982 8-year follow-up revealed that cholesterol intake had been cut by 42%, saturated fat consumption by 28%, total calories by 21%, and there had been a significant reduction in hypertension and cigarette smoking in the intervention group, compared to usual care controls. Although there was also a modest fall in serum cholesterol, there was no effect on coronary heart disease and the disappointing conclusion was **"The overall results do not show a beneficial effect on Coronary Heart Disease or total mortality from this multifactor intervention."**

The WHI (Women's Health Initiative) study was established by NIH in 1991 to address the most common causes of death, disability and impaired quality of life in postmenopausal women. This 15-year $625 million project involved 161,808 healthy postmenopausal women followed at 40 clinical centers that included a Dietary Modification interventional trial. It was designed to evaluate the effect of a low-fat and high fruit, vegetable and grain diet on the prevention of heart disease, breast and colorectal cancers. Despite a modest lowering of cholesterol and diastolic blood pressure, there was no reduction in coronary heart disease in the low fat group.

Did Official Low Fat Guidelines Cause Our Obesity And Diabetes Epidemics?

It certainly seems to have been an important influence. Because of the low fat diet mandate, food manufacturers steadily eliminated or reduced fat as much as possible in all of their products. Supermarkets are now loaded with cookies, cakes, ice cream, soups, other canned foods and almost anything edible in order to display a prominent "Low Fat" and/or "No Cholesterol" label. The tacit implication is that you could eat as much of these low fat versions as you wanted because they were safe, or even healthy. However, removing fat detracted from their taste, so large amounts of fructose had to be added to make them appealing, especially for soft drinks. Fructose was subsequently found to have serious long term adverse effects such as developing metabolic syndrome (hypertension, increased abdominal fat, Type 2 diabetes, elevated triglycerides, low HDL) and increased risk of coronary disease. Many low-fat foods have increased amounts of sugar and other high glycemic index refined carbohydrates that promote obesity and diabetes. To improve shelf life, some also include artificial trans fats that also increase risk of coronary disease.

Nevertheless, low fat foods are still advertised as being "heart healthy." A significant portion of the non-profit AHA (American Heart Association) income, which is now close to $800 million/year, comes from its Heart-Check Certification Program that began in 1995. This allowed companies to advertise their products as "heart healthy" by displaying the AHA red heart with a white check mark logo. The first-year fee was $7,500 per product and $4,500 for annual renewals. Certification now costing up to $700,000 has been extended to menus and restaurants, and the 700 or so certified products are in six categories that include different types of "Extra Lean" meat and seafood, certain nuts and grains, fish with a required level of omega-3 fatty acids, etc. Unfortunately, among those still endorsed are chocolate milk, high sugar breakfast cereals, processed meats full of chemicals and preservatives, as well as other products that are anything but healthy.

It is no coincidence that the present obesity epidemic started precisely after these low fat guidelines were first published in 1980. The steady rise in obesity in the U.S. since then can be seen in Figure 1 from the CDC (Centers for Disease Control).

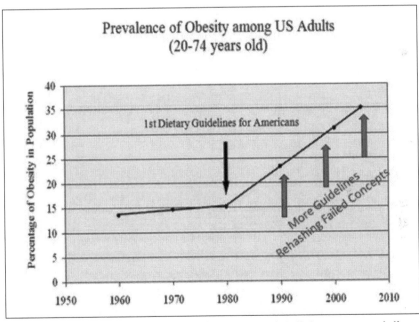

FIGURE 1 **Increase in obesity following 1980 low fat diet recommendations**

Advertising is crafted to be misleading. For instance, Welch's "Healthy Heart" 100 % Grape Juice is a proud recipient of certification, but is sweetened with fructose. An 8-ounce serving contains 36 grams of sugar and 140 calories, about one-third more than the same amount of Coca-Cola. Their Concord Grape Juice Cocktail is only 25% juice and also contains high fructose corn syrup. The Academy of Nutrition and Dietetics, the "world's largest organization of food and nutrition professionals" (formerly the American Dietetic Association or ADA), educates and licenses registered dieticians. Its largest sponsors include over a dozen junk food companies like Coca-Cola, PepsiCo and Mars that provide educational courses claiming that sugar is healthy for children. Coca-Cola spent $3.3 billion on global advertising in 2013 to make people think that all calories are equal, sugared drinks are good for anyone who exercises, celebrity athletes drink them, so you should also. Many ads are targeted to children, who are particularly vulnerable to TV advertising and more apt to crave anything sweet. Coca-Cola advertising increased to an astounding $4.3 billion in 2015 in an attempt to counter growing acknowledgement of its dangerous health effects.

The tragedy is that none of these low cholesterol low fat recommendations had any scientific support. It all began with the 1977 publication "Dietary goals for the United States" by the Select Committee on Nutrition and Human Needs chaired by Senator George McGovern.). The report was written by Nick Mottern, a former labor reporter for *The Providence Journal*, who had no scientific background and no experience writing about science, nutrition, or health. He relied heavily on Mark Hegsted, Professor of Nutrition at Harvard Medical School, who strongly believed that saturated fats from eggs and meat elevated harmful cholesterol levels, in contrast to monosaturated and polyunsaturated fats that might be beneficial. Mottern, a vegetarian, recommended that everyone should limit saturated fat intake to 10% or less, total fat intake should not exceed 30% and carbohydrates should be increased to 60% of daily calories. His report was not well received and there were objections from leading authorities like Rockefeller University's Edward "Pete" Ahrens, and NHLBI Director Robert Levy, both of whom argued that nobody knew if eating less fat or lowering blood cholesterol levels would prevent heart attacks. The American Medical Association warned that the proposed diet raised the "potential for harmful effects" and others described it as a "dangerous public health experiment". Dairy, egg, and cattle industry representatives from farming states, including McGovern's own South Dakota, vigorously opposed the guidelines for other obvious reasons. The McGovern committee was due to expire at the end of 1977, and their report probably would have faded away, but the USDA (United States Department of Agriculture) was anxious to implement their recommendations, since a high carbohydrate-low fat diet would promote the sale of grains.

As a result, in 1980, the USDA and HHS (Health and Human Services) issued their first joint "Dietary Guidelines for Americans", which adopted Mottern's low fat high carbohydrate recommendations. This was the same low fat diet the American Heart Association had previously recommended for middle aged-men men at high risk of heart disease, without any proof that it was effective. A similar diet for everyone in the U.K. was proposed in 1983 but the only basis for this was Keys flawed Seven Countries Study, which stated that coronary heart disease "tended to be related" to serum cholesterol values and that, these in turn "tended to be related" to the proportion of calories provided by saturated fats in the diet.

These USDA and HHS "Dietary Guidelines" are reviewed and revised every five years but despite growing evidence that they were faulty, few changes have been made. The 2010 version claimed that "Lowering the percentage of calories from dietary saturated fatty acids even more, to 7 percent of calories, can further reduce the risk of cardiovascular disease." As in the past, there was no reference to justify this. Moreover, a very recent **thorough meta-analysis of all the relevant randomized clinical trials prior to 1983 found nothing to support any relationship between dietary fat, serum cholesterol and deaths from coronary heart disease**. None of the trials included women and all but one was in middle-aged men with a history of coronary disease, so it was not known how this severe reduction of fat might affect children, women, or men in different age groups. In addition, none of these studies involved restricting saturated and total fat intake to this degree.

The sad fact is that this low fat diet should never have been introduced, and the consequences of this error have been disastrous. As shown in the graph above, only 15% of the population was obese when the low fat guidelines appeared in 1980. This has now increased to 35% in adults, and 17% in children and teenagers. If obesity rates continue on their current trajectories, 50% or more adults could be obese by 2030. And the diet heart idea has even had more catastrophic results.

Why Is There An Epidemic Of Type 2 Diabetes?

Type 2 diabetes was previously called "adult onset diabetes" to distinguish it from childhood, or insulin dependent diabetes. This term has been discarded, as it has been more and more common among adolescents and children, especially Hispanic/Latino and African Americans. It is well established that type 2 diabetes is a frequent complication of obesity, so it is not surprising that the obesity epidemic has been followed by a similar escalation in diabetes. As shown in Figure 2, from 1980 through 2014, the number of Americans with diagnosed diabetes has increased fourfold (from 5.5 million to 22.0 million). 40% of U.S. women and 17% of teenagers are now obese.

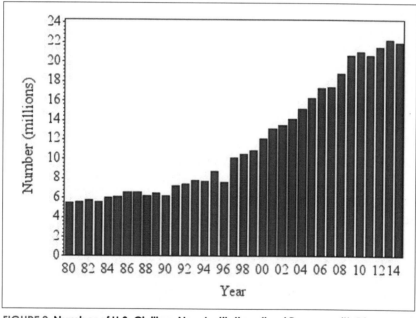

FIGURE 2 **Number of U.S. Civilian, Non-Institutionalized Persons with Diagnosed Diabetes, 1980-2014. (Centers for Disease Control and Prevention, National Center for Health Statistics)**

Type 2 diabetes is a serious condition because of its long-term complications, which include heart disease, stroke, retinopathy, kidney failure and peripheral arterial disease that can lead to amputations.

Why Have The Low Fat And Low Cholesterol Diet Recommendations Persisted?

Although leading authorities pointed out the fallacies and dangers of the diet-heart disease hypothesis and the need to lower cholesterol and LDL as much as possible, they soon found they could not get their views published or funding for their research renewed. One example was George Mann, Professor of Medicine and Biochemistry at Vanderbilt, a renowned nutritionist who was Co-Director of the Framingham Study in the early 1950s. Based on an analysis of the data he came to the conclusion that there was no evidence that higher fat intake or elevated cholesterol increased heart attacks or coronary mortality. His findings were never published since this contradicted what Framingham had been established to approve, and he quit in disgust. He subsequently showed that saturated fat was 66% of total calories for the Maasai in Kenya due to the consumption of large amounts of meat, milk and blood. Yet, heart disease was rare and cholesterol levels were about half those of the average American. In a 1977 *New England Journal of Medicine* editorial entitled "Diet-Heart: End of an Era", Mann documented the lack of relationship between diet and cholesterol levels, the lack of correlation between trends in fat consumption and death rates in the U.S. and the disappointing outcome of the cholesterol lowering trials with clofibrate and niacin. He referred to the American Heart Association and other panelists who had approved the low fat recommendations as "committee men" who essentially rubber stamped everything, and summed the situation up as follows:

The scientific issue was settled by majority votes. Galileo would have flinched. The dietary dogma was a money-maker for segments of the food industry, a fund raiser for the Heart Association, and busy work for thousands of fat chemists... To be a dissenter was to be unfunded because the peer-review system rewards conformity and excludes criticism.

As might be expected, this precipitated an avalanche of criticism from influential organizations, government agencies and their minions, as well as leading cardiologists, all of whom were strong proponents of the lipid hypothesis. Mann was vilified in the press, but these were mostly *ad hominem* attacks rather than any refutation of the supportive evidence he had cited. Although other experts voiced objections similar to Mann's, they were also drowned out by the opposition and had little impact.

What the cholesterol crusaders desperately needed was something to show that lowering cholesterol reduced heart attacks. In 1984, their prayers seem to be answered with the publication of the NIH's LRC-CPPT (Lipid Research Clinics Coronary Primary Prevention Trial) cholestyramine study. Cholestyramine binds to bile acids and since it is not absorbed, it is excreted along with the bile acids and blood cholesterol falls. After three years of screening 480,000 applicants, 3,806 men aged 35-59 with a serum cholesterol over 265 mg/dL and no history of heart disease were recruited. Half were treated with cholestyramine, half received an equally unpleasant tasting placebo and both groups followed a "moderate cholesterol lowering" diet that limited fat intake. It had been predicted that taking cholestyramine daily for seven years would lower LDL cholesterol by 28% and result in a 50% reduction in significant coronary events. At the end of the study, although there was only an 8% fall in total cholesterol and a 12% drop in LDL the sponsors triumphantly claimed a 19% reduction in risk for coronary events in the cholestyramine group. This allowed Basil Rifkind, the director, to claim *"for each 1% reduction in cholesterol, we can expect a 2% reduction in CHD events"*, *implying a causal relationship rather than a statistical association.* The statement was widely circulated in the media, even though it was not valid, since a subsequent review of the data found no difference in CHD events between the two groups. More importantly, 19% was a relative risk reduction. The absolute or actual risk reduction was 1.1% for all coronary events, and for fatal heart attacks, it was only 0.6% and without statistical significance, because the authors had used the one-sided t-test, an incorrect statistical method.

In addition, the cholestyramine study dealt mainly with individuals with familial hypercholesterolemia, a lipid disorder affecting fewer than one in five hundred. It was uncertain that lowering cholesterol would be beneficial for men in other age groups or women of any age, or whether cholestyramine would be safe, or even tolerated. Some men stopped taking the foul tasting four or five packets of cholestyramine after a few days, and many complained of severe constipation and other gastrointestinal complaints due to the lack of bile acids. Most were unable to take the full 24 grams daily, so that relatively few stayed on the required regimen for seven years. With respect to safety, cholestyramine interferes with the absorption of fat-soluble vitamins and numerous common drugs, including Coumadin, Digoxin, Inderal phenobarbital, thiazide diuretics and thyroid. As indicated, there was no statistically significant difference in heart attacks between the two groups and their overall mortality rates were essentially the same. However, there were more deaths from cancer, intestinal disease, stroke, violence and suicide in the cholestyramine group. Little mention was made of this, or the 21 cases and 8 deaths from gastrointestinal cancer in those taking the drug, compared to 11 cases and only 1 death in the control group.

There was so much criticism of this trial that an NIH-sponsored National Cholesterol Consensus Conference was assembled in late 1984 to evaluate the numerous complaints. Although dissenters were allowed to speak briefly, their comments were not included in the final report, which had apparently been prepared in advance with a few blanks to fill in numbers. One of these was 200 mg/dl to indicate that anyone with a cholesterol over this was "at risk", when everyone had previously agreed that the upper limit of normal was 240 mg/dL Prior to that it had been 280 mg/dL and this new arbitrary reduction would put most adult Americans "at risk". The major conclusion of the NIH Consensus Panel published in the *Journal of the American Medical Association* that was widely referred, to was, "**It has been established beyond a reasonable doubt that lowering definitely elevated blood cholesterol levels (specifically, blood levels of low density [LDL] cholesterol) will reduce the risk of heart attacks caused by coronary heart disease.**"

Although the LCR-CPPT was a drug, rather than a diet trial, the investigators and their sponsors made the unwarranted claim that if lowering cholesterol with a medication could prevent heart disease, lowering cholesterol by reducing fat intake would have the same result. This led to an enormous public relations campaign to convince the public as well as physicians that avoiding dietary fat was crucial to prevent and treat coronary disease. The NCEP (National Cholesterol Education Program) was established under the auspices of NHLBI (National Heart, Blood, and Lung Institute) to meet on a recurring basis, review pertinent scientific research and make recommendations about ways to reduce coronary disease. A large "Physicians Kit" was sent to all doctors in America, compiled in part by the American Pharmaceutical Association, whose representatives served on the NCEP coordinating committee. It emphasized the importance of cholesterol screening, the advantages of cholesterol-lowering drugs, the unique benefits of the Prudent Diet and the use of margarine rather than butter. September was designated National Cholesterol Education Month, during which everyone is urged to have their blood cholesterol and other lipids checked and to take steps to correct any abnormalities. These activities were promoted by NIH, NCEP, AHA, USDA, numerous other medical organizations and low fat food manufacturers in an unprecedented, massive advertising blitz.

Manipulating Data, Dirty Tricks And Deceptive Advertising

This evoked even more criticism, that now included some previous lipid hypothesis proponents, like Michael Oliver, who first showed that coronary heart disease patients were more likely to have abnormal levels of blood lipids than matched controls. In a Nutrition Today editorial, George Mann again summed things up:

Saturated fat and cholesterol in the diet are not the cause of coronary heart disease. **That myth is the greatest scientific deception of this century, perhaps of any century.** *The diet-heart hypothesis has been repeatedly shown to be wrong, and yet, for complicated reasons of pride, profit and prejudice, the hypothesis continues to be exploited by scientists, fund-raising enterprises, food companies and even governmental agencies.* **The public is being deceived by the greatest health scam of the century.**....*They have held repeated press conferences bragging about this cataclysmic break-through which the study directors claim shows that lowering cholesterol lowers the frequency of coronary disease. They have manipulated the data or reached the wrong conclusion....The managers at NIH have used Madison Avenue hype to sell this failed trial in the way the media people sell an underarm deodorant.*

This and numerous other complaints were drowned out by the propaganda promulgated by the cholesterol cartel of manufacturers of low fat foods, cholesterol lowering drugs, lipid testing equipment and other vested interests. In addition, anyone who jeopardized their lucrative profits was swiftly and severely punished.

For example, Mann was determined to bring this issue before the public by organizing a conference of leading authorities who supported his views in Washington, D.C. In his invitation, he wrote, "Hundreds of millions of tax dollars are wasted by the bureaucracy and the self-interested Heart Association.... Segments of the food industry play the game for profits. Research on the true causes and prevention is stifled by denying funding to the 'unbelievers'. This meeting will review the data and expose the rascals." When the cholesterol cartel, or "Heart Mafia" as Mann called them, learned about this, they sent out false press releases to speakers and other invitees that the conference had been canceled. Speakers were also phoned and warned that their funding would be canceled or their academic status would suffer if they participated in such an event. Many backed out and the Greenwall Foundation, which had promised to fund this event, also reneged. Mann eventually funded the conference himself, but there were only half- dozen or so speakers, and he told the audience:

*You will see that many of our contributors are senior scientists. They are so for a reason that has become painfully conspicuous as we organized this meeting. Scientists who must go before review panels for their research funding know well that to speak out, to disagree with this false dogma of Diet/Heart, is a fatal error. They must comply or go unfunded. I could show a list of scientists who said to me, in effect, when I invited them to participate: 'I believe you are right, that the Diet/ Heart hypothesis is wrong, but I cannot join you because that would jeopardize my perks and funding.' For me, that kind of hypocritical response separates the scientists from the operators, the men from the boys...Those who manipulate data do not appreciate that understanding the nature of things cannot be permanently distorted – the true explanations cannot be permanently ignored. Inexorably, truth is revealed and deception is exposed.... **In due time truth will come out**. This is the relieving grace in this sorry sequence.*

Kilmer McCully's discovery of the contribution of homocysteine to coronary heart disease suggesting that it could be more important than cholesterol and might be easily prevented by inexpensive B vitamins, also brought swift and vicious retaliation. Funding for research disappeared leading to the loss of his laboratory at

Massachusetts General Hospital. The hospital Director told him to leave and "never to come back" and his Harvard affiliation and tenure were also terminated in 1978. When subsequently interviewed about his research on a TV program, he promptly received a phone call from the Public Affairs Director of the hospital who told him to "shut up" and that "they didn't want the names of Harvard and Massachusetts General Hospital to be associated with my theories." Although obviously well qualified for many positions that were being offered, and despite the fact that he did well on numerous interviews, he was unable to find employment for two years.

When McCully and those who had recommended him made appropriate follow-up inquiries they ran into a stone wall of silence. However, repeated rumors of "poison phone calls" from Harvard began to surface and it was only after a leading Boston attorney threatened a lawsuit that things suddenly changed, and despite previous rejections, he was able to resume his research at the Veterans Administration Hospital in Providence, Rhode Island. Since then, the association between elevated homocysteine and heart attacks, stroke, and accelerated atherosclerosis has been repeatedly confirmed, as well as links to other disorders.

Uffe Ravnskov's book *The Cholesterol Myths* was actually burned on a 1992 Finnish television show because it was a scathing and devastating indictment of the numerous flaws in the lipid hypothesis. Since none of the well documented claims could be refuted, critics resorted to this medieval practice to retaliate. Although Uffe escaped being burned at the stake, his e-mail was later hacked and "spoofed" and he has been harassed in other ways.

Other examples of skullduggery, dirty tricks and deceptive practices could be cited, especially with respect to the safety and efficacy of statins. Cholesterol proponents proclaimed they had now proven their claims with the November 19, 1994 *Lancet* publication of the Scandinavian Simvastatin Survival Study, often referred to as the 4S study. It involved assessing the effect of simvastatin on morbidity and mortality in 4,444 heart attack patients aged 35-70 with elevated cholesterol levels. Half were treated with simvastatin (Zocor) and half with a placebo. At the end of 5.4 years, LDL had been lowered by 35%, cholesterol by 25%, and only 5% in the treated group had died from a heart attack, compared to 8.5% of the placebo controls.

The reduction in nonfatal heart attacks was even more impressive, 15.9% vs. 22.6% in controls and for strokes, it was 2.7% compared to 4.3% for controls. Unlike previous cholesterol lowering drug trials, there was no apparent increase in adverse side effects. Michael Oliver, a leading authority, urged physicians in the *British Medical Journal*, "*Lower patients' cholesterol now! There is no longer any doubt about the benefit and safety of treating hypercholesterolemia in patients who have had a myocardial infarction.*"

The fact is that none of the subsequent statin trials showed similar rewards in patients with a history of heart disease. None of them has succeeded in lowering mortality by more than 2 % and only for patients with previous cardiovascular disease. No trial has succeeded in lowering mortality in people without heart diseases, in women or in senior citizens, so why prescribe them for everyone or put them in the drinking water as some enthusiasts had suggested.

However, as documented in the following chapters data are manipulated in company sponsored drug trials in order to conceal or minimize the adverse side effects of statins or exaggerate their benefits. The results were often presented to physicians in a similarly deceptive fashion as were television and media advertisements to the public. For example, the 42% reduction in risk of cardiac death in the simvastatin study was relative risk, whereas the absolute risk reduction was only 3.5%. The TV commercials for atorvastin (Lipitor) featuring Dr. Robert Jarvik, identified him as the inventor of the artificial heart. Jarvik tells viewers that as a cardiologist, he takes Lipitor and prescribes it for family members. He is shown vigorously and adroitly sculling a boat over a serene lake into the sunset as proof that Lipitor has kept his heart in excellent shape. The facts are that Jarvik is not a cardiologist and could not prescribe anything since he does not even have a medical license. He had no experience sculling and the muscular frame viewers saw rowing away was that of a stunt double who was an expert sculler. Although he made some subsequent revisions, he did not invent the artificial heart and there is no indication that he took Lipitor prior to the guaranteed $1.35 million for serving as pitchman. Pfizer withdrew the ad following a Congressional investigation, but it continued to merchandize Lipitor with some $250 million a year in commercials that generated $11 billion a year in sales, more than any other pharmaceutical in history.

The Relative Risk, LDL "Bad Cholesterol" and HDL "Good Cholesterol" Fiascos

Lipitor print ads featuring Jarvik persisted, such as this *New York Times* commercial "In patients with multiple risk factors for heart disease, LIPITOR REDUCES RISK OF HEART ATTACK BY 36%. * But 36% of what? The asterisk explains this in mice type at the bottom of the page as follows: "That means in a large clinical study, 3% of patients taking a sugar pill or placebo had a heart attack compared to 2% of patients taking Lipitor." The 36% was relative risk and the absolute risk reduction of only 1% was not mentioned. **In other words, if you take Lipitor daily for years, your risk of having a heart attack drops 1%, and this is only if you have risk factors such as family history, high blood pressure, age, low HDL ("good" cholesterol) or smoking**. Another Jarvik/Lipitor Times ad proclaims: "In patients with type 2 diabetes, LIPITOR REDUCES RISK OF STROKE BY 48%* In this instance, the asterisk refers to the following mice type explanation, "That means in a large clinical study, 2.8% of patients taking a sugar pill or placebo had a stroke compared to 1.5% of patients taking Lipitor." The absolute risk reduction here is 1.3% and this is also only in patients at increased risk due to other influences. The fact is that statins increase risk of developing diabetes, and not only do not prevent strokes, but can actually increase those due to bleeding.

The problem here is that lowering cholesterol or LDL ("bad cholesterol) has been accepted as a surrogate for preventing heart attacks, even though this has never been proven. In addition, when most people read that Lipitor reduces risk of stroke by 48%, they think this means it will cut the likelihood of a stroke almost in half. No association between cholesterol levels and the degree of atherosclerosis has ever been found in postmortem studies of the general population, and no clinical or imaging study has found any relation between the degree of cholesterol lowering and improvement. **In one angiography study in which blood cholesterol had been reduced by more than 25% in 26 patients, atherosclerosis was increased in 18 and unchanged in the remainder**. No correlation has ever been found between cholesterol levels and the degree of coronary calcification or peripheral atherosclerosis. High cholesterol does not increase risk for heart attacks in people older than 60, healthy women of any age, nor in patients with diabetes or renal failure. Senior citizens with high cholesterols are protected against cancer, have significantly fewer infections and live longer than low cholesterol controls. At least half of heart attack patients do not have elevated levels of cholesterol or LDL and two studies found that cholesterol and LDL were lower than normal in those admitted for acute myocardial infarction. In one of these in which patients were followed for 3 years, mortality was highest among those with the lowest cholesterols. In familial hypercholesterolemia, there is no correlation between the very high cholesterol (1,000 or more) and LDL levels (over 250) and any increased incidence or severity of coronary disease.

As the insignificance of cholesterol as a cause of coronary atherosclerosis became increasingly obvious, emphasis shifted to LDL as the culprit. This had its origin in the 1984 statement, "*The more LDL there is in the blood, the more rapidly atherosclerosis develops*" by Nobel Laureates Michael Brown and Joseph Goldstein. Nevertheless, the vast majority of statin studies do not show that the degree of atherosclerosis or its severity is related to either LDL levels or the magnitude of their reduction with statins. Lowering LDL "bad cholesterol" as much as possible does not prevent heart attacks in healthy people. Adding ezetimibe, which blocks absorption of cholesterol to simvastatin, resulted in a greater lowering of cholesterol, triglycerides and LDL and significantly raised HDL. However, it showed no reduction in coronary events or mortality and was associated with a possible increase in cancer. Clinical trials of torcetrapib, a drug that raised HDL "good cholesterol" had to be stopped because of an increase in cardiac death rates and hypertension.

But things may be much more complicated, since particle size may determine whether LDL might be good and HDL might be "bad". Light and fluffy LDL particles actually appear to be associated with a lower risk of heart disease, probably because, as documented by Ravnskov and McCully, they participate in the immune system. Furthermore, as indicated previously, elevating HDL with drugs actually increased cardiac mortality and some individuals with very high HDL also have increased atherosclerosis. A recent study suggests that this paradox is due to a genetic defect that produces an excess of large HDL particles that are harmful. Thus, **we now have to contend with bad LDL that is good, and good HDL that is bad**.

Truth Will Out And The Times They Are A Changin, But Is It Too Little, Too Late?

There may be some light at the end of the tunnel, since as Shakespeare noted and George Mann predicted, "truth will out". Faced with overwhelming evidence that a high fat diet did not cause heart attacks, the latest official guidelines finally acknowledge that "cholesterol is not a nutrient of concern for overconsumption", although saturated fat is still limited. And the most recent American College of Cardiology and American Heart Association guidelines have abandoned lowering LDL and cholesterol as much as possible as the goal of statin therapy, since any benefits are unrelated to their concentrations. On the other hand, none of these changes will decrease statin sales since the new recommendations are to treat individuals at high risk rather than high cholesterol. This would include everyone with existing heart disease, an LDL of 190 mg/dL or higher and all type 2 diabetics between 40 and 75 years of age regardless of LDL or cholesterol levels. In addition, anyone aged 40 to 75 with a 10-year risk of heart disease that is 7.5 percent or higher using a risk calculator with arbitrary values based on age, gender, race, cholesterol, HDL, blood pressure and smoking. **As a result, 13 million more Americans will now be eligible for statins, including 97% of senior citizens, despite evidence that this would do more harm than good**, as will be seen in the next chapters. Almost 20% of patients experience statin side effects, and although the vast majority stop taking them, it may be too little and too late for some. A recent study of physically active healthy people who took statins for 90 to 365 days reported that their **risk of developing diabetes and diabetic complications doubled over the next five years compared to controls**. Short term statin use was not associated with any decrease in cardiovascular events, so for healthy people in particular, statins can do more harm than good, especially since type 2 diabetes is a significant risk factor for heart disease.

It would appear that the lipid hypothesis will continue to persist and prevail as long as it remains profitable for statin and low fat food manufacturers and other vested interests. A good example of this are the recently approved PCSK9 inhibitors, Sanofi-Regeneron's Praluent (alirocumab) and Amgen's Repatha (evolocumab). These monoclonal antibodies, which lower LDL by helping the liver to remove it, are indicated for the treatment of heterozygous familial hypercholesterolemia and heart attack and stroke patients who have not been able to lower LDL to satisfactory levels despite maximal statin dosage. The drugs are given by injection every two weeks, or in some cases once a month and were initially projected to cost over $14,000/year, although this may have changed. They are covered by most insurance and Medicare plans but co-payments can vary. The competition is so keen that Sanofi-Regeneron paid $67.5 million to speed up approval of Praluent so that it would be available before Repatha. Both drugs are given as **an adjunct to diet and maximal statin dosage**. No significant adverse effects have been noted but there are no long term follow-up studies, and some clinical trials have shown that neurocognitive side effects are double those in controls, but this is only a 1% absolute risk increase.

The issue here is that these drugs have been approved solely on the basis of their ability to lower LDL rather than reduce or prevent coronary events or mortality, This, despite the fact that lowering LDL or cholesterol as much as possible has been abandoned as a goal of statin therapy. Praluent's hook phrase is "the fall of high cholesterol" and 2-page ads in *Time* and *People* magazines explain that "When diet and the highest tolerated dose of statin are not enough, PRALUENT will make it PLUNGE". It shows a happy middle-aged male whose LDL dropped from 126 to 68. The ad does include in tiny print the following sentence " The effect of Praluent on heart problems such as heart attacks, stroke, or death is not known." This means that patients who had stopped statins because they failed to reduce LDL sufficiently, will be encouraged to resume maximum tolerable doses along with with Praluent injections, even though there is no evidence this will provide any cardiovascular benefits. In addition, once a drug is approved by the FDA as being safe and effective for a specific indication, it can be prescribed for any condition if a physician feels it could be beneficial. It has already been suggested that Praluent should be useful in myocardial infarction and acute coronary syndromes and the 18,000 patient ODYSSEY trial may determine this when the results are released in 2017. As with Humira (adalimumab) and other therapeutic monoclonal antibodies, resistance may develop or there can be adverse immune system responses. Nevertheless, more drugs are in the pipeline. Pfizer's PCSK9 inhibitor, bococizumab has already completed two phase 3 trials showing that is superior to a placebo for lowering LDL, including patients taking statins.

CETP (cholesterol ester transfer) inhibitors, which increase HDL and lower LDL have not lived up to expectations., Lilly's 12,000-patient phase 3 trial with evacetrapib was suddenly halted last October since it showed no reduction in rates of heart attack, stroke, or cardiovascular disease, despite positive effects on lipid levels. Prior to that, Pfizer's $800 million torcetrapib study was discontinued because of increased death rates in the treatment group. Nevertheless, Merck's anacetrapib, which raises HDL and lowers LDL, may be approved in 2017 if there are no safety concerns, regardless of whether it provides cardioprotective benefits.

Why And How This eBook Was Assembled To Honor Uffe Ravnskov And THINCS

In 2014, I was invited by the senior editor of *Expert Review of Clinical Pharmacology* to serve as Guest Editor for their March 2015 special focus issue. These deal with important or controversial issues and generally consist of 7-9 review articles (5000 to 7000 words) and 1 or 2 Editorials (up to 1500 words). The topic I selected was the lipid hypothesis of coronary heart disease, which was not only important but extremely controversial. I had devoted several days to exposing its flaws at the annual International Congress on Stress in Switzerland 2 decades earlier that included George Mann, Bill Stehbens, "Pete" Ahrens, Ray Rosenman, Stewart Wolf and other critical luminaries. The subsequent 2000 publication of Uffe Ravnskov's *The Cholesterol Myths* in English had exposed and convincingly documented numerous additional fallacies. He had also established THINCS (The International Network of Cholesterol Skeptics), which grew to include 100 physicians, scientists and others who opposed the entrenched fatty food and cholesterol cause of heart disease dogma. It was a challenge to draw up a Table of Contents since there was such an embarrassment of riches and so many important facets of this topic that it was difficult to cover everything in the limited space available. I explained this and the editor agreed that I could choose my own format as long as I did not exceed the 80,000-word count limit. My tentative title for this special focus issue was "Why Cholesterol And Lipids Don't Cause Coronary Heart Disease And Statins Are Not The Solution." In addition, it was designed to honor Uffe Ravnskov for his seminal efforts in demonstrating these claims and for his establishment of THINCS, The International Network of Cholesterol Skeptics.

I had an enthusiastic response and in October 2015, submitted 12 papers for peer review. Both the editor and I thought these were of high quality, and were surprised that even after being revised to satisfy peer reviewer concerns, only three were accepted. I attributed this to bias and in some cases ignorance. Fred Kummerow had "too many self-references" despite the fact that he has written extensively about the dangers of trans fats for over 50 years and finally sued the FDA successfully for failure to warn consumers and physicians about this. Others who had previously published papers on their topics were accused of self-plagiarism, an oxymoron, and I was severely reprimanded for questioning the conclusions of Ancel Key's flawed Seven Countries study. Beatrice Golomb's state of the art contribution on what the new recommendations should be for statin therapy had "too many references" and Duane Graveline's account of his global amnesia experience and the thousands of confirmations he received from others about memory loss and neurocognitive statin side effects was anecdotal, not supported by references, and had an excessive number of first person sentences. Even though most of the above authors, as well as Zoe Harcombe, Luca Mascitelli, Mark Goldstein, Uffe Ravnskov and I repeatedly responded to peer review criticisms and suggestions, our revisions were rejected.

The editor explained that she had to abide by the peer review decisions and was obligated to notify the authors of the three satisfactory papers that these could be published in their regular March 2015 issue. She asked if I had any objection to this, since it would no longer have a special focus edition dedicated to Uffe as we had previously agreed. I saw no reason to refuse this request, and these papers apparently attracted more media attention over the next month than this journal usually receives in a year. I was anxious to see the other papers published and an eBook appeared to be the most rapid and cost effective way to disseminate this information.

Most required only minimal revisions to be updated and since there were no space limitations, additional authorities could be invited to participate in this tribute to Uffe. In addition, all income from this eBook will go to defray the expenses of maintaining and expanding the THINCS website. Uffe has funded and performed all these duties since its inception but no longer has the time to devote to this. Fortunately, Andy Harcombe of Columbus Publishing has graciously agreed to take on this additional responsibility.

Authors prefer journals, since books are not indexed in Medline, PubMed or Embase and two of the original group decided to take this route. However, books, and especially eBooks, are increasingly accessible on search engines. Many find that Google retrieves pertinent information more rapidly than a Medline search, and that it is often more comprehensive and up to date. This is especially true when abstracts and keywords are prominently displayed on web sites. We plan to post these on the THINCS and as many other web sites as possible, along with a copy of the Table of Contents and and information on how to obtain the eBook book at a very nominal fee. Another advantage of this is that eBook chapters can be periodically updated to include important new information that is pertinent. The following chapter outlines his numerous contributions, including establishing THINCS, and may help explain why this book has been dedicated to Uffe Ravnskov, MD, PhD.

Paul J. Rosch, MD

Editor
Clinical Professor of Medicine and Psychiatry
New York Medical College
Chairman, The American Institute of Stress
stress124@optonline.net

Chapter Two

On The Origin And Evolution Of THINCS
An interview with Uffe Ravnskov, MD, PhD

Paul J. Rosch, MD

As noted in my Preface, many scientist and physicians, including eminent authorities, have criticized the lipid hypothesis of coronary heart disease. Dr. George Mann, an early Co-Director of the Framingham Study and Professor of Medicine and Biochemistry at Vanderbilt University called it "the greatest scientific deception of this century, perhaps of any century." However, nobody has done more to expose the flaws and dangers of this scam than Uffe Ravnskov, MD, PhD, and members of THINCS (The International Network of Cholesterol Skeptics), an organization he created in 2001. What is particularly noteworthy is that he had no particular background or expertise in nutrition or cholesterol metabolism when he began his investigations and has personally funded this campaign for the past 15 years. I was curious as to why he embarked on this and since I thought this might also be of interest to others, decided to explore this further in the following interview.

PJR: My recollection is it was shortly after receiving your MD from the University of Copenhagen in 1961 that you first became aware of the cholesterol theory of atherosclerosis. You subsequently developed an interest in Internal Medicine and Nephrology, obtained a PhD from the University of Lund in 1973, and entered into private practice in 1980. What was it that made you dispute the role of cholesterol and saturated fat in the pathogenesis of heart disease?

UR: You are right that I heard about the cholesterol hypothesis already in 1961, but I was confident that more wise researchers should show that this idea was without any evidence. Unfortunately I was wrong, but it took more than 25 years before I started my research about this issue. I wanted to become a general practitioner, and I therefore started by working on various types of clinics in Denmark and Sweden in the sixties. At the medical department of a small country hospital in Sandviken, Sweden, two of our patients suffered from postmyocardial infarction syndrome (PMIS), which at that time was treated with cortisone. Both of them died later on, and at the autopsy I found that both of them had a small aneurysm of the heart. I was convinced that two rare phenomena in the same patient couldn't be an accident, and when I sought the literature in the nearby University library I found about a dozen case reports of PMIS. Most of the authors noted in passing the presence of a heart aneurysm, but nothing was mentioned about it in the discussion sections or in the abstracts. Therefore I wrote a paper, where I referred to these papers and warned against treating PMIS with cortisone, because I thought this was what had caused the aneurysm.[1]

I was proud as a pope having published a scientific paper from a small hospital without assistance from my superior. I asked myself if I should devote myself to research instead. About the same time I treated a patient with acute renal failure with peritoneal dialysis, a new method at that time. That the patient survived and regained normal renal function started my interest in nephrology, and half a year later I obtained a temporary job in the Department of Nephrology at the University Hospital in Lund.

The academic level was not impressive in that department, so after some time I moved to the Department of Clinical Chemistry. Assisted by my supervisor Bengt G. Johansson, who was an expert in immune electrophoresis, I published several papers about proteinuria and introduced the albumin/creatinine clearance ratio as a more exact way to measure degree of albuminuria.[2]

When the professor at the nephrologic department retired, I went back. At that time Stephen Zimmerman and his co-workers had published a study of patients with glomerulonephritis (GN) and chronic renal failure, which showed that most of them had been exposed to toxic chemicals, most often hydrocarbons.[3] I became curious, because it is well known that hydrocarbons are tubulotoxic, and in my previous studies I had shown that low-molecular-weight

(LMW) proteins are filtered by the glomeruli and reabsorbed by the tubules, and also that in GN there was a strong, inverse association between LMW proteinuria and glomerular function.[4,5] I realized that tubular damage must be an important factor when renal failure appears in patients with GN.

My first publication in this area was a study of 15 patients with acute poststreptococcal GN. Ten of them had been exposed to organic solvents, either regularly on their work or acutely between the tonsillitis and the start of the GN. One year later renal failure was only present among those who had continued their exposure. I also interviewed 15 patients of the same age and sex, who had had an infection with the same streptococcal type without developing a GN. None of them had an occupation with exposure to solvents or had been exposed during the infection.

My finding was of course highly controversial because all experts "knew" (and still "know") that GN is caused by immunologic damage of the glomeruli, and whereas all my previous papers had been accepted directly, this paper, which I sent to a kidney journal, was rejected after six months without any comments. A referee on *Acta Medica Scandinavica* rejected it as well, but after having corresponded with the editor, it became accepted.[6]

I organized a research group that included experts from Lund, Malmö and Copenhagen in medicine, immunology, pathology and occupational medicine. Occupational hygienists interviewed 150 patients with glomerulonephritis and we got a similar result as that of Zimmerman et al. and our lengthy report was accepted for publication in the *Quarterly Journal of Medicine*. But a serious problem occurred.

Two years before we submitted the paper I discovered that one of my clinical co-workers had falsified a paper, which was going to be included in his doctoral thesis. I tried to stop his dissertation by criticizing it in public, but in vain.

PJR: Why did you do it in public?

UR: Because of my bad manners. As a child I was never told how to behave. My mother wasn't interested in her children, and my father, who rarely was at home, died when I was 8 year old, so I had to learn everything by myself. Perhaps it also explains my disrespect for authorities. What I hadn't learned at that time was, that whistleblowers are not welcome in the academic world.

Shortly afterwards the new professor arrived to our department. She was a good friend with the supervisor of my fraudulent colleague and had cooperated with him for many years previously at the university hospital in Gothenburg. When we had submitted our report, she found some careless mistakes in the text. I asked *QJM* to wait with the publication until we had corrected the errors, but this was not enough. Although the corrections had no influence on the results, the professor accused me for fraud and asked me to leave the department. If not, she would downgrade me and prohibit my research. I found it intolerable and opened therefore a private praxis in Lund in 1980.

PJR: Why didn't you seek employment at another university?

UR: Because she had told most of the Scandinavian professors in nephrology that I was fraudulent. However, I continued my research in nephrology. Totally I succeeded in publishing 20 papers about glomerulonephritis as a private practitioner. What I found was that glomerulonephritis is just as innocent as flu, unless the patient is exposed to tubulotoxic chemicals or drugs. However, according to the general view renal failure in GN is caused by immunological processes in the glomeruli, because numerous animal experiments have succeeded in producing GN with renal failure by injections of various microorganisms or other immunoreactants. What nobody seem to have understood is, that it cannot be produced unless the antigens are mixed with Freund's adjuvant, a tubulotoxic oil mixture, that is able to produce GN by itself.

One of my papers was published in *The Lancet* in cooperation with a statistician and Åke Nordén, professor in general medicine in Lund. We had compared the number of occupations where exposure to organic solvents was unavoidable or likely in the general population and among our patients with GN, and found that it was much more common among the latter.[7] You can read a review of my research about GN on www.ravnskov.nu/GN.

Shortly after the publication of our *Lancet* paper, the subeditor David Sharp told me that my professor had sent a letter in which she claimed that all my papers about GN were fraudulent. I suggested him to ask her about the evidence. He had already done that, but as she had refused, her letter was rejected. Instead she published it in *Acta Medica Scandinavica*, whose editor was a good friend of her. Therefore I asked David Sharp to publish it in *The Lancet* as well together with a short answer from me.[8] I also sent my answer to *Acta Medica Scandinavica*, but whereas her letter was presented with a marked heading; my answer was published half a year later with no heading at all.

PJR: Didn't you react in some way?

UR: Yes of course. I contacted the dean of the medical faculty in Lund and asked him to let neutral experts analyze her accusations. Instead he asked the professor to select two researchers herself and she chose of course two friends of her. One of them was professor in psychology; the other one in nephrology but without any experience about glomerulonephritis or occupational medicine. I sent the dean a protest, but he didn't respond.

Without giving me an opportunity to respond, their first report was sent to a large number of colleagues including the head of the university, who immediately sent a letter back to all of them that he would retract my docent title (assistant professor). However, it was easy for me to show that their criticism was unfounded. A few weeks afterwards the dean and the vice dean came to my practice with many excuses and I kept my docent title as well. What I should have done was of course to sue her for slander, because she had sent her accusations to a large number of international colleagues as well, but at that time I didn't know that.

Another issue of my research was urinary tract infection. I tried for several years to tell Swedish doctors that a lower urinary tract infection in women is an innocent disease, which never result in renal failure, unless the patient has malformations or other defects of the urinary tract, and that more than 50 studies had shown that it could be cured by only three days treatment and even by a single dose of an antibiotic.[9] At that time everybody "knew" that a urinary infection might progress to pyelonephritis and renal failure. Consequently many patients were prescribed antibiotics to use for several months or years.

One of my own observations as a practitioner was, that the main cause of dysuria is soap, not bacteria. Among 31 of my female patients with dysuria, 29 used soap to wash their sexual organs, whereas among 19 women with asymptomatic bacteriuria 13 never used soap and four used it only once a week. I have never got such a strong statistical confirmation in my research – the p-value was <0.000001.[10]

PJR: How did you become interested in the cholesterol hypothesis?

UR: When the cholesterol campaign started in Sweden in the eighties I became much surprised. I had followed the literature about cholesterol superficially, but had never seen anything in support. I became curious. Were the cholesterol researchers just as unwilling to listen to critical voices?

Several researchers had already documented that the cholesterol hypothesis was without scientific support. According to George Mann the villains were the drug and vegetable oil industries, the American Heart Association and the National Institutes of Health. I met him when we organized a meeting in Finland together with several skeptical Scandinavian researchers. He told us that he had been a member of the Framingham research group, but he left it when he realized that they didn't publish results that contradicted the diet-heart idea.

When I started reading the scientific literature about cholesterol I realized that most of the authors were just as blindfolded as those in the area of GN. I have learned that it is easy to publish correctly performed studies as long as they are in line with the accepted dogmas, but it becomes very difficult if they aren't. Consequently most of my papers about GN have been published in non-nephrological journals and I experienced that the same rules were present in the cholesterol field. When I sent a review where I pointed to the many contradictory findings, it was rejected by half a dozen medical journals before it was accepted in *Medical Hypotheses*.[11]

What I also discovered was that many authors who hail the cholesterol hypothesis deliberately mislead their readers. To demonstrate it I checked how the authors of three, major authoritative reviews had referred to the literature. I was shocked. To cite part of the abstract of a paper I published about that issue:

"Only two of twelve groups of controversial papers were quoted correctly, and only in one of the reviews. About half of the papers were ignored. The rest were

quoted irrelevantly; or insignificant findings in favour of the hypothesis were inflated; or unsupportive results were quoted as if they were supportive. Only one of six randomized cholesterol-lowering trials with a negative outcome were cited and only in one of the reviews. In contrast, each review cited two, four, and six non-randomized trials with a positive outcome, respectively."[12]

I have experienced the fraudulent methods used by the cholesterol fanatics more closely myself. In 1993 The National Food Agency in Sweden organized a conference about prevention of cardiovascular disease. I participated together with three cholesterol-critics; one of them was Lars Werkö, head of SBU (the Swedish Agency for Health Technology Assessment and Assessment of Social Services). The other participants were about 40 Scandinavian and British "experts". They used a meta-analysis by the Norwegian statistician Ingar Holme[13] as their main argument for their warnings against saturated fat. I had just published a meta-analysis of all the correctly performed cholesterol-lowering trials in *British Medical Journal*, where I showed that taken together, no benefit was achieved; in fact, total mortality was higher in the treatment groups.[14] I had also included a table of the previous meta-analyses. One of them was the analysis by Holme, and in that paper he had excluded seven trials: most of them with a negative outcome, I wrote to him and asked why. I had also checked his data and found that there were numerous errors; most of them in favor of the diet-heart hypothesis. He admitted most of the errors and promised to correct them in his future publications. However, shortly afterwards he published two meta-analyses which included the same trials and with the same errors.[15,16] Since then he has been a statistical coauthor of more than 40 statin trials.

PJR: You have published several critical books as well. How did you succeed with that?

UR: There were no major problems in the start. My first book was published in 1991 in Swedish and a year later in Finnish. Initially, there was much interest about it in the Scandinavian media. However, when Finnish television aired an interview with me, Finnish researchers critical to my view were asked to comment what I had said without informing me, and at the end of the program, my book was put on fire.

PJR: But as I remember it became much more difficult during the following years

UR: Yes, after the introduction of the statins almost all of my papers were routinely rejected by U.S. and U.K. journals even though all my claims were supported by references to peer reviewed publications.

Later on I was interviewed by the Dutch TV-program Tros Radar. Soon afterwards the leading cholesterol experts in Holland described me in another Dutch TV program as a crackpot, who had been expelled from the universities of Copenhagen and Lund, and that my only contribution to science was a letter, which I had published in 70 different publications. However, the head of Tros Radar called the universities, and when she realized that the experts had lied, she invited them to debate with me on a follow-up program, but they declined: To discuss with a maverick who claims that the earth is flat would be a tremendous waste of time.

PJR: But what about your books?

UR: For several years I tried to find a book agent or a publisher for the English version of my book, but no one was interested. Therefore, I published parts of it on the web. This soon became one of the top ten sites for searches on cholesterol at that time, and I began to receive numerous e-mails from doctors, scientists, patients and journalists who supported my views.

One of them was Mary Enig, a biochemist who for many years had tried to inform the world about the dangerous effects of trans fat. She introduced me to Sally Fallon, president of Weston A. Price Foundation, who published my first book in English, *The Cholesterol Myths; the Fallacy that Saturated Fat and Cholesterol cause Heart Disease.* She also invited me and my wife Bodil to Washington, where she had arranged several talks and radio interviews.

PJR: Please tell me what led to your organization of THINCS. I had long been critical of the lipid hypothesis and devoted several sessions to exposing its flaws at our annual International Congress on Stress in Switzerland starting in 1993. These included presentations by George Mann, Bill Stehbens, "Pete" Ahrens, Ray Rosenman, Stewart Wolf and other authorities, but I was unaware of your contributions. I learned about them from Ray Rosenman, a close friend and Vice President of The American Institute, who urged me to join THINCS, which I did in early 2003. I first met you several months later at the May 2003 annual Weston Price Conference in Virginia, where I was invited to give a presentation titled "Cholesterol Does Not Cause Coronary Heart Disease and Statins Don't Work by Lowering Lipids: The Role of Inflammation and Stress.

By that time there were about 50 members of THINCS, some of whom also participated, including Kilmer McCully (Homocysteine, Vitamins and Vascular Disease), Peter Langsjoen (CoQ10 Depletion From Statins), Leslie Klevay (Copper Deficiency and Coronary Disease) and your talk (High Cholesterol May Protect Against Infections And Atherosclerosis). I had become aware of Duane Graveline's experience, and arranged for his presentation (Transient Global Amnesia – A Side Effect of Statin Treatment) and he quickly joined our group. Eddie Vos, a mechanical engineer and THINCS member also participated, and there may have been others that I did not meet. I was impressed with the quality of these papers as well as their diversity and continue to be astounded by the contributions of subsequent THINCS members, which now exceed one hundred.

UR: To fight alone is not a good idea; in particular if you are working alone as a private practitioner. As you mention, my book and my websites had resulted in several interesting contacts with wise colleagues, who were just as critical to the cholesterol campaign as myself.

Among the members present at the Weston A. Price meeting I would also like to mention the Polish-Australian pharmacologist and toxicologist Bogdan Sikorski. Bogdan worked at TGA, the Australian equivalent to FDA, and according to a recent investigation they had found that about half of all clinical studies and trials were fraudulent. He told me about Jan Kwasniewski, the Polish doctor, who already in the sixties introduced "the optimal diet" in Poland. This was an extreme LCHF diet, by which he said that he had cured many patients from multiple diseases, for instance MS, ALS, Crohn's disease and type 1 and type 2 diabetes. I asked Bogdan, why he hadn't published his findings. Bogdan had asked him the same question. His response was that "No one wants to know!"

One of the early members was Dag Viljen Poleszynski, a Norwegian professor with several academic titles, author of more than 30 popular-scientific books and editor of a magazine about alternative medicine. A few years later Kaare Norum, one of the leading cholesterol fanatics in Norway succeeded in expelling him from the high-school because of his skepticism against the cholesterol campaign.

Many more interesting individuals contacted me, and it gave me the idea to start an electronic network of university people skeptic to the cholesterol hypothesis and the diet-heart idea. At the start our organization included about 40 members with varying backgrounds and hypotheses about the cause of atherosclerosis and cardiovascular disease, but with skepticism as a common denominator. Since then we have had many interesting discussions on the web.

PJR: We next met in 2008 in Gothenburg, where you were the recipient of the Leo-Huss-Walin Prize for independent thinking. I had been invited to give the opening lecture at the Award ceremony, and other THINCS members who presented included Michel de Lorgeril, Peter Langsjoen and yourself. Professors Richard Feinman, Tore Scherstén and Björn Folkow, who were not THINCS members also spoke, and it appeared from the discussion period that most of the audience supported our opinions but were not aware of THINCS. I have been impressed with the large number of other qualified physicians and scientists who share our views, but have not joined THINCS, which does not require any membership fees or other costs. I believe their ranks are increasing and wondered what your experience has been in this regard.

UR: It is very difficult for medical researchers to go against the common view. Almost all research about atherosclerosis and cardiovascular disease is funded by drug companies, and they are generous. Therefore, researchers, who appear on our members list, would immediately lose their financial support and also support and respect from their colleagues. As you know, a paradigm shift in medical science may not happen before most of the leading professors have retired or died.

PJR: This is reminiscent of Max Planck's observation that "*A new scientific truth does not triumph by convincing its opponents and making them see the light, but rather because its opponents eventually* *die, and a new generation grows up that is familiar with it.*" You referred earlier to the difficulty in getting anything published in a peer reviewed journal that was critical of the cholesterol hypothesis or the efficacy and safety of statins. As a result, many frustrated researchers and other have resorted to writing books. Although these are not accessible via Medline, Embase etc., some have become best sellers in their field. The Cholesterol Myths has been out of print for some time, but apparently is available on line at no charge. What prompted you to write *Fat and Cholesterol are GOOD for You!* and *Ignore the Awkward.*

UR: I had been told that many lay people found that The Cholesterol Myths is not too easy to read. Furthermore, due to a different view on the cause of atherosclerosis, Sally Fallon stopped publishing it. To find a new publisher would demand much work, and I therefore allowed it for free. Instead I wrote a shorter and more popular-scientific version. I also found it interesting to tell about the many ways we are fooled by the drug industry and their paid scientist, which was my motive for writing Fat and Cholesterol Are Good for You. However, I have not yet succeeded in publishing a best seller.

PJR: One of the problems is of course that few medical journalists dare to write about the many contradictions to the cholesterol hypothesis.

UR: You are right. I can give you an example. In 2006 I was invited to a conference in London, where supporters and opponents to the cholesterol hypothesis were asked to present their arguments to a large number of British journalists. At the start they were asked whether they were believers or not, and almost all of them voted as believers. At the end of the conference they were asked again, and almost all of them had changed their mind. I was confident that now the journalists should start writing critical articles, but I was wrong – not a single one appeared after our meeting.

PJR: Tell me about the hypothesis about atherosclerosis, which you have presented together with Kilmer McCully.

UR: By reading systematically about the lipoproteins I had learnt, that they participate in the immune system by adhering to and inactivating all kinds of microorganisms. As this fact, documented by more than a dozen research groups was unknown for most researchers I published a review about it.[17] Among the opponents at the meeting with the journalists was our member Malcolm Kendrick. When I listened to his description of the vulnerable plaque, it struck me how it was created; it might simply be a microscopic boil, which starts the formation of an arterial thrombus, when it ruptures.

During the following year I used most of my time to formulate my idea in more detail, but my final manuscript was rejected by nine journals. Here are their responses:

August 3, 2007. *Nature*: "We must decline it on editorial grounds."

August 5, *Nature Medicine*: "We feel the work is better suited for a journal specialized in cardiovascular disease."

August 8, *The Lancet*: "It would be better placed elsewhere."

August 20, *Science*: "Although your analysis is interesting, we feel that the scope and focus of your paper make it more appropriate for a more specialized journal."

September 19, *Journal of Infectious Diseases*: "The manuscript is better suited for a different journal."

March 17, 2008, *Clinical Science*: "Your proposal appears to be more suited to a medical hypothesis journal."

March 26, *Journal of Clinical Investigation*: "We feel the manuscript would not be appropriate for publication in the Journal of Clinical Investigation."

March 31, *Archives of Pathology*: "Unfortunately, your manuscript is not consistent with our current priorities for publication in the Archives."

April 15, *Archives of Internal Medicine*: "After some effort, we have been unable to identify a qualified author for an opposing paper."

A little later I discussed my hypothesis with Kilmer McCully. He bought it immediately because his own hypothesis about homocysteine fits perfectly into mine. He added some sections about the role of homocysteine and as he is a coeditor of *Annals of Clinical and Laboratory Science*, they accepted our paper directly.[18]

PJR: But there were no problems associated with our cancer paper.[19] How come?

UR: A paper written by a retired private doctor outside the academic world is less attractive for editors of a medical journal than a paper authored by one or more professors. I think that my two famous coauthors made our paper more acceptable.

PJR: But although we have presented massive evidence in support of the idea that low cholesterol predisposes to cancer, supporters of statin treatment claim that the statins are protective.

UR: Evidently they haven't read our paper, or they do it on purpose by economical reasons. Their evidence is cohort studies where statin-treated people are compared with untreated. Obviously those on statin treatment may have lived most of their life with high cholesterol and it is well known that many statin-treated patients stop their treatment. As high cholesterol is associated with a lower risk of cancer, this can explain the lower number of cancer, in particular because most of the untreated controls may have lived most of their life with normal or low cholesterol. It is also curious, that none of the authors of these studies have any comments to the fact that several statin trials have resulted in a significant increase of cancer in the treatment groups and the fact that statins are carcinogenic in rodents.

PJR: What do you think about the future? Is it possible to stop this madness in a foreseeable coming?

UR: A difficult question, indeed. Almost 60 years ago Fred Kummerow, previously professor of comparative biosciences and one of our members, described the dangers associated with eating partially hydrogenated oils (trans fatty acids), which has been a major component in many types of margarine for almost hundred years.[20] In 2013 he filed a lawsuit against the FDA, which had ignored his petition sent four years previously calling for ban on artificial trans fats. Two years later FDA reacted and forbid food containing such fats, but they gave the manufacturers a deadline of three years.

Fred succeeded, but to win, you obviously have to become a centenarian, like Fred. He is still active; for instance you can read about his experience in this field published last year in World Nutrition,[21] and he was also a coauthor to a paper that we published recently in Mayo Clinic Proceedings.[22]

PJR: Thus it took almost 60 years for Fred. Do you think the same is valid for you?

UR: Hopefully not. I think that William Stehbens, one of our early members, was the first who questioned the cholesterol hypothesis and it was more than 40 years ago,[23] but when Joseph Goldstein and Michael Brown received the Nobel Price in 1985, everybody became convinced about the role of high cholesterol. But what Goldstein and Brown showed was, that the cellular LDL-receptors of people with familial hypercholesterolemia were less effective as in normal people, not that high cholesterol is the cause of atherosclerosis or coronary heart disease. Since then several of our members have documented, both in medical journals, books and newspapers, that high cholesterol and saturated fat are our good friends. If you search PubMed and Google with the names (in alphabetic order) Michel de Lorgeril, Mary Enig, Duane Graveline, Zoë Harcombe, Malcolm Kendrick, Lesley Klevay, Louis Krut, Peter Langsjoen, Luca Mascitelli, Kilmer MCCully, Harumi Okuyama, Ray Rosenman, Stephanie Seneff, Morley Sutter, Jørgen Vesti Nielsen, Eddie Vos, Glyn Wainwright and our own, the list of references would fill many pages.

However, it is not an easy task to question Nobel Prize winners. My first paper questioning their idea was published 36 years ago,[24] but it made no impact whatsoever. I also sent a kind letter to both of them pointing at the many findings that contradicted their idea, but they never answered. Our recent paper, where we have documented that people above the age of 60 with high LDL-C live the longest,[25] should hopefully open the eyes of many scientists, but I doubt that it is able to stop the cholesterol madness; there is too much money involved. It took almost 60 years for Fred Kummerow to change the view about trans fat; we have only tried for 40. As the great artist Freddie Mercury sang: "The Show Must Go on."

Paul J. Rosch, MD*, Uffe Ravnskov, MD, PhD**

*Clinical Professor of Medicine and Psychiatry
New York Medical College
Chairman, The American Institute of Stress
stress124@optonline.net

** Independent Researcher
ravnskov@tele2.se
www.thincs.org

References

1. Ravnskov U. Aneurysm of the heart and the post-myocardial-infarction syndrome. Acta Med Scand 1968;183:393-5

2. Ravnskov U. On renal handling of plasma proteins. Scand J Urol Nephrol 1973;7 suppl 20. [Thesis]

3. Zimmerman SW, Groehler K, Beirne GJ. Hydrocarbon exposure and chronic glomerulonephritis. Lancet 1975;2:199-201.

4. Ravnskov U, Johansson BG, Göthlin J. Renal extraction of beta2-microglobulin. Scand J Clin Lab Invest. 1972;30:71-5

5. Johansson BG, Ravnskov U. The serum level and urinary excretion of albumin, β2-microglobulin and lysozyme in renal disease. Scand J Urol Nephrol. 1972;6:249-56

6. Ravnskov U. Exposure to organic solvents--a missing link in poststreptococcal glomerulonephritis? Acta Med Scand 1978;203:351-6.

7. Ravnskov U, Lundström S, Nordén Å. Hydrocarbon exposure and glomerulonephritis: evidence from patients' occupations. Lancet 1983;2:1214-6.

8. Bengtsson U. Glomerulonephritis and organic solvents. Lancet 1985;2:566.

9. Ravnskov U. Single-dose treatment of uncomplicated cystitis and asymptomatic bacteriuria-a review. Läkartidningen 1986;83:45-7.

10. Ravnskov U. Soap is the major cause of dysuria. Lancet 1984;1:1027-8.

11. Ravnskov U. An elevated serum cholesterol is secondary, not causal, in coronary heart disease. Med Hypotheses 1991;36:238-41.

12. Ravnskov U. Quotation bias in reviews of the diet-heart idea. J Clin Epidemiol 1995;48:713-719.

13. Holme I. An analysis of randomized trials. Evaluating the effect of cholesterol reduction on total mortality and coronary heart disease incidence. Circulation 1990;82:1916-24.

14. Ravnskov U. Cholesterol lowering trials in coronary heart disease: frequency of citation and outcome. BMJ 1992;305:15-19.

15. Holme I. Cholesterol reduction in single and multifactorial randomized trials. Blood Pressure. 1992;1 (suppl 4):29-34.

16. Holme I. Relation of coronary heart disease incidence and total mortality to plasma cholesterol reduction in randomised trials: use of meta-analysis. Br Heart J 1993;69(1 Suppl):S42-7.

17. Ravnskov U. High cholesterol may protect against infections and atherosclerosis. QJM 2003;96:927-34.

18. Ravnskov U, McCully KS. Vulnerable plaque formation from obstruction of vasa vasorum by homocysteinylated and oxidized lipoprotein aggregates complexed with microbial remnants and LDL autoantibodies. Ann Clin Lab Sci 2009;39:3-16.

19. Ravnskov U, McCully KS, Rosch PJ. The statin-low cholesterol-cancer conundrum. QJM 2012;105:383-8.

20. Johnston PV, Johnson OC, Kummerow FA. Occurrence of trans fatty acids in human tissue. Science 1957;126:698–699

21. Kummerow F. Good health and well-being. My diet [Idea]. World Nutrition 2015;6: 72-78

22. Ravnskov U, DiNicolantonio JJ, Harcombe Z, Kummerow FA, Okuyama H, Worm N. The questionable benefits of exchanging saturated fat with polyunsaturated fat. Mayo Clin Proc. 2014;89:451-3.

23. Stehbens WE. The role of lipid in the pathogenesis of atherosclerosis. Lancet 1975;1:724-7.

24. Ravnskov U. An elevated serum cholesterol is secondary, not causal, in coronary heart disease. Med Hypotheses 1991;36:238-41

25. Ravnskov U, Diamond DM, Hama R et al. Lack of an association or an inverse association between low-density-lipoprotein cholesterol and mortality in the elderly. A systematic review. BMJ Open 2016;6: e010401. doi:10.1136/ bmjopen-2015-01040

Chapter Three

How Dietary Guidelines, Bad Science, Politics And
Profit Have Contributed To The Current Epidemic
of Obesity and Incidence of Heart Disease

Zoë Harcombe, PhD

Abstract

In 1960, 13.3% of United States (US) adults were obese; 44.8% were
overweight.[1] Age adjusted all-cause mortality was 1,339.2 per 100,000
population, a death rate of 1.33%.[2] "Diseases of heart" mortality was
559.0 per 100,000 population, a death rate of 0.56%.[2]

By 2007, 34.7% of US adults were obese; 67.7% were overweight.[1]
Age adjusted all-cause mortality was 760.2 per 100,000 population, a
death rate of 0.76%.[2] Heart disease mortality was 190.9 per 100,000
population, a death rate of 0.19%.[2]

Heart deaths accounted for 42% of all deaths in 1960 and 25% of
all deaths in 2007. Smoking more than halved during this period from
41.9% of US adults in 1965 to 19.7% in 2007.[3]

In fewer than five decades we have witnessed an obesity problem
become an epidemic and failed to reduce heart disease by more than
smoking cessation and advances in medical care facilitated. This
paper argues that this scenario is of our making.

Diet-heart hypothesis

What has become known as the diet-heart hypothesis has its origins in
the works of Russian pathologists at the turn of the twentieth century.
Pre World War I, the works of Ignatowski,[4-6] Stuckey,[7-9] Chalatow,[10]
Wesselkin[11] and Anitschkow[12] established associations between

dietary interventions and fatty deposits/thickening of the intima in rabbits. The dietary interventions involved administering foods of animal origin, as sources of cholesterol and fat, to herbivorous rabbits. Knack questioned the validity of this and discovered that rabbits fed a plant diet with added cholesterol showed no arterial damage while rabbits fed eggs and milk, substances that they cannot digest, did.[13] Anitschkow tested omnivorous rats and found egg yolk administered in milk produced no observable changes in the aortas.[14] Regrettably the herbivore limitations were ignored and the hypothesis of an association between cholesterol in food and indications of heart disease gathered momentum.

In the 1950s, Ancel Keys comprehensively tested the hypothesis that dietary cholesterol increased serum cholesterol levels.[15] Keys concluded that "The evidence - both from experiments and from field surveys - indicates that cholesterol content, *per se*, of all natural diets has *no* significant effect on either the cholesterol level or the development of atherosclerosis in man."[16]

The erroneous notion that dietary cholesterol can increase serum cholesterol prevails with modern dietary advice to avoid egg yolks and seafood specifically and animal foods generally.

Having determined that dietary cholesterol has no significant effect on either the cholesterol level or the development of atherosclerosis in man, Keys maintained the view that diet and serum cholesterol levels were significant determinants of heart disease. At the Mount Sinai symposium, Keys presented a now well-known graph, showing an association between deaths from heart disease per 1,000 US men aged 55-59 and fat calories as a percentage of total dietary intake.[17] Criticisms were made that data were available for 22 countries, showing a scatter plot, rather than a linear relationship.[18] By the time this 1957 retort had been published, the Seven Countries Study had been conceived, planned and was underway.

The Seven Countries Study noted that "Epidemiological studies alone can rarely if ever produce final proof of a causal sequence."[19] Despite acknowledgment of this limitation, positioning the Coronary Heart Disease (CHD) death rate as 42% (of deaths), as opposed to 0.56% (of people), created a sense of urgency: "The urgency of finding means of prevention is sharpest for men in middle age ... Starting with men aged 40 through 59, the follow-up would show CHD causing close to 40% of all deaths in five years."[19]

The introduction to the Seven Countries Study was not explicit about the study hypothesis.[19] The opening chapter stated "By the mid-1950's epidemiological studies had identified two important risk factors in the development of CHD among middle-aged white men in the United States." These risk factors were not stated, but Keys' view that dietary fat and serum cholesterol levels were the prime risk factors were so strongly held at this time, he may have assumed that they did not need clarification.[20]

The Seven Countries study examined 12,770 men, aged 40 through 59 years, in 16 cohorts in Finland, Greece, Italy, Japan, the Netherlands, the United States, and Yugoslavia from 1956 onwards. As the study progressed, dietary fat generally became saturated fat specifically although Keys was unscientifically casual in his use of these terms. The verbatim conclusions were:

- "The incidence rate of CHD tends to be directly related to the distributions of serum cholesterol values."

- "The average serum cholesterol values of the cohorts tended to be directly related to the average proportion of calories provided by saturated fats in the diet."

- "The CHD incidence rates of the cohorts are just as closely related to the dietary saturated fatty acids as to the serum cholesterol level."[21]

The diet-heart hypothesis thus became the tripartite association of saturated fat, serum cholesterol levels and CHD.

Bad Science

The administration and conclusions of the Seven Countries Study made a number of nutritional errors:

1) Animal foods had been exonerated

The only foods that contain dietary cholesterol are of animal origin: meat; fish; eggs and dairy products. Having extensively tested high cholesterol diets with human subjects, with the conclusion that these had no significant impact on serum cholesterol levels or the development of atherosclerosis in man, it follows that animal foods *per se* have no significant impact on serum cholesterol levels or the development of atherosclerosis in man.[15]

All foods, except sucrose and oils, contain protein. Meat and fish are combinations of water, fat and protein. Glycogen in offal aside, meat and fish are void of carbohydrate. Dairy products contain some carbohydrate and eggs have a trace. The macronutrient entirely, or largely, absent in animal foods is carbohydrate. Plant foods are primarily combinations of water, carbohydrate and protein. The macronutrient largely absent in plant foods is fat, although most foods of vegetable origin, from blueberries to oats, have trace to small amounts. The exceptions to these principles are nuts and seeds, containing all three macronutrients in good measure.

Having exonerated animal foods in his human dietary cholesterol studies, the obvious macronutrient for Keys to have studied was carbohydrate, not fat.

2) Carbohydrates were misclassified as fats

Keys did in fact study carbohydrate, but incorrectly classified substances such as cake and ice cream as fat. They contain fat, but are predominantly carbohydrate.[22]

In the most comprehensive write up of the Study, "Seven Countries: a multivariate analysis of death and coronary heart disease", Keys noted: "The fact that the incidence of coronary heart disease was significantly correlated with the average percentage of calories from sucrose in the diets is explained by the inter correlation of sucrose with saturated fat."[23]

Sucrose and fat do not occur naturally together in food; avocado being an exception. This admission thus confirmed i) that processed foods, such as cake and ice cream, were erroneously deemed fat and

ii) that processed foods *per se* could be risk factors for heart disease, not any natural fats contained therein.

3) Fats were misclassified

A nutritional error of the time, which prevails today, was the assumption that fats of animal origin are saturated and fats of plant origin are unsaturated. Every food that contains fat contains all three fats: saturated; monounsaturated and polyunsaturated. There are no exceptions.[24]

Volume VII of the Seven Countries study described rural Italy: "The cuisine of Bologna and Modena is the richest of the regional cuisines of Italy, it is loaded with saturated fatty acids and cholesterol from butter, cream, meats, and eggs."[25] The mention of dietary cholesterol was unnecessary, having been declared to have no impact on serum cholesterol or the development of atherosclerosis in man. The assumption that meats and eggs are "loaded with saturated fatty acids" is incorrect. Sirloin steak, for example, is approximately 71% water, 21% protein, 3% unsaturated fat and 2% saturated fat (trace minerals and rounding error account for 100%).[26] Of the 10 g of fat per 100 g of egg, 37% is saturated, 46% is monounsaturated, and 17% is polyunsaturated.[27]

In the rare dietary references in the Seven Countries Study, Keys complimented vegetable fats, such as olive oil, and denigrated animal fats, such as meat. Keys noted that the Yugoslavian cohort of Dalmatia consumed olive oil "to the exclusion of almost all other fat", while in Slavonia "animal fat, especially pork fat, takes the place of oil in the diet."[28] Keys did not demonstrate the nutritional knowledge that one tablespoon of olive oil[29] has more than three times the total fat and a third more saturated fat than a 100g pork chop.[30] Such nutritional ignorance continues to be widespread more than 30 years later.

The only food group that contains more saturated than unsaturated fat is dairy products.[24] Dairy products have many health benefits being rich in vitamins and minerals, especially the bone nutrients: calcium; vitamin D and phosphorus. The most recent meta-analysis of studies evaluating dairy products and health factors concluded: "The observational evidence does not support the hypothesis that dairy fat or high-fat dairy foods contribute to obesity or cardiometabolic risk."[30]

Dietary Guidelines & Politics

US public health dietary advice was announced by the McGovern Select Committee on Nutrition and Human needs in 1977[31] and was followed by UK public health dietary advice issued by the National Advisory Committee on Nutritional Education in 1983.[32] Dietary recommendations in both cases focused on reducing dietary fat intake; specifically to i) reduce overall fat consumption to 30% of total energy intake and ii) reduce saturated fat consumption to 10% of total energy intake.

The UK nutritional guidelines[32] made reference to the Seven Countries Study, the US committee document[31] did not. There were five Randomized Control Trials (RCTs), examining dietary fat interventions, all-cause mortality and CHD mortality, available to the US committee[33-37] and a sixth was available to the UK review group.[38] None of these RCTs were referenced by either dietary committee. The US Committee publication reported data from the non-randomized, cross-over trial, the Finnish Mental Hospital Study.[39,40]

None of the five RCTs tested the dietary fat recommendations introduced. The sixth, Woodhill,[38] tested the 10% saturated fat recommendation and reported significantly more deaths in the intervention group. The six RCTs, combined in meta-analysis, reported no difference in all-cause mortality and no significant difference in CHD mortality.[41]

The UK Committee on Medical Aspects of Food Policy admitted: "There has been no controlled clinical trial of the effect of decreasing dietary intake of saturated fatty acids on the incidence of coronary heart disease nor is it likely that such a trial will be undertaken."[42]

This was reiterated by Truswell in his 1994 review of the data: "It has been accepted by experienced coronary disease researchers that the perfect controlled dietary trial for prevention of coronary heart disease has not yet been done and we are unlikely ever to see it done."[43]

It was confirmed again by the UK Food Standards Agency in 2009: "The ideal controlled dietary trial for prevention of heart disease has not yet been done and it is unlikely ever to be done."[44]

These facts are not widely known. US and UK citizens believe that government dietary recommendations have been proven; they have not been tested.

The Seven Countries Study disregarded the totality of country data available. It selected countries, which the Mount Sinai presentation showed would concur with a fat-heart hypothesis. It could at best show association and failed to establish this in five cohorts: West Finland; Rome; Crete; Belgrade and Corfu.[45] It made several nutritional errors about dietary fat, cholesterol and carbohydrate and misclassified foods as a result.

Randomized Controlled Trials were not taken into account and they would not have supported the introduced dietary guidelines had they been. Evidence and interviews of the time confirm that the dietary guidelines were political rather than evidential.[46]

Dietary Guidelines and food intake

The primary nutritional impact of dietary recommendations to decrease fat was that carbohydrate intake concomitantly increased. With protein in all foods, with the two exceptions noted, advice to decrease fat/protein necessarily increases carbohydrate/protein, as a proportion of dietary intake, if not as an absolute amount. US dietary guidelines reinforced this inevitable consequence: "Increase carbohydrate consumption to account for 55 to 60 percent of the energy (caloric) intake."[47] The UK publication positioned the carbohydrate recommendation as an opportunity emanating from the fat advice: "The panel sees advantages in compensating for a reduced fat intake with increased fibre-rich carbohydrates (e.g. bread, cereals, fruit and vegetables)."[42]

A United States Department of Agriculture review of dietary recommendations throughout history compared the "Basic four foundation advice" of 1956-70s with the 1984 Food Pyramid guide, which followed the McGovern committee guidelines.[48] The basic four advice was based on four food groups: meat; milk; bread and cereals;

fruits and vegetables. Four portions a day of starchy carbohydrates, such as bread and cereal, were recommended (a slice of bread was given as an example portion). The Food Pyramid named six food groups: dairy products; meat, poultry, fish, eggs, beans and nuts; breads, cereals, rice and pasta; vegetables; fruits; and fats, oils and sweets. Recommended servings of starchy carbohydrates increased to 6-11 daily (a slice of bread remained the example portion size). Fruit servings of 2-4 per day were recommended and sweets were inexplicably featured in the fats and oils food group, thus adding significant amounts of sucrose to starch intake. The addition of recommendations for 3-5 servings of vegetables brought Tanner's obesity advice of 1869 to mind: "Farinaceous and vegetable foods are fattening, and saccharine matters are especially so."[49]

The *Dietary Guidelines for Americans* are issued every five years. Table 2.2 in the most recent edition, 2010, reported dietary intakes for American adults.[50] The main source of calories was grain-based desserts (cakes, cookies, pies, cobblers, sweet rolls, pastries and donuts).Yeast breads (including bagels and rolls, white, whole-wheat and multi-grain) were in second place. Chicken dishes (dominated by take-away fried chicken and chicken nuggets, rather than home-cooked grilled chicken) were in third place. The fourth highest source of calories for US adults was the soda/energy/sports drinks category and alcohol was in fifth place.

The American diet is dominated by processed food. The top 25 sources of calories contained only one listing of natural food: "regular cheese". The milk line entry was reduced fat and thus adulterated: fat, taste, satiety and nutrients having been removed. There were mentions of other real foods, such as fish, eggs and beef, but such categories included processed variants, for example: breaded fish; quiche; and beef noodles.[50]

Analysis of Table 2.2 revealed that carbohydrate based items accounted for 67% of the calorie intake from the most consumed 25 foods and 50% of total adult caloric intake. The carbohydrates were typically the starches recommended in dietary guidelines: bread; cereals; potatoes; rice; and pasta.[50] US Department of Health data confirmed that carbohydrate accounted for approximately 50% of the American adult diet; fat contributed 34% and protein made up the remaining16% and that this had remained stable this (twenty-first) century.[51] Saturated fat intake was 11%. American diets were 4% higher in fat and accordingly lower in carbohydrate than government recommendations, but the dietary guidelines were mostly being achieved.

The primary benefactors of the dietary guidelines were the cereal and grain producers. "[Annual] Per capita use of flour and cereal products reached 200 pounds in 2000 from 138 pounds in the 1970s".[52] Annual per capita intake of sweeteners increased from 123.7lb in the 1970s to 152.4lb in 2000. High fructose corn syrup, Corn Syrup (HFCS) consumption increased almost twelve-fold from 5.5 to 63.8 annual pounds per capita. Salad and vegetable oil intake almost doubled, while annual butter intake remained constant at a relatively insignificant 4.6lb per person. Whole milk consumption in 2000 was almost one third that of the 1970s. Consumption of low-fat milk almost doubled in parallel. Red meat and egg intake fell; white meat intake rose. It cannot be argued that butter, eggs, red meat and whole milk - foods that our grandparents would have relied upon - have caused the obesity epidemic. HFCS, vegetable oils and cereals are implicated.

Vegetable oil producers have also benefitted from the dietary guidelines. Reinforcing nutritional ignorance promoting plant fats as unsaturated and animal fats as saturated, traditional fats such as lard (60% unsaturated[53]) have been rejected in favour of modern processed oils, less stable at cooking temperatures.[54] This switch has been supported by meta-analysis,[55] which included the discredited Finnish crossover trial[39,40] and excluded the two RCTs with significantly more deaths in the diet interventions,[33,38] and contained Aramark and Unilever declarations of interest. The Finnish crossover trial was excluded by Truswell[43] and the definitive Cochrane review,[56] as "inappropriate for assessing effects on cardiovascular events or mortality." The study selection of the Mozaffarian meta-analysis has been questioned,[57] as has the safety of vegetable oils generally.[58]

The misclassification of predominantly carbohydrate foods as saturated fats, made by Keys in 1970,[22] continued decades later. The *Dietary Guidelines for Americans* listed: ice cream; sherbet; frozen yogurt; cakes; cookies; quick breads; doughnuts; margarine; sausages; potato chips; corn chips; popcorn and yeast bread as major sources of saturated fats.[59]

The Executive Summary of the *Dietary Guidelines for Americans* noted the "epidemic of overweight and obesity affecting men, women, and children in all segments of our society" making no connection with the rise in obesity since dietary guidelines were introduced. The introduction reported that 24 million Americans, almost 11% of the adult population, were diabetic and 78 million Americans, 35% of adults were pre-diabetic.[50] This has recently been updated to 29 million diabetics and 86 million pre-diabetics.[60] A recent review in *The Lancet*, estimated that the lifetime risk for developing diabetes was 40.2% for American men and 39.6% for women.[61] Diabetes was correctly described as a condition of high blood glucose levels and impaired glucose metabolism, but the connection between this epidemic, and advising Americans to base their meals on glucose, was not made.

The Executive Summary assumed that calories explain the obesity epidemic: "Americans must decrease the calories they consume and increase the calories they expend." Calories do not explain the obesity epidemic. Notwithstanding that the calorie theory (one pound of fat is 3,500 calories and a deficit of 3,500 calories will elicit a loss of one pound of fat), which has become folk lore, has no evidence base or proof,[45] if it did hold it could not explain the data. Mean daily calorie intake for men was 2,450 in 1971-74 and 2,656 in 2005-2008.[62] Mean daily calorie intake for women was 1,542 in 1971-74 and 1,811 in 2005-2008. The data represented an average increase of five calories per day, year on year, for men and approximately seven calories per day, year on year, over this period for women. If one additional jelly bean could create an obesity epidemic, as Taubes posited, the issue becomes how did we *not* have an obesity epidemic in the millennia since *Australopithecus Lucy*, not how did we since the 1970s.[63]

The calorie theory does not provide motive. It is the gluttony/sloth hypothesis. Researchers at the University of Florida discovered that formerly obese patients would prefer to be normal weight with a major disability (deaf, blind, one leg amputated) than morbidly obese.[64] Expenditure on diet products and services and preparedness to risk death with bariatric surgery,[65] further substantiates the motivation to avoid obesity. It is implausible that the human population maintained normal weight for approximately 3.5 million years and then chose to become greedy and lazy, to the point of epidemic, in a moment in evolutionary terms.

Profit & Food Politics

Natural food production is not lucrative. The 'farm to fork' logistics chain for steak, eggs or apples, is succinct and without opportunity or necessity for 'added value'. Processed food production, and the marketing and advertising that accompanies it, is profitable for many contributors from product concept to promotional toys.

The world's largest processed food and drink company, PepsiCo, had revenues of $66.415 billion in 2013.[66] PepsiCo is the size of Sudan. It is bigger than 65% of the countries of the world.[67] PepsiCo is also a premier sponsor of the American Dietetic Association, which was renamed the Academy of Nutrition and Dietetics in 2012.[68]

Other premier sponsors of American Dietitians are: CoroWise, Cargill; General Mills; Kellogg Company; Mars Incorporated; McNeil Nutritionals; SoyJoy; Truvia sweetener and Unilever. The Academy has the following partners: Abbott Nutrition; Aramark; Coca-Cola; Hershey and the National Dairy Council.[68]

The Commission on Dietetic Registration (CDR) is the credentialing agency for the Academy of Nutrition and Dietetics. Its purpose is to ensure that registered dietitians alone are able to give food and nutrition advice. The CDR was formed in 1969. In 1984 the first registration eligibility reciprocity agreement was signed with the Canadian Dietetic Association. In 1991 registration eligibility reciprocity was extended to foreign countries whose goals were comparable to CDR's. In 1995 the CDR filed registration eligibility requirements and reciprocity agreements with the USA Trade Representative Office and World Trade Organization. By 2013, 89,385 dietitians were registered with the CDR.[69]

47 of the 50 States of America have passed legislation to regulate who is able to provide nutritional advice through licensure, statutory certification or registration.[70,71] The Commission on Dietetic Registration has successfully established a monopoly position for the Academy of Nutrition and Dietetics, which in turn is integrally partnered with the processed food industry. The fake food industry is embedded in our dietary advice; the real food message has no chance of success. Dietetic organisations from Australia to the UK are similarly conflicted.[72-74]

What Does The Future Hold?

To the growing number of real food campaigners, the solution to the obesity and diabetes epidemics and incidence of heart disease is to return to eating the natural foods that we ate before we developed these epidemics. Government food pyramids, plates and dietary guidelines should be torn up and replaced with one message: "Eat real food." Children can and should be taught the difference between real and processed food (fields, not factories). They should reach adulthood knowing that grain-based desserts, yeast breads and chicken nuggets do not constitute a human diet. Banning trans fats and sweeteners, taxing sucrose punitively and any policy that facilitates consumption of real food should be embraced.

Humans need to remember the purpose of food. Food provides essential fats, amino acids, vitamins and minerals vital for survival. The optimal providers of these essential nutrients are natural foods, especially those of animal origin.[24] These are the foods that took us from Neanderthal to rocket scientist.[75] These are the foods we have been told to avoid.

The solution is so obvious that only an understanding of how we got to the current situation can explain why the solution will not be implemented. The erroneous demonization of fat generally and saturated fat particularly, without accurate definition of either term, has been reiterated by successive governments for decades. Admissions of error would harm reputations and could incur compensation claims. Additionally, dietary guidelines have been so lucrative to processed food manufacturers, and pharmaceutical companies treating the concomitant illness, that the resistance to change has been institutionalized. Nowhere more so than in America, with state legislation having granted food conglomerates monopoly access to unsuspecting consumers via dietitians.

The 2015 *Dietary Guidelines for Americans* will be virtually identical to those published in 2010, 2005, 2000, 1995, 1990, 1985 and 1980. The UK has no process for reviewing dietary guidelines and has no impetus to do so. There will be minor shifts in position by governments to distance themselves from advice so wrong that it can no longer be repeated. An example has occurred in the UK with the non-evidence-based five-a-day message having included fruit juice and then having limited fruit juice to one portion and more recently having announced that fruit juice is too sugary to recommend.[76] The processed food industry will also make token changes, especially where changes are to their benefit, for example: making smaller confectionery bars for the same price; replacing butter with cheaper vegetable oils.

The only significant change will emanate from the real food movement, which, facilitated by the internet and social media, is gathering momentum. Low carb high fat (LCHF) is being adopted by increasing numbers of individuals in direct contrast to the low fat high carb (LFHC) government dietary advice. Adoptees are losing weight, gaining health and managing type 2 diabetes with a diet primarily based on meat, fish, eggs and non-starchy vegetables.[77,78] Sweden led the 'underground' trend towards LCHF and this has since been scientifically reviewed and endorsed by authorities.[79]

The US and UK, having been the first to introduce high carbohydrate dietary advice will be the last to change. Their citizens will need to take their health into their own hands.

Peter Cleave was one of many doctors and researchers who testified at the McGovern dietary guidelines committee. Cleave argued: *"For a modern disease to be related to an old-fashioned food is one of the most ludicrous things I have ever heard in my life."*[63] The committee did not find the concept of heart disease being related to natural foods ludicrous and we have had 35 years to experience the consequences.

Zoë Harcombe, PhD

Independent Researcher
www.zoeharcombe.com

References

1. Centers for Disease Control and Prevention. Table 71. Overweight, obesity, and healthy weight among persons 20 years of age and over, by selected characteristics: United States, selected years 1960-1962 through 2005-2008,. In: National Center for Health Statistics, editor.; 2010.

2. Centers for Disease Control and Prevention. Table 26. Leading causes of death and numbers of deaths, by sex, race, and Hispanic origin: United States, 1980 and 2007,. In: National Center for Health Statistics, editor.; 2010.

3. Centers for Disease Control and Prevention. Table 58. Current cigarette smoking among adults 18 years of age and over, by sex, race, and age: United States, selected years 1965-2009,. In: Statistics NCfH, editor.; 2010.

4. Ignatowski AI. Influence de la nourriture animale sur l'organisme des lapins. *Arch Med Exp Anat Pathol* 1908; **20**: 1-20.

5. Ignatowski AI. Changes in parenchymatous organs and in the aortas of rabbits under the influcence of animal protein. *Izvestizy Imperatorskoi Voyenno-Meditsinskoi Akademii (St Petersburg)* 1908; **18**: 231-44.

6. Ignatowski AI. Uber die Wirkung des tierschen Eiweisses auf die aorta und die parenchymatosen organe der kaninchen. *Virchows Arch Pathol Anat Physiol Klin Med* 1909; **198**: 248-70.

7. Stuckey NW. Uber die Veranderungen der kaninchen aorta bei der reichlichen tierischen kost. *Zentralbl Allg Pathol Pathol Anat* 1910; **21**: 668.

8. Stuckey NW. Uber die Veranderungen der kaninchen aorta unter der Wirkung reichlicher tierscher nahrung. *Zentralbl Allg Pathol Pathol Anat* 1911; **22**: 379-80.

9. Stuckey NW. Uber die Veranderungen der kaninchen-aorta bei der futterung mit verschiedenen fettsorten. *Zentralbl Allg Pathol Pathol Anat* 1912; **23**: 910-1.

10. Chalatow SS. Uber das verhalten der leber gegenuber den verschiedenen arten von Speisefett. *Virchows Arch Pathol Anat Physiol Klin Med* 1912; **207**: 452-69.

11. Wesselkin NW. Uber die Ablagerung von fettartigen Stoffen in den Organen. *Virchows Arch Pathol Anat Physiol Klin Med* 1913; **212**: 225-35.

12. Anitschkow N. Über die Veränderungen der Kaninchenaorta bei experimenteller Cholesterinsteatose. *Beitr Pathol Anat* 1913; **56**: 379-404.

13. Knack AV. Uber cholesterinsklerose. *Virchows Arch Pathol Anat Physiol Klin Med* 1915; **220**: 36-52.

14. Anitschkow N. Experimental atherosclerosis in animals. In: EV. C, ed. Arteriosclerosis: A Survey of the Problem. New York: Macmillan; 1933: 271-322.

15. Keys A, Anderson JT, Mickelsen O, Adelson SF, Fidanza F. Diet and Serum Cholesterol in Man: Lack of Effect of Dietary Cholesterol. *The Journal of Nutrition* 1956; **59**(1): 39-56.

16. Keys A, Anderson JT. The relationship of the diet to the development of atherosclerosis in man. In: National Research Council DoMS, ed. Symposium on atherosclerosis. Washington; 1955: 181-96.

17. Keys A. Atherosclerosis: a problem in newer public health. *J Mt Sinai Hosp N Y* 1953; **20**(2): 118-39.

18. Yerushalmy J, Hilleboe HE. Fat in the diet and mortality from heart disease; a methodologic note. *N Y State J Med* 1957; **57**(14): 2343-54.

19. Keys A. Coronary heart disease in seven countries I. The study program and objectives. *Circulation* 1970; **41**(I-1-I-8).

20. Keys A. Prediction and possible prevention of coronary disease. *Am J Public Health Nations Health* 1953; **43**(11): 1399-407.

21. Keys A. Coronary heart disease in seven countries Summary. *Circulation* 1970; **41**(I-186-I-195).

22. Keys A. Coronary heart disease in seven countries XVII. The Diet *Circulation* 1970; **41**(I-162-I-183).

23. Keys A. Seven countries: a multivariate analysis of death and coronary heart disease: Harvard University Press; 1980.

24. Harcombe Z, Baker J, Davies B. Food for Thought: Have We Been Giving the Wrong Dietary Advice? *Food and Nutrition Sciences* 2013; **4**(3): 240-4.

25. Flaminio Fidanza, Vittorio Puddu, Bruno Imbimbo, Alessandro Menotti, Keys. A. Coronary heart disease in seven countries VII. Five-Year Experience in Rural Italy. *Circulation* 1970; **41**(I-63-I-75).

26. United States Department of Agriculture ARS. Beef, bottom sirloin, tri-tip, separable lean only, trimmed to 0" fat, choice, raw [URMIS #2244]. 2013.

27. United States Department of Agriculture ARS. Egg, whole, raw, fresh. 2013.

28. Ratko Buzina, Ancel Keys, Ivan Mohacek, M. Marinkovic, Arpad Hahn, Blackburn H. Coronary heart disease in seven countries V. Five-Year Follow-up in Dalmatia and Slavonia *Circulation* 1970; **41**(I-40-I-51).

29. United States Department of Agriculture ARS. Oil, olive, salad or cooking. 2013.

30. Kratz M, Baars T, Guyenet S. The relationship between high-fat dairy consumption and obesity, cardiovascular, and metabolic disease. *Eur J Nutr* 2013; **52**(1): 1-24.

31. Select Committee on Nutrition and Human Needs. Dietary goals for the United States. First ed. Washington: U.S. Govt. Print. Off.; February 1977.

32. National Advisory Committee on Nutritional Education (NACNE). A discussion paper on proposals for nutritional guidelines for health education in Britain. 1983.

33. Rose GA, Thomson WB, Williams RT. Corn Oil in Treatment of Ischaemic Heart Disease. *BMJ* 1965; **1**(5449): 1531-3.

34. Research Committee. Low-fat diet in myocardial infarction: A controlled trial. *The Lancet* 1965; **2**(7411): 501-4.

35. Medical Research Council. Controlled trial of soya-bean oil in myocardial infarction: Report of a research committee to the Medical Research Council. *The Lancet* 1968; **292**(7570): 693-700.

36. Leren P. The Oslo Diet-Heart Study. *Circulation* 1970; **42**: 935-42.

37. Dayton S, Pearce ML, Hashomoto S, Dixon WJ, Tomiyasu U. A Controlled Clinical Trial of a Diet High in Unsaturated Fat in Preventing Complications of Atherosclerosis. *Circulation* 1969; **40**(1S2): II-1-II-63.

38. Woodhill JM, Palmer AJ, Leelarthaepin B, McGilchrist C, Blacket RB. Low fat, low cholesterol diet in secondary prevention of coronary heart disease. *Advances in experimental medicine and biology* 1978; **109**: 317-30.

39. Turpeinen O, Karvonen MJ, Pekkarinen M, Miettinen M, Elosuo R, Paavilainen E. Dietary prevention of coronary heart disease: the Finnish Mental Hospital Study. *Int J Epidemiol* 1979; **8**(2): 99-118.

40. Miettinen M, Turpeinen O, Karvonen MJ, Pekkarinen M, Paavilainen E, Elosuo R. Dietary prevention of coronary heart disease in women: the Finnish mental hospital study. *Int J Epidemiol* 1983; **12**(1): 17-25.

41. Harcombe Z, Baker JS, Cooper SM, et al. Evidence from randomised controlled trials did not support the introduction of dietary fat guidelines in 1977 and 1983: a systematic review and meta-analysis. *Open Heart* 2015; **2**(1).

42. Committee on Medical Aspects of Food Policy (COMA). Diet and cardiovascular disease: Report of the panel on diet in relation to cardiovascular disease. 1984.

43. Truswell AS. Review of dietary intervention studies: effect on coronary events and on total mortality. *Aust N Z J Med* 1994; **24**(1): 98-106.

44. Food Standards Agency. Letter to Zoë Harcombe. September 25, 2009.

45. Harcombe Z. The Obesity Epidemic: What caused it? How can we stop it? York, UK: Columbus Publishing; 2010.

46. Teicholz N. The Big Fat Surprise. New York: Simon & Schuster; 2014.

47. Carter J.P. Eating in America; Dietary Goals for the United States; Report of the Select Committee on Nutrition and Human Needs US Senate. *Cambridge, MA, USA: MIT Press* 1977.

48. Davis C, Saltos. E. Dietary Recommendations and How They Have Changed Over Time,. In: United States Department of Agriculture ERS, editor. Agriculture Information Bulletin No (AIB-750) 494 pp; 1999.

49. Tanner TH. The Practice of Medicine. Philadelphia: Lindsay & Blakiston; 1869.

50. Department of Health and Human Services (HHS). Dietary Guidelines for Americans. In: Department of Health and Human Services (HHS), editor.; 2010.

51. Wright JD, Wang. C-Y. Trends in Intake of Energy and Macronutrients in Adults From 1999–2000 Through 2007–2008. In: Services USDoHaH, editor.: National Center for Health Statistics; 2010.

52. United States Department of Agriculture ERS. Agriculture Fact Book 2001-2002. In: United States Department of Agriculture ERS, editor. Washington: U.S. Government Printing Office; 2003.

53. United States Department of Agriculture ARS. Lard. 2013.

54. United States Department of Agriculture ARS. Oil, vegetable, sunflower, linoleic (less than 60%). 2013.

55. Mozaffarian D, Micha R, Wallace S. Effects on coronary heart disease of increasing polyunsaturated fat in place of saturated fat: a systematic review and meta-analysis of randomized controlled trials. *PLoS Med* 2010; **7**: e1000252.

56. Hooper L, Summerbell CD, Thompson R, et al. Reduced or modified dietary fat for preventing cardiovascular disease. *Cochrane database of systematic reviews (Online)* 2011; (7): CD002137.

57. Ravnskov U, DiNicolantonio JJ, Harcombe Z, Kummerow FA, Okuyama H, Worm N. The Questionable Benefits of Exchanging Saturated Fat With Polyunsaturated Fat. *Mayo Clinic proceedings Mayo Clinic* 2014.

58. Harcombe Z, Baker J. Plant Sterols lower cholesterol, but increase risk for Coronary Heart Disease. *Online J Biol Sci* 2014; **14**(3): 167-9.

59. Department of Health and Human Services (HHS). Dietary Guidelines for Americans. In: Department of Health and Human Services (HHS), editor.; 2005.

60. Centers for Disease Control and Prevention. National diabetes statistics report: estimates of diabetes and its burden in the United States,: U.S. Department of Health and Human Services, 2014.

61. Gregg EW, Zhuo X, Cheng YJ, Albright AL, Narayan KMV, Thompson TJ. Trends in lifetime risk and years of life lost due to diabetes in the USA, 1985-2011: a modelling study. *The Lancet Diabetes & Endocrinology* 2014.

62. Centers for Disease Control and prevention. Table 69. Mean energy and macronutrient intake among persons 20 years of age and over, by sex and age: United States, selected years 1971-1974 through 2005-2008 In: Statistics NCfH, editor.; 2011.

63. Taubes G. The Diet Delusion. UK: Vermilion; 2009.

64. Rand CS, Macgregor AM. Successful weight loss following obesity surgery and the perceived liability of morbid obesity. *Int J Obes* 1991; **15**(9): 577-9.

65. Flum DR, Salem L, Broeckel Elrod J, Dellinger E, Cheadle A, Chan L. Early mortality among medicare beneficiaries undergoing bariatric surgical procedures. *JAMA* 2005; **294**(15): 1903-8.

66. PepsiCo. Annual Report, 2013.

67. International Monetary Fund. Report for Selected Countries and Subjects. World Economic Outlook., 2014.

68. Academy of Nutrition and Dietetics. Annual Report, 2012.

69. Commission on Dietetic Regulation: the credentialing agency for the Academy of Nutrition and Dietetics. Setting the Standard since 1969, 2014.

70. Commission on Dietetic Regulation: the credentialing agency for the Academy of Nutrition and Dietetics. State Licensure Agency List. 2014. http://www.cdrnet.org/state-licensure-agency-list (accessed 10 October, 2014).

71. Alliance for Natural Health USA. Dietitian Licensure by U.S. State 2010.

72. Dietitians Association of Australia. Annual Report, 2013.

73. British Dietetic Association. Annual Report, 2013-14.

74. British Nutrition Foundation. Annual Report, 2013-14.

75. Gowlett JAJ. What Actually was the Stone Age Diet? *Journal of Nutritional and Environmental Medicine* 2003; **13**(3): 143-7.

76. Mansey K. Obesity tsar calls for tax on juice. The Sunday Times. January 12, 2014.

77. Bazzano LA, Hu T, Reynolds K, et al. Effects of Low-Carbohydrate and Low-Fat Diets: A Randomized Trial Effects of Low-Carbohydrate and Low-Fat Diets. *Ann Intern Med* 2014; **161**(5): 309-18.

78. Feinman RD, Pogozelski WK, Astrup A, et al. Dietary Carbohydrate restriction as the first approach in diabetes management. Critical review and evidence base. *Nutrition (Burbank, Los Angeles County, Calif)* 2014.

79. Hansen A. Swedish health advisory body says too much carbohydrate, not fat, leads to obesity. *BMJ* 2013; **347**.

Chapter Four

The Culprit in Coronary Disease Is *Trans* Fats, Not Cholesterol: But Why Did It Take Decades to Ban Them?

Fred A.Kummerow, PhD

Abstract

Partially hydrogenated vegetable oils (PHOs) have been in the American diet since 1910. More than 50 years ago it was discovered that they contained *trans* fatty acids that were different from natural fatty acids in plant oils and in animal fat. There was growing evidence that the consumption of artificial *trans* fats had negative health effects, including increasing plasma lipid levels. In 2003, the Food and Drug Administration (FDA) ruled that the amount of trans fat in a food item must be stated on the label. In my opinion negative health effects can only be changed by banning artificial *trans* fats. A petition was filed with the FDA in 2009 to ban artificial *trans* fat and followed by a lawsuit in 2013. The decision to ban artificial trans fat was finally realized June 16, 2015. Some of the key issues that explain why it took so long to ban them include:

- Shortening produced from the partial hydrogenation of soybean oil was first thought to be a miracle fat because of the desirable culinary properties.

- It took years to realize that all trans fats did not have the same properties. Artificial trans fatty acids and ruminate *trans* fatty acids have entirely different properties in vivo as well as in vitro. Even small amounts of artificial trans fat affect the prostacyclin synthesis.

- When the amount of artificial trans fat in margarines was lowered the sudden cardiac death rate also showed a decrease.

- When *trans* fats are removed from the food supply, there will be 325,000 less sudden cardiac deaths per year.

Discovery of *trans* fats

Hydrogenation was discovered by Nobel laureate Paul Sabatier in the late 1890s. He worked with hydrogenating only vapors. In 1901, a German chemist named Wilhelm Normann showed that liquid oils could be hydrogenated, and patented the process in 1902[1]. Production of the hardened fat commenced in 1909. Procter & Gamble acquired the US rights to the Normann patent and in 1911 they began marketing the first PHOs (partially hydrogenated oil). Hydrogenated fat began to replace lard in the 1920s. PHOs had desirable culinary properties as they had melting points close to body temperatures and became liquid in the mouth like butter. Prior to 1910, dietary fats consisted of butterfat, beef tallow, and lard. In 1910, no one knew what effect PHOs would have on the health of Americans. The effects *trans* fat in PHOs have on prostacyclin synthesis are now known[2]. The present mix of dietary fat in the marketplace results in less prostacyclin synthesis, which is an important factor in cardiovascular health[3,4]. Prostacyclin is a dominant prostaglandin produced by endothelial cells in arteries and is a potent vasodilator and inhibitor of platelet aggregation and leukocyte adhesion[5]. It limits the response to thromboxane, which is a potent inducer of vasoconstriction and platelet adhesion on the arterial wall and is partially responsible for the interruption of blood flow[6]. The rise of artificial *trans* fats in the diet correlates to the rate of American age-adjusted heart disease-related deaths since 1910[7].

Composition of *trans* fats

It took nearly five decades before the biochemical structure of trans fatty acids were understood. In 1952, the gas chromatography was made available[8] and could identify the components of PHOs. The partial hydrogenation of soybean oil added atoms of hydrogen to 50% of the bonds 9,12 in linoleic acid (n-6) and the bonds 9,12,15 in linolenic acid (n-3), converting them to 50% stearic acid[9]. Forty to fifty percent of the double bonds of fatty acids in n-6 and n-3 were shifted to different positions on the carbon chain making 9 different synthetic *trans fatty* acids and 5 different *cis* fatty acids. These were cis and *trans* isomers of octadecenoic and octadecadienoic acids that are not present in animal fats or plant oils. They interfere with the action of two isoforms a constitutive COX-1and an inducible COX-2 enzyme[4,10]. COX-2 is the enzyme that recognizes the isomers produced during hydrogenation as a foreign substrate and reacts to them by causing inflammation and inhibition of arachidonic acid, which is necessary to make prostacyclin. The 14 synthetic fatty acids were a source of energy but interfered with the conversion of n-6 to arachidonic acid and n-3 to eicosapentaenoic acid[11].

Several studies have called the attention to the *trans* fatty acids (TFAs) present in margarines and shortenings with some success. Samples of tissue obtained from human autopsies were shown to contain up to 14% TFAs[12]. Samples of fat from human placental, maternal, fetal and baby tissue were also examined for the presence of TFAs[13]. While the maternal tissue contained considerable amounts of TFAs, these lipids were not found to any measurable extent in placental, fetal or baby fat[14]. This was also shown in rats that were fed *trans fat*. When the *trans fat* was removed from the diet, their tissue metabolized the *trans fat* and their tissue no longer contained *trans fat*[15]. The results of these studies indicated that the TFAs present in human tissue apparently arise solely from dietary fat, and they do not normally appear in the tissues unless a source of TFAs is included in the diet.

Differences between PHOs and ruminant fats

It was believed by the FDA that partially hydrogenated soybean oil *trans fat* had the same chemical structure and worked the same way in our bodies as natural vaccinic acid[16]. These two *trans* fat sources have entirely different properties *in vitro* as well as *in vivo*.[3] The elaidic acid in PHOs has a double bond at position 9, while the vaccinic acid in ruminant fats is at position 11. The enzymes in the body recognize vaccinic acid (butterfat and beef fat) as the fatty acid that has been in the diet for untold generations.

In vitro and *in vivo* study

An *in vitro* study showed that the fatty acids in partially hydrogenated fat had different properties than fatty acids in animal fat or vegetable oil[17]. *Trans* acids increased the incorporation of $^{45}Ca^{2+}$ into the cells, where as *cis* acids did not incorporate $^{45}Ca^{2+}$ into the coronary artery cells. An *in vivo* study showed that the TFAs inhibited the synthesis of arachidonic acid, a polyunsaturated fatty acid, in the phospholipid membrane of arterial cells[18]. It was concluded that dietary *trans* fat perturbed essential fatty acid metabolism, which led to changes in the phospholipid fatty acid composition in the arterial wall, the target tissue of atherogenesis. Partially hydrogenated fat is a risk factor in the development of coronary heart disease because arachidonic acid is needed to synthesize prostacyclin.

Data from the CDC

Data obtained from the Center of Disease Control (CDC) shows the rate of death started increasing in 1910 and continued until 1968[7], at which time the industry lowered the percentage of trans fat from 44% to 27% and increased the amount of linoleic acid from 8% to 25%[3]. In 1968 the age-adjusted rate of heart disease-related deaths began to decrease[7]. Data from the CDC states that almost 600,000 Americans died of heart disease in 2011, 325,000 of those from sudden cardiac death[19]. The other 275,000 deaths were due to calcification of the coronary arteries to 100% occlusion[3].

Tentative determination to ban PHOs

On November 7, 2013 a tentative determination regarding PHOs was released by the FDA[20]. It stated that PHOs, which are a primary source of industrially-produced *trans* fatty acids or *trans* fat, are not generally recognized as safe (GRAS) for any use in food. The FDA requested comments of scientific data and information on this determination giving 60 days for responses. Before the 60 days were over they extended it another 60 days. That extension was over March 8, 2014. The FDA released this information in the Federal Register on November 8, 2013, "*trans* fats are an integral component of PHOs and are purposely produced in these oils to affect the properties of the oil and the characteristics of the food to which they are added."[20] At zero percent of *trans* fat content in the body, the prostacyclin release from vascular endothelial cells is 38.7 ng/mg of cell protein[3]. Data released in the Federal Register states that in 2012, the average American consumed 2.1 grams of trans fats per day, with the 90% percentile consuming 4.2 grams per day[20]. While consuming 2.1 grams of *trans* fat per day, the arterial cells will release 25 ng/mg cell protein, which is a significant drop from 38.7 ng/mg at zero percent. Consuming 4.2 grams/day of *trans* fat the cells will only release 15.5 ng/mg cell protein[3]. As more grams per day of *trans fat* are consumed, prostacyclin release from vascular endothelial cells to cell protein will decrease, proving an inverse relationship between the two processes. With the determination finalized the food manufacturers are no longer be permitted to sell PHOs without prior FDA approval.

Expert Opinion

The partial hydrogenation of vegetable oils have been shown to have an adverse effect on Americans. The FDA believed that artificial *trans* fats had the same chemical structure and worked the same way in the human body as natural trans fats. It has been shown that this is not true. The FDA finalized their decision to make artificial trans fat non-GRAS giving the industry three years to comply. With this decision more lives will be saved.

Funding for this type of research is difficult to find when one does not believe the mainstream about cholesterol and *trans* fats. The belief that heart disease is not a disease but a somatic response to a simple error involving the effect of *trans* fat in partially hydrogenated oil on prostacyclin synthesis goes against the mainstream. Therefore the present mix of dietary fat in the marketplace results in less prostacyclin synthesis and more sudden cardiac death.

In spite of the fact that the author has found an answer to heart disease and has convinced the FDA to consider making *trans* fats non-GRAS, he still has not received funding to continue his work.

Fred A.Kummerow, PhD

Adjunct Professor, Department of Comparative Biosciences, College of Veterinary Medicine, University of Illinois
fkummero@illinois.edu

References

Papers of special note have been highlighted as:

* of interest
** of considerable interest

1. Wilhelm Normann und die Geschichte der Fetthartung von Martin Fiedler, 2000". 2011-12-20.

2. Kummerow FA, Mahfouz MM, Zhou Q, Masterjohn C. Effects of prostacyclin production. Scandinavian Cardiovascular J. 2013; 47(5): 377-382.
** *This study showed that PHO* trans *fat prevented the synthesis of prostacyclin.*

3. Kummerow FA. Two lipids in the diet, rather than cholesterol, are responsible for heart failure and stroke. Clinical Lipidology 2014;9(2):189-204.
** *This study showed that* trans *fat is half the reason for heart failure and stroke.*

4. Vane J, Bakhle YS, Botting RM. Cyclooxygenase 1 and 2. Annu Rev Pharmacol Toxicol. 1998;38:98-120.

5. Cheng y, Austin SC, Rocca B, et al. Role of prostacyclin in the cardiovascular response to thromboxane A_2. Science 2002;296:539.

6. Mahfouz MM, Kummerow FA. Oxidized low-density lipoprotein (LDL) enhances thromboxane A_2 synthesis by platelets but lysolicithin as a product of LDL oxidation has an inhibitory effect. Prostaglandines Other Lipid Mediat. 2000;62:183-200.

7. CDC: leading causes of death 1900-1908.Available at: www.cdc.gov/nchs/data/lead1900_98.pdf. (Accessed November 2012)

8. James AT, Martin AJ. Gas-liquid partition chromatography: the separation and micro-estimation of ammonia and the methylamines. Biochem J 1952; 52: 238-242.

* *Adaption of the this technique led to the identification of the 14 synthetic fatty acids in* trans *fats*

9. Zalewski S, Kummerow FA. Rapeseed oil in a two-component margarine base stock. JAOCS 1968;45:87-92.

10. Vane JR, Mitchell JA, Appleton I, et al. Inducible isoforms of cycooxygenase and nitric-oxide synthase in inflammation. Proc Natl Acad Sci USA. 1994; 91: 2046-2050.

11. Kummerow FA. The negative effects hydrogenated *trans* fats and what to do about them. Atherosclerosis. 2009; 205: 458-465.

* *This study shows why the 14 synthetic fatty acids should be removed from the food supply.*

12 Johnston PV, Johnson O, Kummerow FA. Occurrence of *trans* fatty acids in human tissue. Science. 1957; 126: 698-699

* *This is the first publication that pointed to the possibility that* trans *fatty acids were harmful.*

13. Johnston PV, Johnson OC, Kummerow FA. Non-transfer of *trans* fatty acids from mother to young. Proc Soc Exp Biol Med. 1957; 96: 760-762.

14. Johnston PV, Kummerow FA, Walton C. Origin of the *trans* fatty acids in human tissue. Proc Soc Exp Bio Med. 1958; 99: 735-736.

15. Johnston PV, Johnson OC, Kummerow FA. Deposition in tissues and fecal excretion of *trans* fatty acids in the rat. J Nutr. 1958; 65: 13-23.

16. Food Labeling: *trans* fatty acids in nutrition labeling, nutrient content claims and health claims. Finale rule. Fed Reg 2003; 68: 41433-41506.

17. Kummerow FA, Zhou Q, Mahfouz MM. Effects of *trans* fatty acids on calcium influx into human arterial cells. Am J Clin Nutr. 1999; 70: 832-838.

18. Kummerow FA, Zhou Q, Mahfouz MM, et al. *trans* fatty acids in the phospholipid of arterial cells. Life Sci. 2004; 74(22): 2707-2723.

* *The* trans *fatty acids present in phospholipids transferred from female pigs to their piglets.*

19. Jain M. Explaining why so many cases of cardiac arrest strike in the morning. Presented at the national meeting of the American Chemical Society 2013;Sept 6-11.

20. Tentative Determination Regarding Partially Hydrogenated Oils; Request for Comments and for Scientific Data and Information. US Government. Federal Register. Docket No. FDA-2013-N-1317. 11/08/2013;78(217): 67169-67171.

Chapter Five

Industrial Control of Guidelines for Lipid Nutrition

Harumi Okuyama, PhD, Peter H. Langsjoen, MD,
Alena M. Langsjoen, MS, Naoki Ohara, PhD

Abstract

During the past half century, lipid nutrition has been strongly affected by the cholesterol hypothesis which states that increasing the intake of linoleic acid (ω-6) while reducing cholesterol and saturated fat is effective in lowering blood cholesterol and thereby reduces coronary heart disease. Even after the accumulation of enough evidence which indicate the fall of the hypothesis, pharmaceutical and food industries continue to advocate the risks of cholesterol and saturated fats, possibly to secure the profits of cholesterol lowering drugs and foods. Farming and livestock industries are closely associated with each other through seed oils. The established framework in the agricultural field involves seed oils containing linoleic acid and toxic components which might endanger human health when ingested chronically in large amounts. So far, industrial people, administration and associated scholars have been trying to hide the harmful aspects of vegetable fats and oils. In this review we emphasize that the safety of some vegetable fats and oils is an urgent problem to be addressed, and international collaborative research is necessary, to solve the problem rather than try to hide the facts from general public.

Introduction

After World War II, when the production of grains exceeded the levels that suffice human demands, excess grains began to be fed to livestock. Grains such as corn, soybean and rapeseed were chosen because of good productivity, amino acid score and other nutrient contents. However, since these grains contain too much oil for the health of herbivores, the oils were expressed. The remaining grains' meal was fed to livestock and the oils to humans. Such agricultural changes occurred from around 1965 toward 1975 in Japan, and some Western industrialized countries preceded Japan by several years. These industrial and nutritional changes were supported and accelerated by Keys' and Hegsted's equations published in the 1950's proclaimed that elevating polyunsaturated to saturated fatty acid ratio of ingested foods and reducing cholesterol intake are effective ways to lower plasma cholesterol levels and thereby reduce cardiovascular disease (CVD).

What we would like to emphasize here is that this agricultural and nutritional framework has been maintained firmly up to now, and any changes affecting this framework would cause conflict of interest among exporting countries (India, EU, USA, Canada) and importing countries (China, Japan, Mexico) of the seed oils. For example, evidence that excessive intake of linoleic acid causes many chronic diseases (Okuyama H et al., 1996) would be disadvantageous to the grain producers and food industry producing high linoleic acid foods, similarly to how critical evaluations of cholesterol lowering drugs are not welcomed by statin-related industries.

When scientists cannot reach agreement through publications, and the general people cannot judge scientists' discussions, people tend to seek the recommendations from authoritative organizations such as World Health Organization (WHO) and Food and Agriculture Organization (FAO) in the United Nations. However, more than half of the budget of WHO comes from global industries and the presence of routes for specialists from industry to express their opinions as those of WHO are officially established? Therefore, serious questions arise as to whether the guidelines from these organizations are based on scientific evidence without being affected by their budget supporters. More specifically, The Codex Alimentarius from WHO/FAO is a set of international standards for food labeling and safety.

TABLE 1 Codex General Standard for the Labelling of Prepackaged Foods, specified for fats and oils, and Our Proposal for Classification of Fats and Oils.

Codex Classification

Except for those ingredients listed in section 4.2.1.4, and unless a general class name would be more informative, the following class names may be used.

Name of Classes	Class Names	Additional Remarks
Refined **oils** other than olive	Vegetable oil	Hydrogenated or partially hydrogenated as appropriate
	Animal oil	—
Refined **fats**	Vegetable fat	—
	Animal fat	Pork fat, lard and beef fat shall always be declared by their specific names

Our proposal for the classification of fats and oils

Name of Classes	Class Names	Remarks
Vegetable fats and oils	Soybean oil, rapeseed oil, perilla oil, hydrogenated soybean oil etc.*	Type of fats and oils should be clarified
Animal fats and oils	Butter, lard, beef fat, fish oil, hydrogenated fish oil etc.	

* A type of oil with a significant difference in fatty acid compositions may be classified as, e.g., high-oleic or high-linoleic safflower oil, and fractionated oil as high-oleic or high-palmitic palm oil.

According to the "CODEX GENERAL STANDARD FOR THE LABELLING OF PREPACKAGED FOODS (CODEX STAN 1-1985, refined oils other than

75

olive oil are classified either as "vegetable oil" or "animal oil" (Table 1.), and refined fats as vegetable fat or animal fat. It is noted that the animal fat shall always be declared either as pork fat, lard and beef fat. In contrast, all types of vegetable oils could be labeled as vegetable oil.

This standardization of labeling of fats and oils does not appear to be scientific. Lard is a purified pork fat and there is no need to differentiate these two; the pork fat should be replaced with butter with fatty acid and minor component compositions significantly different from those of beef fat. Moreover, we have emphasized that various vegetable oils differ not only in their fatty acid compositions but also in minor components which exert significantly different physiological activities (Okuyama H, 2007a). Codex Alimentarius, just issued last year from WHO/FAO as labeling standard for packaged foods, does not appear to be evidence-based, but to be skewed by the influence of seed oil exporting countries and associated industry people who do not want to discuss the nutritional differences among different types of vegetable fats and oils (more detail in the sections II and II).

In Japan, committee members selected by the government tend to depend too much on the guidelines from WHO and world-leading medical societies of the US, simply translating them to people rather than evaluating and judging the available information by themselves. Currently, it is time for the general public to realize that nutritional and medical guidelines from the so-called authoritative organizations are likely to be seriously skewed by industry-supported scholars.

I. Fall of the cholesterol hypothesis, which has not been accepted by WHO and AHA

I-1. "The Cholesterol Myths" showing evidence against the "Cholesterol hypothesis"

A pioneering book by Uffe Ravnskov, "The Cholesterol Myths" was published in 2000. He collected many lines of evidence that contradict the cholesterol hypothesis defined above. In many countries, there have been scientists who disagree with the cholesterol hypothesis, but they encounter difficulties in publishing their opinions in established medical journals. Ravnskov directed a group of these people gathered under THINCS, The International Network of Cholesterol Skeptics. In the meantime, the mainstream scientists supported by the related industries continued to maintain their belief in the cholesterol hypothesis, ignoring opinions from THINCS, and the two groups' arguments have not been on the same wavelength. Why have the scientific arguments on the cholesterol hypothesis continued for so long after the fall of the hypothesis became clear? The answer is probably simple; there are scientists who derive great benefits by laying smoke screens on the criticisms and prolonging the arguments or they lack the ability to critically evaluate the presented data.

Because of the onset of unethical problems associated with the reports on clinical trials performed mainly by industry-associated scientists, a penal regulation for performing clinical trials came into effect in the EU in 2004, which was quite effective in changing the evaluation of cholesterol-lowering medications; randomized controlled trials of statins revealed no significant beneficial effects for the prevention of coronary events despite significant decreases in LDL-cholesterol levels (de Lorgeril M, 2008). Even now, scientists continue to claim that benefits of statins (prevention of CVD) outweigh their adverse effects (onset of diabetes and other adverse effects) based on meta-analyses of clinical papers published both before and after 2004. However, we did not adopt conclusions from meta-analysis of clinical papers including those published before 2004, mainly in 1990s', as reliable when we published a new cholesterol guideline 2010 (Okuyama H, 2011).

I-2. Fighting with the cholesterol guidelines issued from medical societies in Japan – high cholesterol level is a predictor of longevity

Japanese cholesterol guidelines for the prevention of CVD used to be issued from the Japan Atherosclerosis Society (JAS) supported by 9 related medical societies (JAS guideline). At the end of the last century, when the tentative guidelines were opened for discussion, the contents were essentially the same as those in ATP III (Adult Treatment Panel III) from the National Institute of Heart, Lung and Blood Institute,

USA. In 2001, we challenged these guidelines by pointing out that the risk of high cholesterol level is variable depending on the populations examined; the relative risk of high cholesterol for CVD is as high as >5 when the population or subpopulation includes a high proportion of familial hypercholesterolemia (FH), but no positive associations or even inverse associations are seen between these parameters when the proportion of FH is lower; e.g., among general populations over 40~50 years of age (Okuyama H, 2007; Japanese edition in 2002). The Japan Atherosclerosis Society and related medical societies have been ignoring our proposal, and have continued to publish new guidelines based on "the lower, the better hypothesis" in 2007 and 2012, regardless of our new guidelines in 2010, and the latest guidelines by Hamazaki T et al., 2015.

During the past couple of decades, biological and pharmacological researches on statin actions have been rapidly in progress. Analyzing such results, we reached the conclusion that statins stimulate atherosclerosis and heart failure (Okuyama H, 2015). As the latest message from us forwarded to medical societies is gaining increasing number of supportive comments among internet information, we are optimistic in reaching an agreement among the world medical societies on the cholesterol guidelines for the prevention of CVD, diabetes and other lifestyle-related diseases, that is, high plasma cholesterol is a predictor of longevity and statin-applicable cases are extremely restricted, if any.

I-3. Dietary lipids with high ω6/ω3 ratios as a major risk of CVD and other lifestyle related diseases

During the last century, large-scale dietary intervention trials based on the cholesterol hypothesis were performed and were unsuccessful. Helsinki Mental Hospital study (Miettinen M, 1972) is often cited as a successful trial, but it was a 6-year crossover study, which is too short a time to estimate the effects of dietary lipid intervention on CVD. In the Helsinki Businessmen study (Strandberg TE, 1991), increased mortality rates for CVD and all causes became clearer after 10 years of dietary intervention that was essentially based on the cholesterol hypothesis (Fig. 1). Thus, we should not cite the Helsinki Mental

Hospital study as the one that showed the effectiveness of increasing polyunsaturated/saturated ratios and reducing cholesterol intake for the prevention of CVD; The Helsinki Businessmen study revealed that it is in fact the opposite.

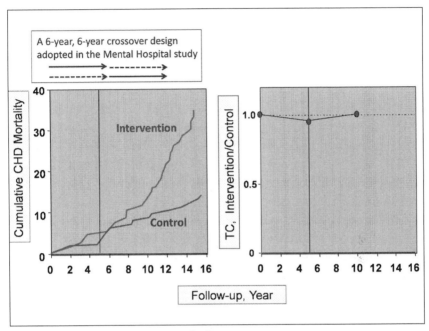

FIGURE 1 **Helsinki Businessmen study**

This is the first long-term (15 years) dietary intervention trial. For the beginning 5 years, hypocholesterolemic and hypotensive drugs were used, and dietary intervention was continued throughout the 15 years. Plasma cholesterol levels at 10 years of intervention were similar between the control and intervention groups (Strandberg, 1991). In the inserted square, the 6-year, 6-year crossover study schedule of the Helsinki Mental Health study (Miettinen M, 1972) is shown for comparison.

We would like to introduce an early example of papers that were distorted by industrial influence. The Helsinki Businessmen study was extended to 28 years (essentially it was 18 years, 3 years extension from the initial study of 15 years) (Strandberg TE, 1995), and new groups were added for the analysis beside the control and intervention groups; Low risk group, Excluded group, Refused group, and Dead in 1974 group. However, adding these new groups with background data much different each other is not rational even though the authors claim that multivariate adjustment was performed. The conclusion starts with "The traditional risk factors (smoking, blood pressure, and cholesterol) are significantly associated with 28-year mortality". However, the data do not support this statement. We interpret that only the Control and Intervention groups are to be compared in this trial. The death rates during the 18 years in the control group (n=610) and intervention group (n=612) were 31.1 and 63.7 (coronary heart disease); 1.6 and 26.1 (violent death, not natural death); 106.6 and 155.2 (all- cause deaths). We suspect that the above conclusion is a result of compromise among people in different fields.

The latest paper on large-scale dietary intervention based on the cholesterol hypothesis was published recently (Ramsden CE , 2013; Sydney Diet Heart study), which observed that substituting dietary linoleic acid in place of saturated fats increased the rate of death from all causes, coronary heart disease and cardiovascular disease. Based on the results, the Editorials of British Medical Journal softly criticized American Heart Association's advisory that higher [than 10 % of energy] intakes [of ω-6 PUFAs] appear to be safe and may be even more beneficial may be misguided (Calder P, 2013).

Long term ingestion of lipids with high $\omega6/\omega3$ ratios increase arachidonate/EPA ratio or arachidonate/(EPA+DHA) ratio of membrane phospholipids, and over production of ω-6 eicosanoids is the major cause of CVD, many types of cancer and other allergic, inflammatory diseases currently prevailing (Lands WEM, 2005; Okuyama H, 2007b, Ottoboni A, 2013). Nutritional, pharmacological, and gene technological means have been used to reach this conclusion.

Now it is clear why WHO and other organizations cling to the cholesterol hypothesis when scientific evidence warns of the prevalence of "excessive linoleic acid syndrome" (Okuyama H, 1996). Industrial power from countries exporting seed oils enriched with $\omega6$ fatty acids and the production of foods enriched with such seed oils incomparably outweighs the power of scientific evidence. Guidelines advising an increase in linoleic acid (ω-6) intake far above its essential amounts (1 energy %) are not evidence based, and are likely to be affected by industrial interests; the intake of 2 to 3 energy % is enough (International Society for Study of Fatty Acids and Lipids, ISSFAL).

II. Regulation of industrial *trans* fat based on inconsistent lines of evidence

II-1. Similarity of industrial and ruminant trans fats in physicochemical, biochemical and hypercholesterolemic properties

WHO and Food and Drug Administration (FDA, USA) have taken the initiative in excluding partially hydrogenated vegetable oils from our food and setting an upper limit of industrial *trans* fat at below 1 en%. Many Western countries appear to follow the WHO regulation, but the Japanese government decided not to set legal regulation of *trans* fat. This is because the average intake of *trans* fat was 0.7 en% a decade ago, now it is 0.3 en % and before long it is expected to be negligible. Situations are similar worldwide because alternative oil, palm oil, is available at much lower costs, and the shift from margarine to palm oil is clearly seen in the US (Fig. 2).

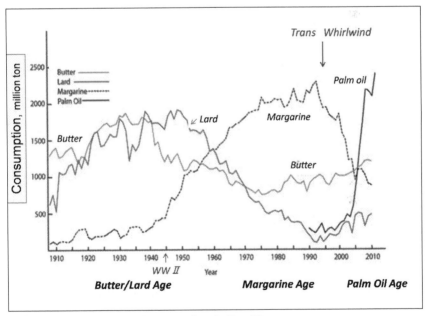

FIGURE 2 **Trends of Fat Consumption in the US**

WWII, the end of the World War II. Data taken from http://www.cnpp.usda. gov/USFoodSupply-1909-2010.

The necessity of regulating *trans* fat intake was based on reports that ingestion of *trans* fat elevates plasma LDL-C/HDL-C ratio and thereby increases CVD events. However, high LDL-C/HDL-C ratio is not a causative factor for CVD as explained in section I and elsewhere (Okuyama H, 2011; Hamazaki T, 2015).

In the regulations of Western countries industrial *trans* fat in partially hydrogenated oils is the target but not ruminant *trans* fat in foods of ruminant animal origin. This difference came from different physiological effects on CVD and diabetes in epidemiological studies as shown in Fig. 3.

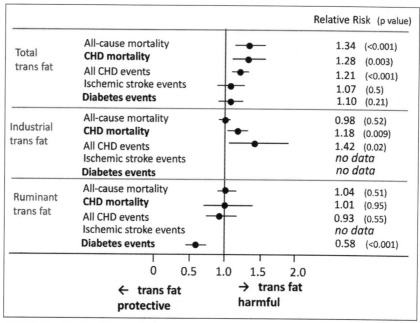

FIGURE 3 **Effect of the types of *trans* fat intake on CVD and diabetes**

Data from de Souza RJ, 2015.

Interestingly, industrial *trans* fat intake was positively associated with CHD mortality but not ruminant *trans* fat. Moreover, ruminant *trans* fat intake was inversely associated with diabetes but not total *trans* fat intake. Unfortunately, data for the correlation of industrial *trans* fat intake and diabetes are not shown. This set of data in Fig. 3 is enough to convince people that industrial *trans* fat and ruminant *trans* fat must be regulated separately, but this raises a serious question. What is the difference between the two types of *trans* fats?

Trans octadecenoic acids (18:1) consisted of 17 positional isomers with a *trans* double bond located at 2 to 17 position numbered from the carboxyl terminus, and the major isomers of the two types of *trans* fats and respective melting points are shown in Fig. 4.

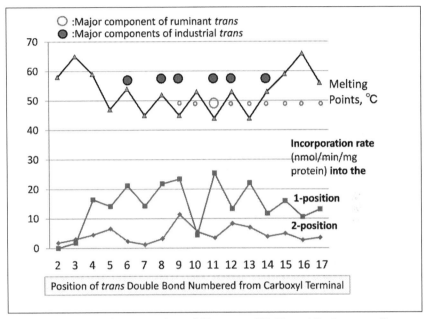

FIGURE 4 *Trans* octadecenoic acid isomers (18:1) and their properties

Respective melting points and incorporation rates into the 1 and 2-positions of phospholipid by acyl-CoA:lysophosphatidylcholine acyltransferase system in rat liver microsomes are presented (Okuyama H, 1972).

Although each isomer has slightly different physicochemical and biological properties (Fig. 4), those of major industrial *trans* isomers and ruminant *trans* isomers as a whole are relatively similar, and no crucial difference to account for the observed difference in the effects on CVD and diabetes (Fig. 3) could be found from Fig. 4. Consistently, both industrial and ruminant *trans* fat exhibited similar effects on plasma lipid levels in human studies; ruminant *trans* fat exhibited even greater activity to elevate LDL-C level and TC/HDL-C ratio (Fig. 5).

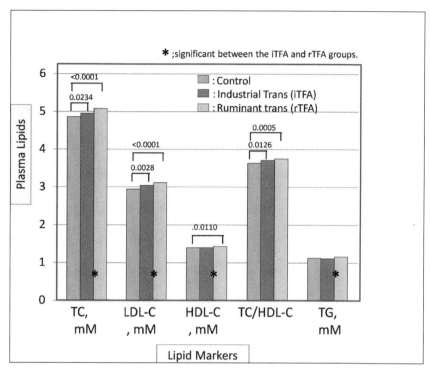

FIGURE 5 Randomized, controlled study comparing the effects of industrial and ruminant _trans_ fats on plasma lipid levels in healthy volunteers

Healthy participants (n=106, 47±10.8 years of age, BMI=28.5±4.0) were randomly assigned for a 24 days cross-over trial. Control diet (33 en% lipid) was supplemented with 3 en% industrial trans fat (iTFA), 3 en% ruminant trans fat (rTFA, vaccenic acid), or 1 en% c9,t12-CLA (conjugated linoleic acid). Data taken from Gebauer SK, 2015.

US Department of Agriculture (USDA) has the facility and experience to perform dietary intervention trial controlling whole nutrients, and concluded that ruminant _trans_ fat should also be included in the regulation of _trans_ fat. In fact, the data shown in Fig. 5 are apparently inconsistent with the results shown in Fig. 3, which raises a possibility that factor(s) other than _trans_ fat per se may be involved in the differential correlation of the two types of _trans_ fats with CVD and diabetes (Fig. 3), which will be explained in section II-3.

II-2. Safety of the alternative oil, palm oil, is of serious concern

Palm oil was chosen in the US, Japan and UK as the alternative to hydrogenated vegetable oils. Earlier, palm oil was not used as food but purification methods were improved, and now is the second most consumed vegetable oil in Japan. However in animal experiments, palm oil exhibited unusual survival shortening activity in mice (Fig. 6). Although this research report was published from National Food Research Institute Japan, and the experiment was stopped half way in, the results raise a serious concern on the safety of palm oil that should not be overlooked.

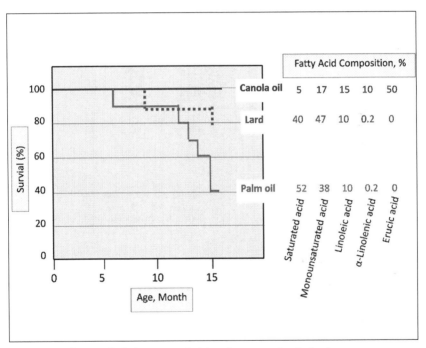

FIGURE 6 **Effects of dietary vegetable oils on survival of mice**

Diet containing 6 w/w % of oil was fed to male ICR mice (n=10 in each group). Data taken from Suzuki H, 1991.

Colon carcinogenesis is known to be promoted by linoleic acid (ω-6) and suppressed by α-linolenic acid (ω-3). The arachidonic acid (ω-6) cascade is involved in colon carcinogenesis, and anti-inflammatory drugs and genetic manipulation to suppress this cascade are effective in suppressing the carcinogenesis in animal experiments. Palm oil is not rich in linoleic acid but colon carcinogenesis was greatly promoted by dietary palm oil (Fig. 7) (Narisawa T, 1991). Similarly, unusual hyperinsulinemia of palm oil observed in diabetic mice (Ikemoto S, 1996) and stroke-stimulating activity observed in SHRSP rats were not accounted for by its fatty acid composition.

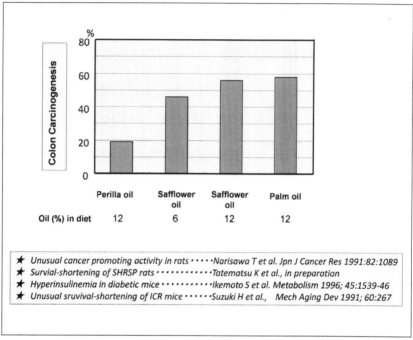

FIGURE 7 Palm oil used as an alternative to hydrogenated oils is not safe – colon cancer-promoting activity and some adverse effects

See text for explanations. Data taken from Narisawa T, 1991.

These results from animal experiments raise serious questions on the safety of palm oil, and does not support the industry guided shift from butter and lard to palm oil. As noted above, this shift is going to be completed before long in Japan. The oil and seed oils meal industries as well as associated administrative people in Japan have made no efforts to inform people of the potential health hazards.

II-3. Vitamin K$_2$ inhibitors rather than industrial trans fat as a causative factor of CVD and DM

Soybean oil and canola oil are rich in vitamin K1. When ingested, its side chain with one double bond is cleaved off to form vitamin K3, and then geranylgeranyl group with 4 double bonds (a prenyl intermediate in cholesterol biosynthesis) is inserted to form vitamin K2. (Fig. 8). In various tissues including brain, vitamin K2 level is higher than K1 and serves as a cofactor for enzymes to γ-carboxylate, the glutamyl residue of proteins. Statins inhibit the supply of geranylgeranyl residue and warfarin inhibits the reactivation of oxidized vitamin K1.

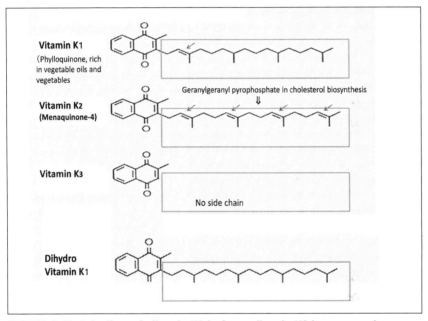

FIGURE 8 **Metabolism of vitamin K1 to form vitamin K2 in mammals**

See text for explanations.

Industrial hydrogenation of canola and soybean oils produces not only *trans* fat but also the dihydro form of vitamin K1 (dihydro-VK1), the side chain of vitamin K1 with one double bond being hydrogenated (Fig. 8). The dihydro-VK1 is not converted to vitamin K2, and inhibits the vitamin K2 dependent processes in human, e.g., bone homeostasis (Booth SL, 2001; Shea MK, 2009).

Recently, research on vitamin K2-dependent reactions is rapidly in progress, revealing the role of several proteins such as protein C, S, Z, matrix Gla protein, and osteocalcin (Ocn) in addition to well-known coagulation proteins. Intercellular Gla protein is γ-carboxylated and acquires the ability to bind calcium and thereby inhibit artery and kidney calcification. Undercarboxylated osteocalcin (uc-Ocn) is synthesized in osteoblasts in the bone, γ-carboxylated form c-Ocn, is accumulated in the matrix phase of bone. When osteoclasts work, acidic conditions are produced to convert c-Ocn to uc-Ocn (Shea MK, 2009; Oury F, 2013). Both c-Ocn and un-Ocn are excreted from the bone serving as bone-derived hormones in various organs as shown in Fig. 9. It is important to realize that inhibition of vitamin K2-dependent processes affects functions of most organs of the body through the bone-derived hormone, osteocalcin.

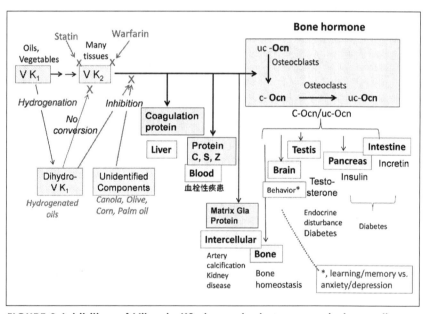

FIGURE 9 Inhibition of Vitamin K2-dependent processes induces diverse disorders

Partially hydrogenated soybean oil as well as canola and some other oils exhibits vitamin K$_2$-deficiency symptom such as hemorrhagic property, decreased platelet counts and kidney lesions (Okuyama H, 2007a; Hashimoto Y, 2014). Both c-Ocn and uc-Ocn from the bone are supposed to work on various target organs (Oury F, 2013).

We have been studying the effects of long-term feeding of vegetable oils in the stroke prone SHR (SHRSP) rat. As compared with soybean oil, canola oil and partially hydrogenated soybean oil and some other relatively common oils shortened the survival of SHRSP rats by accelerating cerebral bleeding, decreasing platelet counts, damaging kidney, and decreasing tissue testosterone levels, some of which are known to occur under vitamin K2-deficiency. Together with the findings by Booth SL, 2001, Shea MK, 2009 and Ito A., 2011, dihydro vitamin K1 was proposed as the active principle in hydrogenated soybean oil to shorten the survival of SHRSP rats (Okuyama H, 2007a).

Canola oil contains no dihydro-VK_1, but unidentified active principle in the oil exhibited similar inhibiting activity toward the vitamin K_2-dependent protein, osteocalcin; both exhibited decreased suppressive activity in the bone morphogenetic protein (BMP)-induced ectopic bone formation in mice (Hashimoto Y, 2013).

Coming back to the WHO regulation of industrial *trans* fat, we pointed out the following problems:

1. Elevation of LDL-C/HDL-C cannot be a causative factor of CVD because statins and statins plus CETP inhibitor therapies lower this ratio but exert no significant beneficial effect on CVD,

2. Industrial and ruminant *trans* fats elevate TC/HDL-C ratios similarly (Fig. 5), but only the industrial trans fat was positively associated with CHD mortality (Fig. 3),

3. Beneficial effect of ruminant *trans* fat, but possibly not industrial *trans* fat, for diabetes has not been explained (Fig. 3).

Instead, we interpret that industrial *trans* fat is the surrogate marker, and coexisting dihydro-vitamin K1 is the active principle to inhibit the vitamin K_2-dependent activation of matrix Gla protein and osteocalcin, thereby accelerating artery and kidney calcification. Similarly, ruminant *trans* fat is the surrogate marker of vitamin K_2 because both ruminant *trans* fat and vitamin K_2 are rich in beef, milk and cheese. In fact, vitamin K_2 intake but not vitamin K_1 intake was inversely associated with mortality rates for all causes and CHD in

Rotterdam study (Geleijnese JM, 2004), and similar association has been noted with metabolic syndrome markers (Shea MK, 2009).

The two different interpretations for the adverse effects of *trans* fat (Fig. 10) bring about definitive impact on human health. If the industrial *trans* fat per se is the active principle and the effect is only on CVD as explained in the WHO guidelines, the alternative oil, zero-*trans* palm oil, is ready to substitute for hydrogenated oils. In fact, industry people are trying to accelerate the shift from hydrogenated oil to palm oil as the latter is available at much lower costs, and sooner or later *trans* fat problems will disappear from media world (Fig. 10).

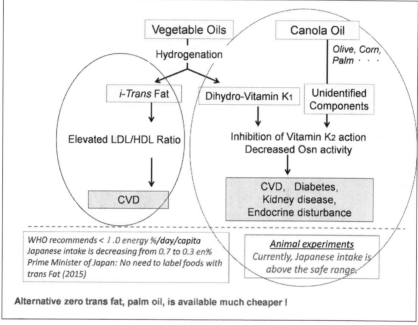

FIGURE 10 **Two different interpretations for the adverse effects of hydrogenated oils on CVD**

See text for explanations.

Contrarily, if our interpretation (Fig. 10) is applicable to food industry, the adverse effects of canola oil and some other vegetable oils need to be solved or human intake of these oils should be reduced (more details in section III).

III. Improved rapeseed quality and its toxicity

III-1. A historical overview of the improvement of rapeseed quality

According to a review by Schmid A and Schmid H, 1992, rapeseed has been planted in central Europe mainly for lighting but rarely for eating. However, rapeseed cake was recognized in 1980s' to cause toxicity in hen and ruminant animals, the problem of which was apparently solved by setting upper limits of rapeseed meal to be fed to livestock (Fig. 11).

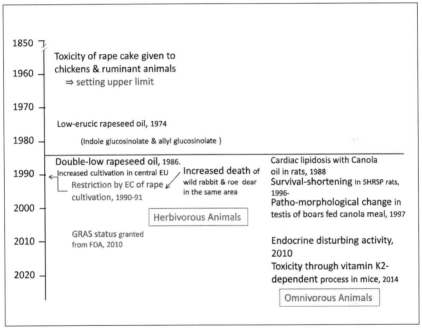

FIGURE 11 **Toxicity of rapeseed (Canola) in mammals and the administrative steps taken**

See text for explanations.

Erucic acid with 22 carbon chain and one double bond is an active constituent of rapeseed to cause lipidosis in the heart. Other toxic components are indole-glucosinolate, allyl-glucosinolate (Fig. 12) and their metabolites such as isothiocyanates, thiocyanates, nitriles, anti-thyroid agent (goitrin), S-methylcystein sulfoxide and dimethyl disulfide. These components affect many tissues but noteworthy are the rapeseed blindness and behavioral disorder (psychosis) observed in herbivores.

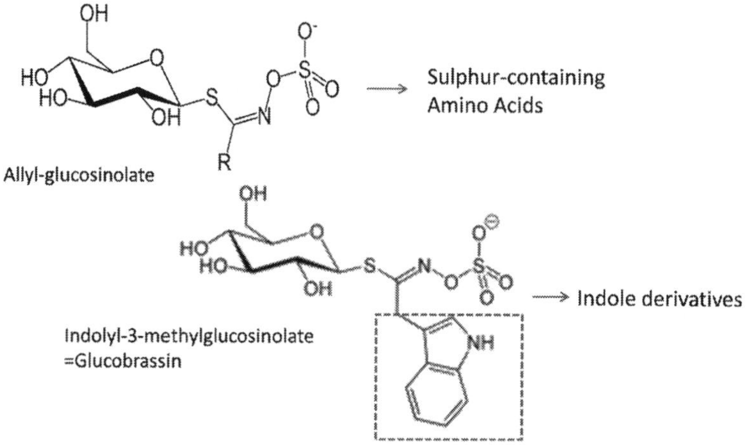

Isothiocyanates: hepatic injury, hemorrhage, epithelial cell and membrane injury
Dimethyldisulfide from SMCS: hemolysis, jaundice due to hepatic injury
Thiocyanates: rape blindness, psychosis, locomotive disorder ⇒ *BSE?*

FIGURE 12 Glucosinolates as toxic materials of rapeseed oil

See text for explanations.

In 1974, low-erucic rapeseed variety was selected and then a double-low rapeseed with much lower levels of glucosinolate was established in 1986, and canola was used as a brand name for a double-low cultivar. Then, the cultivation of double-low rapeseed increased in central Europe. Along with this increase, the numbers of wild rabbit and roe dear decreased significantly in this area, and the European Commission restricted the rapeseed cultivation in 1990-91. Even the double-low rapeseed does not appear to be safe in herbivores (Schmid A, 1992). It is difficult to understand why anyone would think it safe to consume seeds capable of killing wild rabbits and deer. Wild animals are by their nature much more healthy and robust than domestic or laboratory animals.

A Putative Story on Mad Cow Disease and Rapeseed

The rapeseed toxic components caused the so-called rapeseed blindness and behavioral disorder (psychosis) in herbivores, which is similar to BSE (bovine spongiform encephalopathy or mad cow disease) and CWD (chronic wasting disease) of wild deer shaped (fed) with grains to raise large antlers in northern America. The area where wild deer migrate is said to overlap with the area where wild rapeseed grows. These are the part of the observations for the proposal that rapeseed rather than an infectious prion may be the cause of mad cow disease and chronic wasting disease, and we support that this proposal is still considered valid. This theory lacks objective evidence but there may be additional hidden evidence. As a matter of fact, no positive correlation has been found between meat and bone meal (MBM) and BSE in Japan.

Despite these observations, we find no advice from the EC regarding the safety of double-low rapeseed oil, and US Food and Drug Administration later granted GRAS (generally regarded as safe) status to rapeseed oil for human use (2010). It is said that the Canadian government spent US$50 million to get it approved (Foodprints • Health & Nutrition. The Inconvenient Truth About Canola Oil. Original article at: http://www.smallfootprintfamily.com/the-inconvenient-truth-about-canola-oil#ixzz3xVciuab9).

III-2. Toxicity of double-low rapeseed oil and some other vegetable oils

In omnivorous animals, canola oil was reported to cause lipidosis in the rat heart (Magnuson BA, 1988). However, various reasons were presented to minimize the impact of this finding. For example, the proportion of saturated fatty acids is relatively small in canola oil and no statistically significant lipidosis was observed when animal fats were given together with canola oil. Humans in general ingest relatively large amounts of animal fats so that the impact of canola oil induced lipidosis would be negligible in humans. Of course, dilution of canola oil with animal fats would result in reduced degree of lipidosis, but this does not ascertain the safety of long-term canola oil ingestion in humans. Apparently this problem seemed to be solved or covered up.

About a decade later, our group (Huang MZ, 1996) encountered an unexpected result; dietary canola oil and evening primrose oil greatly shortened the survival of stroke-prone, spontaneously hypertensive (SHRSP) rats compared with soybean oil, perilla(seed) oil and fish oil (Fig. 13). Fatty acid composition of oils does not account for the difference, and we postulated the presence of unidentified component(s) rather than fatty acids and phytosterols, because the free fatty acid fractions obtained after alkaline or lipase hydrolysis of canola oil exhibited no significant activity. Hydrogenation of canola was expected to lessen the toxicity but it augmented it.

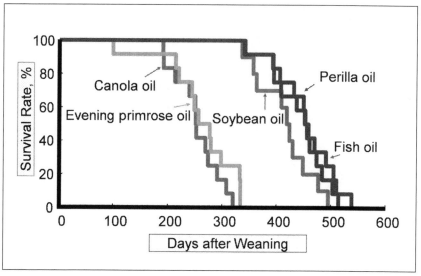

FIGURE 13 **Effects of dietary oils on survival of stroke prone SHR rats**

SHRSP rats (n=12/group) were fed a diet containing 10% (w/w) oil from weaning under ad lib conditions. Data taken from Huang MZ, 1996.

Dr. Lands WEM, former Professor, University of Michigan, advised one of us (HO) to see Dr. Bear-Rogers J, Health Canada and report the results to FDA (USA) and Ministry of Health and Welfare, Japan, so this was done around 1995.

Dr. Bear-Rogers is a very sincere, respectable scientist. Her group started experiments to confirm our experiments, informed us that olive oil and corn oil also exhibited survival shortening activity in SHR rats, and then she quit her positon at Health Canada. One of the successors of the team, Dr. Ratnayake WM (2000) proposed that phytosterols may be the active principle (Ratnayake WM, 2000b), but olive oil was exceptional; it contains little phytosterol but shortened the survival comparably.

A research group supported by the Ministry of Health and Welfare Japan repeated the experiments but no action has been taken so far regarding the use of canola oil. Another ministry of Japan recommended and supported the cultivation of rapeseed, and every spring the fields filled with yellow flowers show up in newspapers emphasizing the ecological approach that the meal is used for livestock, oil for school children and flowers for sightseeing. We have emphasized that rapeseed oil should not be consumed, especially by children.

So far, canola, palm, olive, corn, high-oleic safflower, high-oleic sunflower, evening primrose oil, and partially hydrogenated soybean and traditional rapeseed oil have been shown to shorten the survival of SHRSP rats, and they are likely to contain unidentified inhibitor of vitamin K2-dependent processes. Animal fats such as butter and lard are safer in this animal model (Fig. 14).

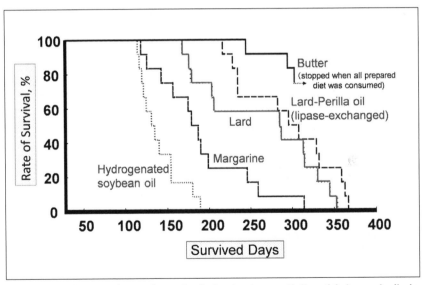

FIGURE 14 Comparison of survival-shortening activity of fats and oils in SHRSP rats

A diet supplemented with 10 (w/w) % of fat was fed to SHRSP rats (n=12 in each group). Data taken from Tatematsu K, 2004.

These chronic adverse effects observed in animal experiments are not easy to be examined in clinical trials. Therefore, the dose-response relationship in animal experiments is important to extrapolate the results to human nutrition. The survival-shortening activity of canola oil is dose-dependent, and a diet containing 6 energy % of oil still exhibited statistically significant activity. Currently, lipid energy % of ingested foods are around 25-35 % in most industrial countries, roughly half is vegetable oils in which more than 40 % is canola oil in Japan. Not only canola oil but also several other vegetable oils and hydrogenated oils exhibit comparable survival-shortening activities. Therefore, current Japanese intake of such oils is likely to be above the safe range without multiplying with the safety coefficient usually applied in toxicology field for the presence of species difference and difference among individuals (0.1 x 0.1). In Western countries where butter is still one of the major lipids consumed, the impact of these vegetable oils may be weaker. However, the EU seems to be one of great exporters and consumers of rapeseed.

The publications reporting these toxic effects of vegetable oils in rodents are listed in Table 2. Most of these reports are PubMed cited. Very importantly, however, the results of these publications, as well as adverse effects of high-linoleic vegetable oils, have been disregarded by WHO and major medical societies worldwide that are possibly supported by globally associated industries. Thus, the information unfavorable to the industry tends to be screened from the general public.

TABLE 2 **Adverse activities of dietary rapeseed (canola) oil and hydrogenated soybean oil compared with perilla (seed) oil, soybean oil, linseed oil, butter and lard in rodents**

Publication	Animal	Major Results	Control oil
Huang MZ, Biol Pharm Bull 1996; 19:554-7	SHRSP rat	Survival-shortening was dose- dependent, associated with cerebral bleeding, anal smudge and weight loss	Perilla oil, microbial oil

Huang MZ, Lipids 1997; 32:745-51.	SHRSP rat	Canola, high-oleic safflower, high-oleic sunflower, olive and evening primrose oil shortened the survival	Perilla oil, soybean oil
Miyazaki M, Lipids 1998; 33:655-61	SHRSP rat	Hydrogenated soybean oil shortened the survival; toxic material was formed during hydrogenation	Soybean oil
Miyazaki M, Nutr Res 1998; 18: 1049-56	SHRSP rat	Hydrogenation of canola and soybean oil did not reduce the toxic effect	Soybean oil
Miyazaki M, Biochim Biophys Acta 2000; 101-10	SHRSP rat	Canola and safflower oil accelerated kidney injury	Soybean oil
Naito Y, Toxicol Lett 2000;116:209-15	SHRSP rat	Canola oil induced shortening of blood coagulation time and increased fragility in erythrocyte membranes	Soybean oil
Ratnayake WM, Lipids 2000; 35: 409-20	SHRSP rat	Canola and low-sulfur canola, olive oil and corn oil shortened the survival. Phytosterol content was inversely associated with survival.	Soybean oil and other types of oils
Ratnayake WM, J Nutr 2000; 130:1166-78.	SHRSP rat	High concentration of phytosterols make the cell membrane more rigid, which might be a factor contributing to the shortened life span.	Soybean oil, olive oil
Ogawa H, Clin Exp Pharmacol Physiol 2003; 30:919-24.	SHRSP rat	Five times more phytosterol was necessary to reproduce the activity of canola	Soybean oil

Naito Y, Toxicology. 2003; 187:205-16.	SHRSP rat	Promotion by canola oil of hypertension-related deterioration in organs was proposed to be related to shortened life span	Soybean oil
Tatematsu K, J Nutr 2004; 134: 1347-52	SHRSP rat	Survival of offspring was affected by the diet that mothers took (2 generational study)	Soybean oil
Tatematsu K, Food Chem Toxicol 2004; 42:1443-51	SHRSP rat	Factor(s) other than phytosterol, and tocopherol status is critical for the toxicity	Soybean oil
Tatematsu K, J Health Sci. 2004; 50:108-11	SHRSP rat	Butter, lard and ester-exchanged lard- perilla were safer than canola	Butter
Ohara N, Food Chem Toxicol 2006; 44:952-63	SHRSP rat	Toxicity and phytosterol were partially separated by CO_2 supercritical extraction method	Soybean oil
Okuyama H, Lipids 2007; 42:821-5 (review)	SHRSP rat	Dihydro-vitamin K1 was proposed to be one of active principles in hydrogenated oils	Soybean oil
Ohara N, Food Chem Toxicol. 2008; 46:2573-9.	SHRSP rat	Supercritical CO_2 extraction produced a safe fraction, though it failed to separate clearly the causative substances.	Soybean oil
Ohara N, Food Chem Toxicol. 2009; 47:157-62	Wistar/ Kyoto rat	Canola oil elevated BP, increased plasma lipids, activated G-6-P DHase, decreased platelet, shortened coagulation time and induced anomaly in the kidney	Soybean oil

Okuyama H, J Toxicol Sci 2010; 35:743-7	SHRSP rat	Testosterone-lowering activities of canola and hydrogenated oil were detected	Soybean oil
da Coata CA, Horm Metab Res 2013; 45(9):652-4	Rat	Canola impaired pancreatic functions	Soybean oil
Hashimoto Y, Toxicol Reports 2014; 1:955-62.	Mouse	Canola and hydrogenated soybean oil accelerated ectopic bone formation	Soybean oil
Cai J, Nutr Neurosci. 2014 May 26	SHRSP rat	Canola accelerated cerebral breeding and decreased platelet counts	Perilla oil

III-3. Principles of rapeseed toxicity and their physiological activities

Two kinds of glucosinolate, allyl- and indolyl-glucosinolate, and their metabolites have been identified as the major components exerting adverse and beneficial effects (Fig. 12). One of metabolites, S-methylcystein sulfoxide (SMCS) is an anemic factor observed in lamb and cow, and thiocyanates cause rape blindness and psychosis (behavioral disorder) (Schmid A, 1992). Indole carbinol, a metabolite of indolyl glucosinolate, is polymerized under acidic conditions of stomach, and a dimer, di-indolylmethane, is a ligand of Ah receptor which binds with allyl hydrocarbon such as dioxin (Bjeldanes, 1991).

Most glucosinolate metabolites identified so far are hydrophilic, and are expected to be washed out during the production of cooking oils. However, di-indolylmethane is likely to be in oil. The survival-shortening factor (s) is hydrophobic and alkaline- or lipase-sensitive, which may suggest the presence of hydrophobic moiety in the molecule. Recently, oil expression is being replaced by hexane extraction in industrial vegetable oil production. Then, the hydrophobic toxic factor would move to oil and the meal for livestock would be safer than before.

Even though the survival-shortening factor(s) in canola and some other oils have not been identified yet, its physiological activities have been clarified to the extent that cannot be disregarded. The mechanisms of action are similar, at least in part, to dihydro-vitamin K1 in hydrogenated soybean oil in that they interfere with vitamin K2 functions, one of the target organs of which is the testis (Fig. 9).

III-4. Endocrine disturbing activity of some vegetable oils

Based on the results from DNA microarray analysis, tissue steroid hormone levels were determined. In the serum and testis, testosterone contents of the canola oil group were significantly lower than in the soybean oil group but not corticosterone and dihydrotestosterone contents (Fig. 15) (Okuyama H, 2010).

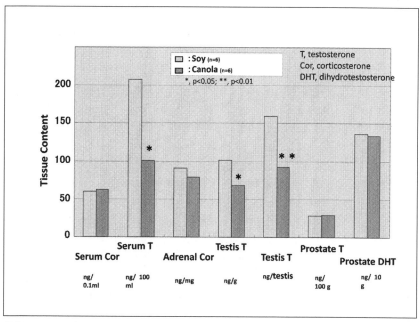

FIGURE 15 Tissue steroid hormone contents in SHRSP rats fed a diet supplemented with canola or soybean oil

SHRSP rats were fed a conventional diet supplemented with canola or soybean oil (Soy, 10 w/w%; 22 en %) from weaning (n=12 in each group). Data taken from Okuyama H, 2010.

In view of the importance of the observed endocrine disturbing activity of canola oil, experiments were repeated adding partially hydrogenated soybean oil group (Fig. 16). Both canola and hydrogenated soybean oil with a comparable survival-shortening activity lowered serum and testis testosterone contents, which was associated with altered survival of the second generation (Tatematsu K, 2004b).

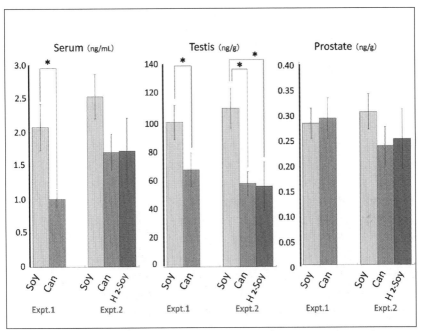

FIGURE 16 **Effects of dietary oils on tissue testosterone contents in SHRSP rats**

*Conditions for Expt. 1 were the same as in Fig.15 In Expt. 2, three groups with additional partially hydrogenated soybean oil (H2-Soy) group were compared. (Data taken from Okuyama H, 2010). *, p<0.05*

Dioxins have been recognized as the most powerful endocrine disturbing substances. The dose of dioxins to lower testosterone level in animal experiments is >200 fold higher than the amounts average Japanese currently ingest (0.69 pg/kg body weight/day in 2012). However, the difference between these two doses is much smaller in the case of vegetable oils, and in fact, both are comparable (~6 en%). The mechanisms of vegetable oils to lower testis testosterone, and affect behavioral pattern through inhibition of vitamin K_2-dependent biochemical pathways have been gradually revealed. Osteocalcin synthesized in osteoblasts is γ -carboxylated to form c-Ocn, which is stored in the matrix phase of the bone. When osteoclasts are activated, acidic conditions are produced to decarboxylate c-Ocn to form uc-Ocn. Currently, it is believed that both c-Ocn and uc-Ocn are secreted from the bone, taken up by Leidig cells in the testis, modify gene transcription and stimulate testosterone production, and the testosterone stimulates spermatogenesis in the spermatocytes (Oury F, 2011).

It is interpreted that dihydro-vitamin K_1 in the hydrogenated oils and unidentified components in canola and some other oils with properties similar to dihydro-vitamin K_1 induce tissue vitamin K2-deficiency, resulting in disorder of testis functions. Testis hypertrophy observed in canola meal fed boars, as compared with soybean meal (Rotkiewicz T, 1997), may be relevant to altered steroid hormone levels, just as both deficiency and overdosing of iodine induce thyroid hypertrophy. Admitting to make a leap from animal studies to humans, it may be noteworthy that vitaminK_2-deficient populations (Geleijnese JM, 2004; Geleijnese JM, 2011) as well as testosterone deficient populations (Khaw KT, 2007) exist in the contemporary societies generally eating enough foods, and that young men's sperm properties are poorer than those of a few decades ago (Iwamoto T, 2005; Anderson A-M, 2008).

Another endocrine disturbing substance is gossypol that is present in both the meal and oil from cotton seeds, which may have been clinically used in the case of one-child policy in an Asian country. A couple of decades ago, using cottonseeds for livestock was stopped in the Western countries, which is possibly associated with disorders of sexual cycle of cattle. Sooner or later, the production of cottonseed oil increased in Japan. Altogether, we propose that excessive intake of some kinds of vegetable fats and oils should not be disregarded when analyzing environmental factors causing endocrine disturbance.

IV. Industrial impacts on lipid nutritional guidelines for the prevention of lifestyle-related diseases

Lipid nutrition is involved in chronic diseases such as atherosclerotic CVD, diabetes, cancer, and other allergic, inflammatory diseases.

Various fats and oils of animal and vegetable origin are characterized by their fatty acid compositions and minor component compositions. Animal experiments have been performed extensively since the latter half of the last century, and observational clinical studies followed. However, large-scale randomized, controlled studies on fats and oils in humans are limited. This is mainly because profits do not accompany the demonstration of new functions of known foods. Therefore, at present, lipid nutrition must be based mainly on basic research and observational human studies.

Fatty acid compositions of cellular lipids are known to differ among organs, but those of an organ are relatively similar among different species. For example, DHA is particularly rich in retinal lipids in mammals as well as in frogs and fish. This **high organ-specificity and relatively low species specificity** is one of the reasons to rely on animal experiments, although there may be cases when species' differences must be taken into consideration. In this chapter, we summarize briefly the results of nutritional evaluation of fats and oils, independently of the evaluation by authoritative organizations.

IV -1. Excessive linoleic acid (ω-6) syndrome

First, long-term ingestion of ω-6 fatty acids in the absence of competing amounts of ω-3 fatty acids leads to membrane phospholipids with elevated arachidonate (ω-6)/EPA (ω-3) ratio or arachidonate (ω6)/(EPA+DHA) (ω3) ratio, resulting in elevated inflammation. Persistent inflammation caused by stimulation of arachidonate cascade is a possible major cause of atherosclerotic diseases, cancer of adenocarcinoma type, and other allergic, inflammatory disease, which has been proven by nutritional, pharmacological and gene technological means as described in section I and elsewhere (Okuyama H, 1996, 2007; Kang JX, 2008).

Obviously, the above notion is disadvantageous to seed oil exporting countries and industries producing high-linoleic foods. In order to maintain the agricultural framework of farming and livestock industry, consuming all the oils produced annually is desirable. Accordingly, the guidelines for the prevention of coronary heart disease issued from WHO and AHA (American Heart Association) still do not accept the positive associations with excessive intakes of vegetable oils with high ω6/ω3 ratios and lifestyle-related diseases. It is very difficult for us to believe that these guidelines were prepared simply based on scientific evidence.

- **WHO**: Prevention of cardiovascular diseases: guidelines for assessment and management of total cardiovascular risk, WHO Press, 2007

- **2013 AHA/ACC guideline on lifestyle management to reduce cardiovascular Risk**: Eckel RH, Jakicic JM, Ard JD et al. Circulation. 2014; 129(25 Suppl 2):S76-99.

IV -2. Intentional regulation of trans fat

People welcomed the regulation of industrial *trans* fat led by WHO and FDA. However, some epidemiological studies were inconsistent with the causative role of dietary *trans* fat for atherosclerosis. Moreover, clinical study demonstrating comparable cholesterol-elevating activities of both industrial and ruminant *trans* fats (Fig. 5) is inconsistent with the regulation targeting industrial *trans* fat only as described above.

Another aspect is that statins are effective in lowering LDL-C/HDL-C ratio, and statin plus cholesterol ester transport protein (CETP) inhibitor combination is more effective, but they are ineffective in reducing CHD significantly, and a clinical trial with the latter increased all-cause mortality. Therefore, we wonder how the so-called authoritative organizations such as WHO and FDA can keep claiming that reducing industrial *trans* fat is effective for the prevention of CHD. The majority of citizens is not informed of this scientific evidence and simply follows the guidelines from such organizations.

We would like to point out that alternative oil, *trans*-free palm oil, is available much cheaper than hydrogenated vegetable oils, and the industry people may have advocated the shift from *trans* fat to palm oil using the cholesterol hypothesis. However, palm oil is not a safe vegetable oil as explained above. The Japanese administration appears to have approved the use of "vegetable fat or edible fat" instead of "palm oil" for labeling packaged foods because palm oil had previously been used only for industrial purposes, e.g., soap production. Currently, palm oil holds the second position among vegetable fats and oils consumed in Japan, the number one being canola oil (>40% of the total). Consumers cannot tell what kind of fats and oils are included in packaged foods when edible oil or vegetable oil is approved for labeling. Another intentional (or unintentional) aspect of industrial *trans* fat bashing is associated with double-low rapeseed oil. Linking the industrial *trans* fats only to LDL-C/HDL-C and CVD, the problems of adverse activities of some other vegetable oils were probably expected to be ignored by critical eyes.

IV -3. Double-low rapeseed oil - disregarded or hidden toxicity

A cultivar of rapeseed low in toxic erucic acid and glucosinolates was established in around 1986, and its cultivation area was increased in the central area of EU, then increased death of wild rabbit and roe deer was noted. The European Commission restricted the cultivation area of the double-low variety (Schmid A, 1992). Another step taken worldwide was to set the upper limit of rape meal to be fed to livestock. However, no other regulations appear to have been issued worldwide.

The toxic substance(s) in canola oil is hexane-soluble, hence the effects may not be confined to herbivores. In fact, the toxic effects were observed in many organs of rats and boars as explained above, although the active component(s) has not been identified. It happened to us that both canola oil and hydrogenated soybean oil exert their toxicity at least partly through inhibition of vitamin K_2-dependent processes as dihydro-vitamin K_1 does (Hashimoto Y, 2014). In a DNA microarray analysis, the genes that were up- or down-regulated by canola oil and hydrogenated soybean oil, as compared with soybean oil, agreed >90% in the rat testis.

One of toxic activities of canola is endocrine disturbance and we are surrounded by vegetable oils with environmental hormone activities (Fig. 17). Japanese are particularly in danger of endocrine disturbing oils (Iwamoto T, 2006; Anderson A-M, 2008), because vegetable oils/ animal fats ratio of ingested foods is high and canola oil and vegetable fats and oils with similar activities comprises the major parts of all fats and oils. Behavioral changes, altered development of sexual characteristics, and increased neuronal disorders, if it is occurring in Japan, are suspected to be associated with lipid nutrition.

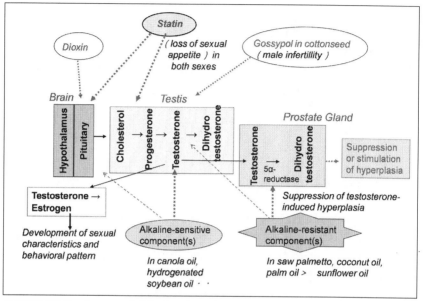

FIGURE 17 Environmental Endocrine Disturbing Substances

Alkaline-sensitive component(s) (vitamin K$_2$-inhibiting) is presumed to be present in canola and some other vegetable oils. Alkaline-resistant component(s) in some tropical fats is known as inhibitor(s) of 5α-reductase to form dihydroxy testosterone.

IV -4. Codex General Standard for the Labelling of Prepackaged Foods - FAO/WHO, 2010

According to this standard, fats and oils are classified by the difference in melting points as usual, and each is classified into animal and vegetable. "Partially hydrogenated" is used as appropriate, and animal fats are to be defined as pork fat, lard or beef fat.

This classification is apparently rational but all types of vegetable oils can be labeled solely as "vegetable oil", regardless of the difference in the fatty acid and minor component compositions. As pointed out by us and many other scientists (Table 2), differential physiological and nutritional effects have been reported for different vegetable oils.

It cannot be a simple mistake of the Codex committee to disregard all these adverse effects of some types of vegetable oils (Table 2), and here we feel the presence of intentional tactics of the food industry. We propose that labelling the type of vegetable oils is essential for consumers to choose foods.

Concluding remarks

Cholesterol hypothesis has been examined by randomized, controlled trials (RCT) to reveal that raising the polyunsaturated/saturated ratio of ingested foods and reducing cholesterol intake are rather detrimental for the prevention of CVD and reduction of all-cause mortality. Observational clinical studies as well as basic studies that are consistent with this interpretation have been reported. Interestingly, some vegetable fats and oils share a common mechanism with statins and warfarin to disturb tissue vitamin K_2-dependent processes, and osteocalcin-regulated functions of various organs. Thus, vegetable oils with high ω-6/ω-3 ratios and vegetable fats and oils with stroke-stimulating activities were proposed to be causatives of CVD, diabetes, kidney disease and other lifestyle-related diseases; dietary cholesterol and animal fats are evaluated to be relatively safe.

Based on these observations and interpretations, we propose that most lipid nutritional guidelines from authoritative organizations should be reevaluated simply based on available evidence and without disregarding reports demonstrating adverse effects.

Harumi Okuyama, PhD[*], Peter H. Langsjoen, MD[**], Alena M. Langsjoen, MS[**], and Naoki Ohara, PhD[***]

[*] *Professor Emeritus, Nagoya City University, and Institute for Consumer Science and Human Life, Kinjo Gakuin University*
okuyamah@kinjo-u.ac.jp

[**] *Clinical Cardiology Practice, Tyler, Texas, USA*
peterlangsjoen@cs.com
alilangsjoen@cs.com

[***] *School of Pharmacy, Kinjo Gakuin University*

References

Andersson A-M, Jørgensen N, Main KM et al. Adverse trends in male reproductive health: we may have reached a crucial 'tipping point'. Int J Androl 2008; 31: 74–80.

Bjeldanes LF, Kim JY, Grose KR et al. Aromatichydrocarbon responsiveness -receptor agonists generated from indole-3-carbinol in vitro and in vivo: comparisons with 2,3,7,8-tetrachlorodibenzo-p-dioxin. Proc Natl Acad Sci U S A. 1991; 88:95437.

Booth SL, Lichtenstein AH, O'Brien-Morse M et al. Effects of a hydrogenated form of vitamin K on bone formation and resorption. Am J Clin Nutr 2001; 74:783-90.

Cai J, Jang JY, Kim J et al. Comparative effects of plant oils on the cerebral hemorrhage in stroke-prone spontaneously hypertensive rats. Nutr Neurosci 2014 May 26. [Epub ahead of print]

Calder PC. Old study sheds new light on the fatty acids and cardiovascular health debate. BMJ 2013; 346:f493.

da Costa CA, Carlos AS, de Sousa Dos Santos A et al. High-fat diets containing soybean or canola oil affect differently pancreas function of young male rats. Horm Metab Res. 2013; 45:652-4.

de Souza RJ, Mente A, Maroleanu A et al. Intake of saturated and trans unsaturated fatty acids and risk of all-cause mortality, cardiovascular disease, and type 2 diabetes: systematic review and meta-analysis of observational studies. BMJ. 2015; 351:h3978.

Dam V, Dalmeijer GW, Vermeer C et al. Association Between Vitamin K and the Metabolic Syndrome: A 10-Year Follow-Up Study in Adults. J Clin Endocrinol Metab. 2015; 100:2472-9.

De Lorgeril M, Cholesterol Menasonges et Propagande, Thierry Souccar Editions, France, 2008

Gebauer SK, Destaillats F, Dionisi F et al. Vaccenic acid and trans fatty acid isomers from partially hydrogenated oil both adversely affect LDL cholesterol: a double-blind, randomized controlled trial. Am J Clin Nutr 2015; 102:1339-46.

Geleijnse JM, Vermeer C, Grobbee DE et al. Prevalence of vertebral fractures, vascular calcifications, and mortality in warfarin treated hemodialysis patients. Curr Vasc Pharmacol. 2015; 13(2):248-58.

Geleijnse JM, Vermeer C, Grobbee DE et al. Dietary intake of menaquinone is associated with a reduced risk of coronary heart disease: the Rotterdam Study. J Nutr 2004; 134:3100-5.

Gerstein HC, Miller ME, Byington RP et al. Effects of intensive glucose lowering in type 2 diabetes. N Engl J Med. 2008; 358(24):2545-59.

Hamazaki T, Okuyama H, Ogushi Y et al. Towards a Paradigm Shift in Cholesterol Treatment. A Re-examination of the Cholesterol Issue in Japan. Ann Nutr Metab. 2015; 66 Suppl 4:1-116.

Hashimoto Y, Mori M, Kobayashi S et al. Canola and hydrogenated soybean oils accelerate ectopic bone formation induced by implantation of bone morphogenetic protein in mice. Toxicology Reports 2014; 1:955–962

Huang MZ, Naito Y, Watanabe S et al. Effect of rapeseed and dietary oils on the mean survival time of stroke-prone spontaneously hypertensive rats. Biol Pharm Bull. 1996; 19:554-7.

Huang MZ, Watanabe S, Kobayashi T et al. Unusual effects of some vegetable oils on the survival time of stroke-prone spontaneously hypertensive rats. Lipids. 1997; 32:745-51.

Ikemoto S, Takahashi M, Tsunoda N et al. High-fat diet-induced hyperglycemia and obesity in mice: differential effects of dietary oils. Metabolism 1996; 45:1539-46.

Ito A, Shirakawa H, Takumi N et al. Menaquinone-4 enhances testosterone production in rats and testis-derived tumor cells. Lipids in Health and Disease 2011, 10:158, http://www.lipidworld.com/content/10/1/158

Iwamoto T, Nozawa S, Yoshiike M et al. Semen quality of 324 fertile Japanese men. Hum Reprod 2006; 21:760-5.

Kang JX. A transgenic mouse model for gene-nutrient interactions. J Nutrigenet Nutrigenomics. 2008;1(4):172-7.

Khaw KT, Dowsett M, Folkerd E et al. Endogenous testosterone and mortality due to all causes, cardiovascular disease, and cancer in men: European prospective investigation into cancer in Norfolk (EPIC-Norfolk) Prospective Population Study. Circulation. 2007; 116:2694-701

Lands WEM, Fish, Omega-3 and Human Health, 2nd Edition. AOCS Publishing; 2nd edition, 2005.

Magnuson BA, Schiefer HB, Crichlow EC et al. Effects of various high-fat diets on myocardial contractility and morphology in rats. Drug Nutr Interact 1988; 5:213-26.

Miettinen M, Turpeinen O, Karvonen MJ et al. Effect of cholesterol-lowering dieton mortality from coronary heart-disease and other causes. A twelve-yearclinical trial in men and women. Lancet. 1972; 2(7782):835-8.

Miyazaki M, Huang MZ, Takemura N et al. Free fatty acid fractions from some vegetable oils exhibit reduced survival time-shortening activity in stroke-prone spontaneously hypertensive rats. Lipids. 1998; 33:655-61.

Miyazaki M, Huang MZ, Watanabe S et al. Early mortality effect of partially hydrogenated vegetable oils in stroke-prone spontaneously hypertensive rats (SHRSP). Nutr Res 1998; 18: 1049-56.

Miyazaki M, Takemura N, Watanabe S et al. Dietary docosahexaenoic acid ameliorates, but rapeseed oil and safflower oil accelerate renal injury in stroke-prone spontaneously hypertensive rats as compared with soybean oil, which is associated with expression for renal transforming growth factor-beta, fibronectin and renin. Biochim Biophys Acta. 2000; 1483:101-10.

Naito Y, Konishi C, Ohara N. Blood coagulation and osmolar tolerance of erythrocytes in stroke-prone spontaneously hypertensive rats given rapeseed oil or soybean oil as the only dietary fat. Toxicol Lett 2000; 116:209-15.

Naito Y, Nagata T, Takano Y et al. Rapeseed oil ingestion and exacerbation of hypertension-related conditions in stroke prone spontaneously hypertensive rats. Toxicology 2003; 187:205-16.

Narisawa T, Takahashi M, Kotanagi H et al. Inhibitory effect of dietary perilla oil rich in the n-3 polyunsaturated fatty acid alpha-linolenic acid on colon carcinogenesis in rats. Jpn J Cancer Res 1991; 82:1089-96.

Ogawa H, Yamamoto K, Kamisako T et al. Phytosterol additives increase blood pressure and promote stroke onset in salt-loaded stroke-prone spontaneously hypertensive rats. Clin Exp Pharmacol Physiol. 2003; 30:919-24.

Ohara N, Naito Y, Nagata T et al. Exploration for unknown substances in rapeseed oil that shorten survival time of stroke-prone spontaneously hypertensive rats. Effects of super critical gas extraction fractions. Food Chem Toxicol. 2006; 44:952-63.

Ohara N, Kasama K, Naito Y et al. Different effects of 26-week dietary intake of rapeseed oil and soybean oil on plasma lipid levels, glucose-6-phosphate dehydrogenase activity and cyclooxygenase-2 expression in spontaneously hypertensive rats. Food Chem Toxicol. 2008; 46:2573-9.

Ohara N, Naito Y, Kasama K et al. Similar changes in clinical and pathological parameters in Wistar/Kyoto rats after a 13-week dietary intake of canola oil or fatty acid composition-based interesterified canola oil mimic. Food Chem Toxicol 2009; 47:157-62.

Okuyama H, Lands WE, Gunstone FD et al. Selective transfers of trans-ethylenic acids by acyl coenzyme A. Phospholipid acyltransferases. Biochemistry 1972; 11:4392-8.

Okuyama H, Kobayashi T, Watanabe S. Dietary fatty acids--the N-6/N-3 balance and chronic elderly diseases. Excess linoleic acid and relative N-3 deficiency syndrome seen in Japan. Prog Lipid Res. 1996; 35(4):409-57.

Okuyama H, Yamada K, Miyazawa D et al. Dietary lipids impacts on healthy ageing. Lipids. 2007; 42(9):821-5. (2007a)

Okuyama H, Ichikawa Y, Sun YJ et al. Prevention of Coronary Heart Disease-from the cholesterol hypothesis to ω6 to ω3 balance, Karger, Basel, 2007 (2007b)

Okuyama H, Ohara N, Tatematsu K et al. Testosterone-lowering activity of canola and hydrogenated soybean oil in the stroke-prone spontaneously hypertensive rat. J Toxicol Sci. 2010; 35(5):743-7.

Okuyama H, Hamazaki T, Ogushi Y et al., New Cholesterol Guidelines for Longevity 2010, World Rev Nutr Diet 2011; 102:124-36.

Okuyama H, Langsjoen PS, Hamazaki T et al. Statins stimulate atherosclerosis and heart failure-pharmacological mechanisms. Expert Rev Clin Pharmacol 2015; 8:189-99.

Ottoboni A, Ottoboni, F. The Modern Nutritional Diseases: Heart disease, stroke, type-2 diabetes, obesity, cancer and how to prevent them. 2nd Edition. Fernley, NV: Vincente Books; 2013, p. 1-289.

Oury F, Sumara G, Sumara O et al. Endocrine regulation of male fertility by the skeleton. Cell. 2011; 144:796-809.

Oury F, Khrimian L, Denny CA et al. Maternal and offspring pools of osteocalcin influence brain development and functions. Cell. 2013; 155(1):228-41

Ramsden CE, Zamora D, Leelarthaepin B et al. Use of dietary linoleic acid for secondary prevention of coronary heart disease and death: evaluation of recovered datafrom the Sydney Diet Heart Study and updated meta-analysis. BMJ 2013; 346:e8707. doi: 10.1136/bmj.e8707.

Ratnayake WM, Plouffe L, Hollywood R et al. Influence of sources of dietary oils on the life span of stroke-prone spontaneously hypertensive rats. Lipids 2000; 35:409-20.

Ratnayake WM, L'Abbé MR, Mueller R et al. Vegetable oils high in phytosterols make erythrocytes less deformable and shorten the life span of stroke-prone spontaneously hypertensive rats. J Nutr 2000; 130:1166-78.

Ravnskov U, The Cholesterol Myths, New Trends Pub Inc, 2000

Rotkiewicz T, Bomba G, Falkowski J et al. Studies on a long-term use of rapeseed products in diets for boars. Pathomorphological changes in the reproductive system, liver and thyroid gland. Reprod Nutr Dev. 1997; 37:675-90.

Schmid A, Schmid H. Rapsvergifting wildlebender Pflanzenfresser. Tierärztl Prax 1992; 20:321-5

Shea MK, Gundberg CM, Meigs JB et al. Gamma-carboxylation of osteocalcin and insulin resistance in older men and women. Am J Clin Nutr. 2009; 90(5):1230-5.

Strandberg TE, Salomaa VV, Naukkarinen VA et al. Long-term mortality after 5-year multifactorial primary prevention of cardiovascular diseases in middle-aged men. JAMA 1991; 266(9):1225-9.

Strandberg TE, Salomaa VV, Vanhanen HT et al. Mortality in participants and non-participants of a multifactorial prevention study of cardiovascular diseases: a 28 year follow up of the Helsinki Businessmen Study. Br Heart J 1995; 74:449-54.

Suzuki H, Yamazaki M, Arai S et al. Effect of lard, palm and rapeseed oils life conservation in aged mice. Mech Ageing Dev 1991; 60(3):267-74.

Tatematsu K, Fuma SY, Nagase T et al. Factors other than phytosterols in some vegetable oils affect the survival of SHRSP rats. Food Chem Toxicol 2004; 42:1443-51. (2004a)

Tatematsu K, Fuma SY, Satoh J et al. Dietary canola and soybean oil fed to SHRSP rat dams differently affect the growth and survival of their male pups. J Nutr. 2004; 134:1347-52. (2004b)

Tatematsu K, Hirose N, Ichikawa Y et al. Nutritional evaluation of an inter-esterified perilla oil and lard in comparison with butter and margarine based on the survival of stroke-prone spontaneously hypertensive (SHRSP) rats. J. Health Sci. 2004; 50:108-11.(2004c)

Troy LM, Jacques PF, Hannan MT et al. Dihydrophylloquinone intake is associated with low bone mineral density in men and women. Am J Clin Nutr 2007; 86:504–8.

Chapter Six

Why The Lipid Hypothesis Of Coronary Heart Disease Is Fallacious And Dangerous

Paul J. Rosch, MD, Uffe Ravnskov, MD, PhD

Not everything that can be counted counts, and not everything that counts can be counted.

– Albert Einstein

Abstract

The lipid hypothesis postulates that decreasing blood cholesterol significantly reduces future coronary events. It is based on experiments showing that feeding saturated fat and cholesterol to rabbits raised cholesterol and produced fatty arterial deposits similar to those seen in people. Subsequent support seemingly came from epidemiologic studies showing a correlation between saturated fat, cholesterol levels and deaths due to CHD (coronary heart disease), but after scrutinizing these reports, they appeared to be heavily biased. Furthermore, trials to lower cholesterol by restricting saturated fat not only failed, but some reported an increase in coronary deaths. Cardioprotection from reducing cholesterol and LDL levels due to statin therapy was demonstrated in men with existing coronary disease, but it is now apparent that this and other alleged benefits result from pleiotropic effects unrelated to lipid lowering. In addition, there are growing concerns about significant side effects that have been suppressed in drug company sponsored studies or are starting to surface with long-term follow-up.

How The Cholesterol Hypothesis Of Coronary Atherosclerosis Originated

Cholesterol crystals were first identified in bile and gallstones by the French physician and chemist François Poulletier de la Salle around 1769[1]. Towards the end of the century, Antoine Francois de Fourcroy found these crystals to be identical to those obtained from adipocere, a waxy material in the fat of putrefied corpses.[2] In 1815, Michel Eugène Chevreul isolated and purified the crystallized material from gallstones and named it cholesterin, from the Greek *chol* for bile plus *stereos* for solid.[3] This was changed to cholesterol when it was subsequently found to be a sterol, and the chemical suffix *ol* for alcohol was added[4]. M.F. Boudet confirmed the presence of cholesterol in human blood in 1833[5], and ten years later, J. Vogel suggested that cholesterol was present in arterial plaque[6].

The term atheroma, from the Greek *ather* (gruel or paste) and *oma* (lump) had been coined by the Swiss physiologist Albrecht von Haller in his 1755 monograph, *Opuscula Pathologica* to describe arterial plaque with a yellowish pustular core that was more common in the elderly[7]. In 1856, the renowned pathologist Rudolph Virchow confirmed that atheroma were age related and was the first to demonstrate that atherosclerotic plaque contained cholesterol[8]. However, he did not believe that cholesterol caused plaque, which he referred to as *endarteritis deformans* to emphasize it resulted from an irritative process that injured the intimal lining of arteries. The cholesterol deposits came later.

Virchow's celebrated contemporary, Karl Rokitansky, also described inflammatory cells in atheroma, but believed they came from healing and resorption of thrombi rather than inflammation[9]. Felix Marchand, another German pathologist, coined the term atherosclerosis, from the Greek *sclerosis* (hard) in 1904 to describe a hardening process of atheroma that started in the inner lining of arteries[10]. This was to distinguish it from arteriosclerosis, (hardening of the arteries), which had been introduced in 1829 by the French pathologist Jean Lobstein to describe stiffening and thickness of the arteries[11]. Arteriosclerosis was thought to be due to a loss of elasticity in the muscular portion of the artery with aging that was often associated with calcification[12]. However, since calcification of atheroma also occurs, atherosclerosis and arteriosclerosis were often viewed as synonyms and are still often used interchangeably.

There was relatively little concern about either condition since CHD was not a significant problem, and prior to 1920, less than 10% of all deaths were due to heart disease. Most likely the reason was that the disease CHD was unknown to most doctors and they therefore put another diagnosis on the death certificate. Up to the early seventies CHD mortality increased steadily, but part of the increase was probably the introduction of ECG in the thirties and of aspartate aminotransferase (ASAT) and alanine aminotransferase (ALAT) in the sixties allowing a more correct diagnosis in many patients. However, the increasing use of hydrogenated fatty acids in margarine may have played a role.

Interest in the role of cholesterol began when there were a series of mysterious deaths in a Russian battalion during the early 20th century war with Japan. It was investigated by A. I. Ignatowski, Professor of Medicine at the Imperial Military Medical Academy in St. Petersburg, who determined it was due to a shipment of polluted meat. To prove this, he fed tainted meat to rabbits, and although none died, autopsies revealed an increase in fatty deposits in several arteries[13]. He thought this was consistent with the theory of Ilya Mechnikov, a Nobel Prize recipient who had previously proposed that an excess of dietary protein accelerated hardening of the arteries and other aspects of the aging process. Ignatowski fed rabbits a protein rich diet of meat, egg and milk that caused cholesterol deposits in the aorta reminiscent of atherosclerotic plaque in people that seemed to confirm Mechnikov's "protein toxicity" theory and published his findings in 1909[14].

The following year, Adolph Windaus, a German physician and chemist, who later received a Nobel Prize, reported that atheroma in human aortas contained 6 times more free cholesterol than healthy arteries, and over 20 times more cholesterol ester[15]. These observations made a great impression on Nikolai Anitschkow, who had just graduated from the same St. Petersburg Military Medical Academy. He suspected that it was cholesterol and fat rather than protein in the diet that caused these atheromatous lesions, and with the assistance of Semen Chatalov, a medical student at the Academy, he showed that simply feeding rabbits purified cholesterol obtained from egg yolks dissolved in corn oil could reproduce the identical changes Ignatowski described[16]. In their 1913 paper, they reported that the earliest lesions appeared in the aortic arch and had vacuolated cells containing cholesterol[17].

However, Anitschkow's research was relatively unknown to Western scientists until he published an English review of the issue in 1933[18]. Nor did this attract much attention until 1950, when John Gofman emphasized the importance of Anitschkow's discovery that feeding cholesterol to rabbits promptly led to atherosclerosis. Gofman and coworkers utilized a powerful ultracentrifuge to analyze the hypercholesteremic serum samples of their cholesterol-fed rabbits and identified two distinct layers or compartments. One that was located at the top of the serum sample was designated low-density lipoprotein cholesterol (LDL) and the fraction deposited at the bottom of the test tube was called high-density lipoprotein cholesterol (HDL)[19,20]. They also claimed that LDL was responsible for the rapid progression of atherosclerosis in human beings. This precipitated an avalanche of studies, including the research of Michael Brown and Joseph L. Goldstein that led to the development of statins and a Nobel Prize "for their discoveries concerning the regulation of cholesterol metabolism"[21].

In a 1958 editorial, Dr. William Dock, a renowned cardiologist who was then Chairman of the Department of Pathology at Stanford University Medical School, wrote in an editorial, "Thus the early work of Anichkov bears comparison with that of Harvey on the circulation and of Lavoisier on the respiratory exchange of oxygen and carbon dioxide"[22]. Dock also compared the significance of Anitschkow's research to Koch's discovery of the tubercle bacillus. And a recent ranking of "Cardiology's Ten Greatest 20th Century Discoveries" listed the top three as 1) The Electrocardiogram, 2) Preventive Cardiology and the Framingham Study, 3) The "Lipid Hypotheses" and Atherosclerosis[23]. Small wonder that those who dispute the dangers of cholesterol and the panacea-like properties of statins have a steep uphill battle against powerful adversaries who are intent on preserving their profits by perpetuating this dogma.

The Lipid Hypothesis

Note that the above authors used the term "Lipid Hypotheses", which implies that there was more than one such theory of the etiology of atherosclerosis. This is not surprising since by the 21st century, the lipid hypothesis was often confused with the diet-heart hypothesis or was referred to as "the cholesterol controversy"[24]. The term "lipid hypothesis" had also been used earlier by Steinberg and others, but came into common usage following a 1976 paper by E.H. "Pete" Ahrens Jr. from Rockefeller University's Center for Prevention of Premature Arteriosclerosis[25]. He defined the lipid hypothesis as follows:

The Lipid Hypothesis is the postulate, based on Framingham and similarly derived data, that reducing the level of plasma cholesterol in an individual or in a population group will lead to a reduction in the risk of suffering a new event of coronary heart disease. It is a premise based on the undisputed fact that people with higher plasma cholesterol levels have more and earlier coronary heart disease than do those with lower cholesterol levels; but the premise has not yet been proved true to the satisfaction of epidemiologists and biostatisticians or of the medical community at large. The Lipid Hypothesis, then, is simply an inference derived from accepted facts; though the hypothesis has been put to the test repeatedly in the past two decades, completely satisfactory evidence has not yet been advanced either pro or con.

Ahrens emphasized that this statistical association did not prove that cholesterol caused heart disease and that the lowering of cholesterol was a relative rather than an absolute risk reduction.

The Diet-Heart Idea

The "diet-heart" concept probably originated from a study published in 1953 by Ancel Keys, the director of the Laboratory of Physiological Hygiene at the University of Minnesota. According to Keys, fat food was the culprit. His proof was a diagram, which showed that the intake of fat food and the death rates from CHD followed each other closely in six countries. The six points on the diagram lay as on a string with Japan at the lower left corner and the US in the upper right[26]. However, as pointed out by Yerushalmy and Hilleboe four years later[27], data were available from 22 countries at that time, and if all the data were included, the strong association disappeared.

But Keys returned with a new study named Seven Countries[28]. In cooperation with local doctors, scientists and health authorities he selected sixteen local populations in the Netherlands, Yugoslavia, Finland, Japan, Greece, Italy and the US. Men between the age of 40 and 59 were studied and anything, which might conceivably cause CHD, was investigated. The men were followed for about five years, and all heart symptoms and all deaths were recorded. In his previous study he claimed that the intake of total fat was important, but in this new study, no association was found between the total fat intake and CHD. Instead his conclusion from this gigantic project was that what best predicted the number of heart attacks was how much animal fat people ate. Heart attacks were common in countries where people ate considerable amounts of animal fat, whereas they were rare in countries where intake was much lower.

However, many contradictory findings were ignored. For instance, CHD mortality was three times more common in eastern than in western Finland, although the difference between the intake of saturated fat in each area was minimal. In Greece, CHD mortality was 6-7 times higher on the island Corfu than on Crete although their intake of saturated fat was also identical; if anything, it was a little higher on Crete. Furthermore, including all 16 districts, intake of saturated fat was weakly related to CHD mortality but not to major ECG abnormalities at entry. The latter observation is evidently more relevant because whereas local doctors wrote the death certificates, American experts evaluated the ECG findings. In spite of these obvious biases, the study was widely heralded as the definitive proof of a causal link between SFA (saturated fat) intake and CHD. As Keys triumphantly proclaimed, "No other variable in the mode of life besides the fat calories in the diet is known which shows such a constant relationship to the mortality rate from coronary or degenerative disease."

Using intricate mathematical manipulations of laboratory study results - including his own - Keys created a formula to predict what happens to cholesterol levels when people eat different types of diets. According to his complicated formula, cholesterol goes up if you eat saturated fat and goes down if you consume a lot of polyunsaturated fat, the dominating fat in most vegetables oils[29].

It is simply impossible to draw any valid conclusions from Keys' studies and many observational studies have also shown that neither dietary cholesterol or saturated fat cause high cholesterol. For instance, males in some African tribes who consumed twice as much saturated fat as their counterparts in other countries had the lowest cholesterol levels ever seen in healthy people, and heart disease was rare[30]. Furthermore, no study has found an association between the intake of dietary cholesterol and its level in the blood[30,31].

Raymond Reiser, an American professor in biochemistry, was the first to question the association between saturated fat and cholesterol based on a thorough review of 40 trials[32]. He pointed out several types of methodological and interpretational errors: For instance, instead of natural saturated fat, many authors had used vegetable oils saturated by hydrogenation, a process that also produces trans fatty acids. We now know that trans fatty acids indeed cause cholesterol levels to go rise, and that trans fats can cause CHD. Furthermore, few researchers have looked at saturated fat intake as the only variable. If they changed the intake of saturated fat, they also changed the intake of monounsaturated or polyunsaturated fats, or both, mostly in the opposite direction. Russell Smith, a psychologist and statistician, who later reviewed over 2,000 studies on the link between dietary fat and cholesterol, was particularly critical[33]:

The word "landmark" has often been used to describe Ancel Keys Seven Countries Study, commonly cited as proof that the American diet is atherogenic. The dietary assessment methodology was highly inconsistent across cohorts and thoroughly suspect. In addition, careful examination of the death rates and associations between diet and death rates reveal a massive set of inconsistencies and contradictions..It is almost inconceivable that the Seven Countries study was performed with such scientific abandon. It is also dumbfounding how the NHLBI/ AHA alliance ignored such sloppiness in their many "rave reviews" of the study... In summary, the diet-CHD relationship reported for the Seven Countries study cannot be taken seriously by the objective and critical scientist".

The Arguments for the Diet-Heart Idea

There was not much interest in cholesterol until the 1950's when CHD became the leading cause of death in the U.S. Due to Ancel Keys' studies it was widely assumed that elevated cholesterol was the culprit. Further support came from the Framingham study based on a 6-year follow-up analysis of over 4,000 healthy men and women aged 31-65. They found that serum cholesterol measured at the start was significantly higher among those who had suffered from CHD during the observation period[34]. This was reinforced by the 1977 McGovern Senate Committee on Nutrition report that focused on avoiding saturated fats to lower cholesterol levels[35]. The problem was that the Prudent Diet and other attempts to lower heart attack risk by following these recommendations were embarrassing failures. No dietary experiment had been able to reduce heart mortality by avoiding saturated fat[32,36]. Even when combined with other cardioprotective lifestyle-changing measures the diet was ineffective.

One of them was the Multiple Risk Factor Intervention Trial (MRFIT). This was a randomized primary prevention trial funded by the National Heart and Lung Institute to test whether multiple risk factor intervention would prevent deaths from CHD in high-risk men[37]. Over 360,000 asymptomatic men aged 35-57 were screened to select those in the top 15% of potentially modifiable risk factors based on Framingham equations. Almost 13,000 with no history or evidence of heart disease were recruited and half of them were given dietary recommendations to lower blood cholesterol, antihypertensive drugs to lower blood pressure, and counseling for exercising and cigarette smoking cessation. The other half was referred to their usual source of medical care. However, as described in chapter 7, it was a gigantic failure. No benefit was achieved, although their intake of cholesterol was halved and their intake of saturated fat was lowered by 25%, no benefit was achieved.[38]

That a reduction of saturated fat is meaningless appears also appears to be confirmed by two major observational studies. The World Health Organization's Monitoring of Trends and Determinants in Cardiovascular Disease (MONICA) epidemiologic project was undoubtedly the largest study ever designed to explore the relationship between "risk factors" and cardiovascular disease[39]. It began in 1971 as a collaborative effort involving thirty-two centers in twenty-one countries that monitored approximately ten million men and women aged 25-64 for ten years.

The MONICA study also failed to find a link between Framingham risk factors and CHD mortality, and it thoroughly debunked the diet-heart hypothesis. All the countries in the top eight for saturated fat consumption had lower death rates for heart disease than all of the eight countries that consumed the least fat. For example, the French consumed three times as much saturated fat compared to Azerbaijan but had one-eighth the rate of heart disease deaths. Heart disease mortality in Finland was four times greater than in Switzerland, even though saturated fat consumption was similar. Researchers noted a significant rise and subsequent fall in coronary death rates over the past five decades that could not be explained, but there was again no correlation with changes in diet or Framingham risk factors of cholesterol, hypertension and smoking.

Most physicians are familiar with the Framingham and Seven Countries Study, but few are aware of MONICA, although it is far and away the largest study of its kind. In meta-analyses involving data for some sixty-two other prospective epidemiological studies, the combined total number of pooled subjects was 1.24 million. MONICA had eight times more but its data was not included based on arbitrary eligibility criteria established by the authors.

The other major study with contradictive results was the Women's Health Initiative (WHI) study in 1991 established by NIH to address the most common causes of death, disability and impaired quality of life in postmenopausal women. It was a 15-year multi-million-dollar project involving 161,808 healthy postmenopausal women and 40 clinical centers. Its focus was on strategies to prevent heart disease, breast and colorectal cancers by observational studies and the following three interventional clinical trials; Hormone Therapy, Calcium/Vitamin D and Dietary Modification. The Dietary Modification component evaluated the effect of a low-fat and high fruit, vegetable and grain diet on the prevention of CHD, breast and colorectal cancers. Study participants followed either their usual eating habits or the dietary regimen noted above. The results indicated that despite some reduction in cardiovascular risk factors such as blood lipids and diastolic blood pressure, there was no significant reduction in the risk of CHD or stroke in the cohort that restricted fat and increased fruit, vegetables and grain[40,41].

The Arguments for the Lipid Hypothesis

From the beginning researchers were frustrated by their inability to find a natural product or drug to reduce cholesterol levels. The cholesterol-lowering properties of nicotinic acid (Vitamin B3) were discovered in 1955 but the drug was ineffective in preventing fatal heart disease and the side effects were intolerable.

Triparanol (MER/29), an amine compound approved in 1959, was the first drug that inhibited cholesterol synthesis[42], but in contrast to statins, it blocked enzymes at the final stages of synthesis. However, it was withdrawn 3 years later because of skin lesions, impotence, cataracts, neuropathy and other serious side effects[43]. Not unexpectedly, the same side effects have been described after statin treatment as well. Probucol (Lorelco), an antioxidant, was approved to lower cholesterol in 1982 but was also withdrawn because of side effects and lack of efficacy[44].

Clofibrate, which had been marketed in England since 1958, was approved in the U.S. in 1967 as Atromid-S. Its mechanism of action was not clear, cholesterol-lowering effects were not impressive, and it was discontinued in 2002 because of increased risk of cancer, liver, gall bladder and pancreatic disease[44].

Other more potent and less toxic fibrates such as gemfibrozil (Lopid) and fenofibrate (Tricor) are still available and are primarily used as adjunctive therapy to lower triglycerides and LDL, although none of them have been able to lower heart or total mortality. None of these cholesterol-lowering therapies were popular since they had significant side effects, none of them were able to prevent mortality and there was little proof that they reduced coronary events[36,44].

A more promising candidate was cholestyramine (Questran), an anion-exchange resin that binds bile acids in the gastrointestinal tract and prevents their reabsorption. As a result, blood cholesterol falls because more of it is converted to bile acids in the liver to replenish their loss. In 1973, the NIH initiated its Lipid Research Clinics Coronary Primary Prevention Trial (LRC-CPPT) in 3800 asymptomatic middle-aged men with cholesterol levels over 265 mg/dl that were largely due to an elevated LDL. It was predicted that after 7 years, Questran would lower coronary morbidity and mortality by 50 %[45,46]. But, as described in chapter 7, this was not the case. The differences in outcome between the two groups were not statistically significant.

Despite this, the results were triumphantly proclaimed as definitive proof of the lipid hypothesis. As a result, The National Cholesterol Education Program was promptly launched, and focused on lowering

LDL by diet and drugs to less than 100 mg/dl, cholesterol to under 200 mg/dl, and increasing HDL to 40 mg/dl or higher[47]. These recommendations were soon endorsed by leading authorities as well as the National Heart, Lung, and Blood Institute, American College of Cardiology Foundation and the American Heart Association. The Centers for Disease Control has issued periodic updates since then identifying additional risk factors and therapies[48]. September was also proclaimed "National Cholesterol Education Month", during which everyone is urged to obtain a lipid profile.

However, a meta-analysis of the cholesterol-lowering trials published before the introduction of the statins found that they did not lower CHD mortality and that they had increased total mortality[36]. Furthermore, the reason for the widespread belief in such trials was that several with a negative outcome had been excluded in the previous meta-analyses[36]. Consequently, skepticism about the benefits of cholesterol lowering therapy increased[49], but this changed with the advent of statins.

In 1994, the Merck trial 4S was published[50]. A total of 4444 men and women with a previous heart attack were treated, half of them with simvastatin, the other half with a placebo. After 5.4 years, 8.5 percent had died from a heart attack in the control group, compared with 5 percent in the treatment group. For the first time a cholesterol lowering trial had succeeded in lowering the risk of both fatal and nonfatal CHD, and even total mortality. The results were heralded in the British Medical Journal: "Lower patients' cholesterol now! There is no longer any doubt about the benefit and safety of treating hypercholesterolemia in patients who have had a myocardial infarction."

However, the improvement included men only; the number of women who had died from a heart attack was in fact higher in the statin group, although not with statistical significance. Furthermore, none of the numerous statin trials that have been published later have succeeded in lowering CHD mortality to that extent; at most it has been lowered by 2 %.

Few are aware that in 1991, Merck had already published EXCEL, the first primary-preventive statin trial[51], but as can be seen in chapter 7, it was a complete failure. In fact, no primary-preventive statin trial has ever succeeded in prolonging the life for the participants, and no trial, whether primary or secondary preventive, has succeeded with that for women. There is also a serious problem with statin treatment. All authors have claimed that adverse effects are mild and rare, but as detailed in other chapters, this is very far from the truth.

Everyone is entitled to their own opinions and theories, but not their own facts. And the facts are that the conclusions based on all the studies cited above are erroneous. The cholesterol feeding studies were done in rabbits, which are herbivorous, and dietary cholesterol is foreign to them. When these experiments were repeated in rats and baboons, no atherosclerotic lesions were produced, and no study has found any association between the intake of saturated fats and degree of atherosclerosis in man[30]. What is also ignored is the result from the 30-year follow-up of the participants in the Framingham study. What the authors found was that for each 1 % drop in cholesterol, there was actually an 11 % **increase** in coronary and total mortality[52].

Some of the cholesterol-lowering trials succeeded in preventing various types of nonfatal cardiovascular events, but at the expense of numerous significant side effects, and as mentioned above, several trials with a negative outcome were excluded from the reviews.

Why Measuring Cholesterol and LDL Is A Waste Of Time And Money

The NIH, American Heart Association and other authorities constantly advise everyone from children to the elderly of the importance of knowing your "cholesterol numbers". Lipid theory proponents still maintain that coronary atherosclerosis is initiated when LDL infiltrates and accumulates in the intima of vessels and activates the endothelium to attract leukocyte adhesion molecules and chemokines[53,54]. The fact is that several observational studies have shown that high total or LDL-cholesterol is not a risk factor for CHD[55-60] and that on average these values are lower than normal in patients with acute CHD.[61]

Many studies have also shown that high cholesterol is not a risk factor for senior citizens; in fact, at least 19 studies have shown that old people with high LDL-cholesterol iive the longest[62]. No association between cholesterol levels and the degree of atherosclerosis has ever been found in postmortem studies of the general population either, and no clinical or imaging study has found any relation between the degree of cholesterol lowering and improvement[63]. Moreover, at least nine studies of people with familial hypercholesterolemia (FH) have shown that LDL-cholesterol in those with heart disease is not significantly higher than in those without[64-72], and the cerebral arteries of people with homozygotic FH are not more atherosclerotic than those of other people[73]. Most likely, CHD in people with FH is caused by an increased level of various coagulation factors, some of which have also been inherited.[74-81]

So why bother measuring total or LDL-cholesterol? Their benefit in patients with existing heart disease is most likely due to immunomodulatory, anti-inflammatory, anticoagulant and other diverse pleiotropic effects. As a result, statin therapy guidelines have abandoned lowering LDL as a goal and replaced it with an arbitrary 10-year risk assessment that would make tens of millions of additional individuals eligible for treatment. These include all diabetics and many healthy people over the age of 50, despite the fact that statins cause diabetes and provide no protection for anyone who does not have CHD.

In that regard, it is important to reemphasize that cholesterol, hypertension, and smoking are not risk "factors", which implies a causal relationship, but rather risk "markers" that are merely statistical associations. There are hundreds of similar correlations, including a deep earlobe crease, potbelly, premature vertex baldness, or living in Glasgow. All of these are associated with an increased risk for CHD. But that does not mean that plastic surgery, a tummy tuck, hair transplant, or moving to Honolulu will lessen the likelihood of a heart attack.

Inflammation

During the last few years, there has been increased interest in inflammation as a causal factor of atherosclerosis[82,83], as expressed below by Dr. Peter Libby, Chief of Cardiovascular Medicine at Brigham and Women's Hospital, which is affiliated with Harvard Medical School

Recent advances in basic science have established a fundamental role for inflammation in mediating all stages of this disease from initiation through progression and, ultimately, the thrombotic complications of atherosclerosis. These new findings provide important links between risk factors and the mechanisms of atherogenesis. Clinical studies have shown that this emerging biology of inflammation in atherosclerosis applies directly to human patients. Elevation in markers of inflammation predicts outcomes of patients with acute coronary syndromes, independently of myocardial damage. In addition, low-grade chronic inflammation, as indicated by levels of the inflammatory marker C-reactive protein, prospectively defines risk of atherosclerotic complications, thus adding to prognostic information provided by traditional risk factors.[84]

The culprit is described as "low-grade chronic inflammation, as indicated by levels of the inflammatory marker C-reactive protein", which has been used to assess the severity of acute inflammation for over 80 years. But what is the nature of this low-grade inflammatory process that does not respond to antibiotics? Virchow was very specific when he wrote:[8]

*We cannot help regarding the process as one which has arisen out of irritation of the parts stimulating them to new, formative actions; so far therefore it comes under **our ideas of inflammation**, or at least of those processes which are extremely **nearly allied to inflammation**... We can distinguish a stage of irritation preceding the fatty metamorphosis, comparable to the stage of swelling, cloudiness, and enlargement which we see in other inflamed parts. I have therefore felt no hesitation in siding with the old view in this matter, and in admitting an inflammation of the inner arterial coat to be the starting point of the so-called atheromatous degeneration.* (emphasis added)

Note that Virchow did not believe cholesterol caused atherosclerosis. The initiating factor was irritation and the cholesterol deposits came later. As indicated by the highlighted words, he was careful not to label this irritative process inflammation, because 2,000 years earlier, Celsus had defined inflammation as heat, pain, redness and swelling (*calor, dolor, rubor,* and *tumor*), to which Virchow later added disturbance of function (*functio laesa*). All of these were acute signs and symptoms that could be seen or felt, such as a pus-filled skin boil. In contrast, this was a chronic, indolent, hidden and silent process whose presence could only be verified by microscopic examination. This was not inflammation as defined by Celsus, but rather some prophlogistic process that had similar elements of swelling and cloudiness.

It has also been proposed that CRP causes coronary atherosclerosis, in addition to being a better risk marker than LDL, as indicated below.

Traditionally, CRP has been thought of as a bystander marker of vascular inflammation, without playing a direct role in the CVD. More recently, accumulating evidence suggest that CRP may have direct proinflammatory effects, which are associated with all stages of atherosclerosis. In our recent study, the results demonstrate that monocytes exhibit an enhanced production of interleukin-6 (IL-6) in response to CRP, and this response is significantly inhibited by simvastatin in a dose-dependent manner. This may be of important interest in the connection between CVD and CRP. Based on this evidence, we hypothesize that CRP is not only an inflammatory marker but also a direct cause of CVD, and treatments that reduce CRP should be of benefit for primary and secondary prevention of CVD. Administration of several agents, especially statins has been showed to modify CRP concentrations with a concurrent fall in cardiovascular events. Our clinical investigation suggested that treatment with a single high-dose or a short-term common dose of simvastatin could rapidly reduce CRP level.[85]

However, the results from the JUPITER trial (see chapter 7) contradict this idea, because although LDL-C was reduced by 50% and CRP was 37% lower in the treatment group, the number of fatal heart attacks was higher[86].

Moreover, reducing inflammation does not reduce heart disease. The powerful non-steroidal anti-inflammatory drug Vioxx was taken off the market because it caused heart attacks, and other anti-inflammatory drugs have had the same effect[87]. Furthermore, steroids like cortisone are extremely potent anti-inflammatory agents, but are more likely to cause cardiovascular problems than prevent them. Aspirin does have anti-inflammatory effects, but its cardioprotective benefits are more likely due to its antiplatelet and anticoagulant effect. In our view, and as proposed in chapter 11, inflammation can result from infection of the arterial wall.

Despite the trend to replace LDL with CRP as the cause of coronary atherosclerosis, a majority of researchers and physicians still maintain that high LDL is the perpetrator. Many believe this is due to the clout of the Cholesterol Cartel of statin, low fat food and lipid testing equipment manufacturers, who are intent on preserving their profits, and fund and oversee favorable clinical trials and meta-analyses. Most authors of these reviews and the organizations they represent are recipients of largesse from drug companies or have other conflicts of interest. As H.L. Mencken noted, "*It is difficult for a man to understand something when his income depends on not understanding it.*"

Conclusion

The list of observations and experiments that contradict the diet-heart idea and the lipid hypothesis is almost endless and it gets longer every year. In spite of this the cholesterol lowering campaign has continued uninterrupted along with a growing collection of adverse side effects. Dietary recommendations to replace saturated fat with foods rich in sugar and other carbohydrates have created a worldwide epidemic of obesity and type 2 diabetes. Moreover, millions of additional healthy people are now being urged to take statins that may convert over 20% of them to patients suffering from muscular weakness and pain, diabetes, impotency, various types of cerebral dysfunction, neuropathy, cataract, kidney damage and cancer.

However, there is an increasing recognition among many researchers that saturated fat and dairy products are beneficial and are not the cause of coronary atherosclerosis. Many feel that the new guidelines for statin therapy are a dangerous public health experiment, since they could put millions of healthy people at risk for serious side effects, with no proof they will provide cardiovascular or other benefits. In an article in the December 2014 issue of JAMA-Internal Medicine appropriately entitled "Prevention Guidelines Bad Process, Bad Outcome, Dr. Steven Nissen chairman of the department of cardiovascular medicine at the Cleveland Clinic, former president of the American College of Cardiology, and a leading researcher and staunch advocate of statin therapy, wrote *"The ACC and AHA should promptly revise the guidelines to address the criticisms offered by independent authorities"*[88].

With respect to the future, it is not likely that the lipid hypothesis will fade away. Although trials showing that drugs designed to raise HDL (the "good cholesterol") had to be halted due to increased cardiac mortality, this is still being pursued. Scientists recently created a synthetic molecule that "mimics" HDL and allegedly reduces plaque buildup in mice.[89] There is also continued interest in cholesterylester transfer protein (CETP) inhibitors, some of which have effects on both LDL and HDL[90] as discussed in chapter 1. And despite the irrelevance of lipid levels, monoclonal antibodies to lower LDL are being developed for patients on statins who have not obtained optimal benefits. These PCSK9 inhibitors are given by injection every 2 to 4 weeks, with an anticipated initial cost of $6,000 to $7000/year.[91]

The preliminary results from PCSK9 inhibitor trials were not encouraging. These trials have been too short (11 months in an evolocumab trial[92] and 80 weeks in an alirocumab trial)[93]. In addition, 7% and 30% respectively, discontinued anti-PCSK9 therapy. Although these drugs lower cholesterol more than 50%, any benefits were minimal. In the evolocumab trial the absolute benefit as regards CVD and unknown mortality was 0.1% and there was no benefit at all with respect to acute myocardial infarction and stroke. In the alirocumab trial the absolute benefit for CHD and unknown mortality was 0.6%, and fatal or nonfatal ischemic stroke occurred more often in the treatment group (0.6% vs. 0.3%). Nevertheless, both drugs were recently approved and are being hyped in deceptive ads, as noted in Chapter 1.

It would be wise to heed the adage that *"Those who do not learn from the mistakes of history are doomed to repeat them"*. With regard to the iconoclastic opinions expressed in this paper, we would remind the reader of Arthur Schopenhauer's contention, *"All truth passes through three stages. First, it is ridiculed. Second, it is violently opposed. Third, it is accepted as being self-evident"*, as well as Max Planck's observation, *"A new scientific truth does not triumph by convincing its opponents and making them see the light, but rather because its opponents eventually die, and a new generation grows up that is familiar with it."* Only time will tell if this will be the fate of the lipid hypothesis.

Key Issues

- No study of unselected individuals has found any association between total or LDL-cholesterol and the degree of atherosclerosis

- No study has documented that a high intake of cholesterol influences its serum level

- Almost all observational studies have shown that a high intake of saturated fat does not raise cholesterol

- Laboratory experiments concerning the effect of dietary lipids on blood lipids are biased

- All cohort and case-control studies have found lack of an association between a high intake of saturated fat and CHD

- No dietary trial has succeeded in lowering CHD mortality by reducing the intake of saturated fat

- Many studies have shown that high t-C or LDL-C is not a risk factor for middle-aged and elderly people

- All studies have shown that high cholesterol is not a risk factor for women

- Before the introduction of the statins, no cholesterol-lowering drug trial has succeeded in prolonging the life for the participants.

- The statins have only been able to lower heart mortality in people with heart disease and the effect is minimal

- As no cholesterol-lowering trial has found a dose-related exposure-response, the small benefit from statin treatment must depend on other effects

- The small benefit from statin treatment is outweighed by their many serious adverse effects

- There is no clinical evidence that, the new cholesterol-lowering drugs the PSCK9-inhibitors are able to lower the risk of CVD.

Paul J. Rosch, MD, Uffe Ravnskov, MD, PhD***

* *Clinical Professor of Medicine and Psychiatry*
New York Medical College
Chairman, The American Institute of Stress
stress124@optonline.net

** *Independent Researcher*
ravnskov@tele2.se
www.thincs.org

References

1. Dam H. Historical introduction to cholesterol. In: Chemistry, Biochemistry and Pathology (R. P. Cook, ed.) pp. 1–14, 1958; Academic Press, New York.

2. Gibbons GF. From gallstones to genes: two hundred years of sterol research. A tribute to George J. Schroepfer Jr. Lipids 2002;37:1153-62.

3. Chevreul ME. "Recherches chimiques sur les corps gras, et particulièrement sur leurs combinaisons avec les alcalis. Sixième mémoire. Examen des graisses d'homme, de mouton, de boeuf, de jaguar et d'oief" (Chemical researches on fatty substances, and particularly on their combinations Sixth memoir. Study of human, sheep, beef, jaguar and goose fat). Annales de Chimie et de Physique. 1816;2:339-72.

4. Olson RE. Discovery of the lipoproteins, their role in fat transport and their significance as risk factors. J Nutr 1998; 128 (2 Suppl): 439S–43S.

5. Boudet M. F. Nouvelle recherches sur la composition du serum du sang humain. Ann. Chim Phys 1833;52:337–48.

6. Popjak G.; In: Lipids: Chemistry, Biochemistry and Nutrition; Mead J. F., Alfin-Slater R. B., Howton DR, Popjak G., Eds. 1986; Plenum Press: New York, p. 29.

7. Haimovici H, DePalma RG et al (eds.) Vascular Surgery, Principles and Techniques, 3rd ed. Appleton and Lange, 1989; Norwalk CT. p.161.

8. Virchow R. Phlogose und thrombose im gefassystem. Gesammelte abhandlungen zur wissenschaftlichen medicin. Frankfurt: Meidinger Sohn and Co; 1856:458.

9. Rokitansky K: The Organs of Circulation: A Manual of Pathological Anatomy. Vol IV. Philadelphia, Blanchard & Lea, 1855.

10. Schwartz CJ, Mitchell JR. The morphology, terminology and pathogenesis of arterial plaques. Postgrad Med J 1962; 38:25-34.

11. Lobstein J. Traité d'Anatomie Pathologique, vol 2. 1829; Levrault, Paris.

12. Long ER. Development of our knowledge of arteriosclerosis. In: Blumenthal HT ed. Cowdry's Atherosclerosis. 1967; Charles C. Thomas, Springfield IL. pp. 5-20.

13. Ignatowski, A. I. Changes in parenchymatous organs and in the aortas of rabbits under the influence of animal protein. Izvestizy Imperatorskoi Voyenno-Meditsinskoi Akademii (St. Petersburg). 1908;18:231-244.

14. Ignatowski, A. I. Uber die Wirkung des tierschen Eiweisses auf die aorta und die parenchymatosen organe der kaninchen. Virchows Arch Pathol Anat Physiol Klin Med 1909;198:248-70.

15. Windhaus, A. Uber der Gehalt normaler und atheromatöser Aorten an Cholesterol und Cholesterinester. Zeitschrift Physiol Chemie 1910;67:174-6.

16. Anitschkow, N. Über die Veränderungen der Kaninchenaorta bei experimenteller Cholesterinsteatose. Beitr Pathol Anat 1913;56:379-404.

17. Anitschkow N, Chatalov S. Über experimentelle Cholesterinsteatose und ihre Bedeutung für die Entstehung einiger pathologischer Prozesse. Zentralbl Allg Pathol

1913; 24:1–9. [On experimental cholesterin steatosis and its significance in the origin of some pathological processes. Reprinted in Arteriosclerosis 1983;3:178–82]

18. Anitschkow, N. Experimental atherosclerosis in animals. In: EV Cowdry, ed. Arteriosclerosis: A Survey of the Problem. 1933: New York: Macmillan, New York pp. 271-322.

19. Gofman JW, Lindgren F. The role of lipids and lipoproteins in atherosclerosis. Science 1950;111:166–71.

20. Gofman JW, Jones HB, Lyon TP et al. Blood lipids and human atherosclerosis. Circulation 1952; 5:119-34.

21. Goldstein JL, Brown MS. Familial hypercholesterolemia: identification of a defect in the regulation of 3-hydroxy-3-methylglutaryl coenzyme A reductase activity associated with overproduction of cholesterol. Proc Natl Acad Sci U S A. 1973;70:2804–8.

22. Dock W. Research in arteriosclerosis; the first fifty years. Ann Intern Med 1958;49:699–705.

23. Mehta NJ, Khan IA. Cardiology's 10 Greatest Discoveries of the 20th Century. Texas Heart Inst J 2002;29:164-71.

24. Steinberg D. The Pathogenesis of Atherosclerosis. An interpretive history of the cholesterol controversy, Part V: The discovery of the statins and the end of the controversy. J. Lipid Res 2006;47:1339-51.

25. Ahrens EA. The management of hyperlipidemia: Whether, rather than how. Ann Intern Med 1976;85:87-93.

26. Keys A. Atherosclerosis: A problem in newer public health. J Mount Sinai Hosp NY 1953;20:118-39.

27. Yerushalmy J, Hilleboe HE. Fat in the diet and mortality from heart disease. A methodologic note. NY State J Med 1957;57:2343-54.

28. Keys A. Coronary heart disease in seven countries. Circulation. 1970;41((suppl 1):1-211.

29. Keys A, Anderson JT, Grande F. Prediction of serum cholesterol responses of men to changes in fats in the diet. Lancet 1957;2:959-966.

30. Ravnskov U. The questionable role of saturated and polyunsaturated fatty acids in cardiovascular disease. J Clin Epidemiol 1998;51:443-460.

31. Ravnskov U. A hypothesis out-of-date: The diet-heart idea. J Clin Epidemiol 2002;55:1057-63.

32. Reiser R. Saturated fat in the diet and serum cholesterol concentration: a critical examination of the literature. Am J Clin Nutr 1973;26:524-55.

33. Smith RL. Diet, Blood Cholesterol and Coronary Heart Disease: A Critical Review of the Literature. Santa Monica, CA. Vector Enterprises Inc; 1991;4-47-4-49.

34. Kannel WB, Dawber TR, Kagan A et al. Factors of risk in the development of coronary heart disease--six year follow-up experience. The Framingham Study. Ann Intern Med 1961;55:33-50.

35. U.S. Senate Select Committee on Nutrition and Human Needs. Dietary Goals for the United States, 2nd ed. Washington, DC, U.S. Government Printing Office, 1977.

36. Ravnskov U. Cholesterol lowering trials in coronary heart disease: frequency of citation and outcome. BMJ 1992;305:15-9.

37. Multiple Risk Factor Intervention Trial Research Group. Multiple risk factor intervention trial: risk factor changes and mortality results. JAMA 1982;248:1465-77.

38. Gorder DD, Dolecek TA, Coleman GG et al. Dietary intake in the Multiple Risk Factor Intervention Trial (MRFIT): nutrient and food group changes over 6 years. J Am Diet Assoc 1986;86,744-58.

39. Stewart AW, Kuulasmaa K, Beaglehole R, for the WHO MONICA Project. Ecological analysis of the association between mortality and major risk factors of cardiovascular disease. The World Health Organization MONICA Project. Intern J Epidemiol 1994;23:505-16.

40. Howard BV, Van Horn L, Hsia J, et al. Low-fat dietary pattern and risk of cardiovascular disease: the Women's Health Initiative Randomized Controlled Dietary Modification Trial. JAMA 2006;295:655–66.

41. Howard BV, Curb JD, Eaton CB, et al. Low-fat dietary pattern and lipoprotein risk factors: the Women's Health Initiative Dietary Modification Trial. Am J Clin Nutr 2010;91:860–74.

42. Blohm TR, MacKenzie RD. Specific inhibition of cholesterol biosynthesis by a synthetic compound (MER-29). Arch Biochem Biophys 1959;85:245–9.

43. Laughlin RC, Carey TF. Cataracts in patients treated with Triparanol. JAMA 1962; 81:339-40.

44. Ravnskov U. The Cholesterol Myths. 2000. New Trends publishing, Washington DC Freely available at www.ravnskov.nu/CM.

45. Lipid Research Clinics Program. The Lipid Research Clinics Coronary Primary Prevention Trial results, I: reduction in the incidence of coronary heart disease. JAMA 1984;251:351-64.

46. Lipid Research Clinics Program. The Lipid Research Clinics Coronary Primary Prevention Trial results, II: the relationship of reduction in incidence of coronary heart disease to cholesterol lowering. JAMA 1984;251:365-74.

47. Public Health Rep 1986;101:2-3.

48. National Cholesterol Education Program. Executive Summary of the Third Report of the National Cholesterol Education Program (NCEP) Expert Panel on Detection, Evaluation, and Treatment of High Blood Cholesterol in Adults (ATP III). May 2001 NIH Publication No.01-3670.

49. Smith GD, Song F, Sheldon TA. Cholesterol lowering and mortality: the importance of considering initial level of risk. BMJ 1993;306:1367-73.

50. Scandinavian Simvastatin Survival Study Group. Randomised trial of cholesterol lowering in 4444 patients with coronary heart disease: the Scandinavian Simvastatin Survival Study (4S). Lancet 1994;344:1383-9.

51. Bradford RH, Shear CL, Chremos AN et al. Expanded Clinical Evaluation of Lovastatin (EXCEL) study results. I. Efficacy in modifying plasma lipoproteins and adverse event profile in 8245 patients with moderate hypercholesterolemia. Arch Intern Med 1991;151:43-9.

52. Anderson KM, Castelli WP, Levy D. Cholesterol and mortality. 30 years of follow-up from the Framingham study. JAMA 1987;257:2176-80.

53. Shishehbor M, Bhatt DL. Inflammation and atherosclerosis. Curr Atheroscler Rep 2004:31-9.

54. Hansson GK, Robertson AK, Söderberg-Nauclér C. Inflammation and atherosclerosis. Annu Rev Pathol 2006;1:297-329.

55. Kannel WB, Castelli WP, Gordon T. Cholesterol in the prediction of atherosclerotic disease. Ann Intern Med 1979:90:85-91.

56. Nissinen A, Pekanen J, PorathnA et al. Risk factors for cardiovascular disease among 55 to 74 year-old Finnish men: a 10-year follow-up. Ann Med 1989;21:239-40.

57. Dagenais GR, Ahmed Z, Robitaille NM et al. Total and coronary heart disease mortality in relation to major risk factors - Quebec cardiovascular study. Can J Cardiol 1960;6:59-65.

58. Simons LA and coworkers. Risk factors for coronary heart disease in the prospective Dubbo study of Australian elderly. Atherosclerosis 1995;117:107-18.

59. Daviglus ML, Stamler J, Pirzada A et al. Favorable cardiovscular risk profile in young women and long-term risk of cardiovascular and all-cause mortality. JAMA 2004;292:1588-92.

60. Petursson H, Sigurdsson JA, Bengtsson C et al. Is the use of cholesterol in mortality risk algorithms in clinical guidelines valid? Ten years prospective data from the Norwegian HUNT 2 study. J Eval Clin Pract 2012;18:927-8.

61. Sachdeva A, Cannon CP, Deedwania PC et al. Lipid levels in patients hospitalized with coronary artery disease: an analysis of 136,905 hospitalizations in Get With The Guidelines. Am Heart J. 2009;157:111-7.

62. Ravnskov U, Diamond D, Hara R et al. Lack of an association or an inverse association between low-density-lipoprotein cholesterol and mortality in the elderly. A systematic review. BMJ Open, in press.

63. Ravnskov U. Is atherosclerosis caused by high cholesterol? QJM 2002; 95: 397-403.

64. Wiklund O, Angelin B, Olofsson SO et al. Apolipoprotein(a) and ischaemic heart disease in familial hypercholesterolaemia. Lancet 1990;335:1360-3.

65. Tato F, Keller C, Schuster H, et al. Relation of lipoprotein(a) to coronary heart disease and duplexsonographic findings of the carotid arteries in heterozygous familial hypercholesterolemia. Atherosclerosis 1993;101:69-77.

66. Vuorio AF, Turtola H, Piilahti KM, et al. Familial hypercholesterolemia in the Finnish north Karelia. A molecular, clinical, and genealogical study. Arterioscler Thromb Vasc Biol 1997;17:3127-38.

67. Real JT, Chaves FJ, Martínez-Usó I, et al. Importance of HDL cholesterol levels and the total/ HDL cholesterol ratio as a risk factor for coronary heart disease in molecularly defined heterozygous familial hypercholesterolaemia. Eur Heart J 2001;22:465-71.

68. Cenarro A, Artieda M, Castillo S. A common variant in the ABCA1 gene is associated with a lower risk for premature coronary heart disease in familial hypercholesterolaemia. J Med Genet 2003;40:163–8.

69. Jansen AC, van Aalst-Cohen ES, Tanck MW et al. The contribution of classical risk factors to cardiovascular disease in familial hypercholesterolaemia: data in 2400 patients. J Intern Med 2004;256:482-90.

70. Skoumas I, Masoura C, Pitsavos C et al. Evidence that non-lipid cardiovascular risk factors are associated with high prevalence of coronary artery disease in patients with heterozygous familial hypercholesterolemia or familial combined hyperlipidemia. Int J Cardiol 2007;121:178-83.

71. De Sauvage Nolting PR, Defesche JC, Buirma BJ et al. Prevalence and significance of cardiovascular riskfactors in a large cohort of patients with familial hypercholesterolaemia. J Intern Med 2003;253:161-8.

72. Hu M, Lan W, Lam CW, et al. Heterozygous familial hypercholesterolemia in Hong Kong Chinese. Study of 252 cases. Int J Cardiol 2013;167:762-7.

73. Postiglione A, Nappi A, Brunetti A et al. Relative protection from cerebral atherosclerosis of young patients with homozygous familial hypercholesterolemia. Atherosclerosis 1991;90:23-30.

74. Nordøy A, Brox JH, Holme S, Killie JE, Lenner RA. Platelets and coagulation in patients with familial hypercholesterolemia (type IIa). Acta Med Scand. 1983;213:129-35.

75. Aviram M, Brook GJ. The effect of human plasma on platelet function in familial hypercholesterolemia. Thromb Res 1982;26:101-9.

76. Sugrue DD, Trayner I, Thompson GR, et al. Coronary artery disease and haemostatic variables in heterozygous familial hypercholesterolaemia. Br Heart J 1985;53:265-8.

77. DiMinno G, Silver MJ, Cerbone AM, et al. Increased fibrinogen binding to platelets from patients with familial hypercholesterolemia. Arteriosclerosis 1986;6:203-1.

78. Jansen AC, van Aalst-Cohen ES, Tanck MW et al. Genetic determinants of cardiovascular disease risk in familial hypercholesterolemia. Arterioscler Thromb Vasc Biol 2005;25:1475-81.

79. Huijgen R, Kastelein JJ, Meijers JC. Increased coagulation factor VIII activity in patients with familial hypercholesterolemia. Blood. 2011;118(26):6990-1.

80. Narverud I, Iversen PO, Aukrust P, et al. Maternal familial hypercholesterolaemia (FH) confers altered haemostatic profile in offspring with and without FH. Thromb Res. 2013;131:178-82.

81. Sebestjen M, Zegura B, Guzic-Salobir B, Keber I. Fibrinolytic parameters and insulin resistance in young survivors of myocardial infarction with heterozygous familial hypercholesterolemia. Wien Klin Wochenschr 2001;113:113-8.

135

82. Shishehbor M, Bhatt DL. Inflammation and atherosclerosis. Curr Atheroscler Rep 2004;6:131-9.

83. Hansson GK, Robertson AK, Söderberg-Nauclér C. Inflammation and atherosclerosis. Annu Rev Pathol 2006;1:297-329.

84. Libby P, Ridker M, Maseri A. Inflammation and atherosclerosis. Circulation 2002;105:1135–43.

85. Li JJ, Fang CH. C-reactive protein is not only an inflammatory marker but also a direct cause of cardiovascular diseases. Med Hypotheses 2004;62:499-506.

86. Ridker PM, Danielson E, Fonseca FA et al. Rosuvastatin to prevent vascular events in men and women with elevated C-reactive protein. N Engl J Med 2008;359:2195-207.

87. Johnsen SP, Larsson H, Tarone RE et al. Risk of hospitalization for myocardial infarction among users of rofecoxib, celecoxib, and other NSAIDs: a population-based case-control study. Arch Intern Med 2005;165:978-84.

88. Nissen SE. Prevention Guidelines Bad Process, Bad Outcome. JAMA Intern Med. 2014;174:1972-3.

89. Zhao Y, Black AS, Bonnet DJ, et al. In vivo efficacy of HDL-like nanolipid particles containing multivalent peptide mimetics of apolipoprotein A-I. J Lipid Res 2014;55:2053-63.

90. Mohammadpour AH, Akhlaghi F. Future of cholesteryl ester transfer protein (CETP) inhibitors: a pharmacological perspective. Clin Pharmacokinet 2013; 52:615-26.

91. Dadu RT, Ballantyne CM. Lipid lowering with PCSK9 inhibitors. Nat Rev Cardiol 2014; 10:563-75.

92. Sabatine MS, Giugliano RP, Wiviott SD et al. Efficacy and safety of alirocumab in reducing lipids and cardiovascular events. N Engl J Med. 2015;372:1500-9.

93. Robinson JG, Farnier M, Krempf M et al. Efficacy and safety of evolocumab in reducing lipids and cardiovascular events. N Engl J Med 2015;372:1489-99.

Chapter Seven

Historical Perspective on the Use of Deceptive
Methods in the War on Cholesterol

David M. Diamond, PhD, Uffe Ravnskov MD, PhD

Abstract

For over half a century dietary and pharmacological approaches aimed at preventing cardiovascular disease (CVD) have mainly been based on the hypothesis that elevated cholesterol is atherogenic and that its lowering with diet or drugs will reduce the degree of atherosclerosis and the risk of CVD. We have reviewed the literature on this topic and have found numerous ways by which the supporters of this hypothesis have succeeded in misleading the readers. In fact, an abundant number of studies have shown that the cholesterol hypothesis is unable to satisfy any of Bradford Hill's criteria for causation. We have also described how the directors of the clinical trials have succeeded in minimizing the pervasiveness of the adverse effects of statin treatment. Overall, the half century long war on cholesterol has been counterproductive because the financial victory for food and drug companies in attacking cholesterol has come at the cost of impaired health for the masse.

Introduction

The reputed role of high serum cholesterol as a risk factor in CVD has been a source of controversy and debate for decades. This debate has been described as a war between the advocates, who view high cholesterol as a causal agent in coronary heart disease (CHD)[1,2] against the skeptics, who consider cholesterol a vital component of cell

137

metabolism which is not atherogenic[3-11]. The advocates' main thesis is based primarily on three components: 1) the presence of cholesterol in atherosclerotic tissue; 2) an association between high levels of serum cholesterol and CHD; and 3) cholesterol-lowering trials with drugs that appear to lower the risk of cardiovascular disease (CVD). Skeptics, by contrast, have emphasized that the advocates have failed to demonstrate evidence of a causal link between cholesterol and CHD. Moreover, as we describe in this chapter, the appearance of an improvement in CVD outcomes with cholesterol reduction is an illusion, one created by the directors of the trials using deceptive statistical means.

An absence of an association between cholesterol levels and the degree of atherosclerosis was first described in 1936[12], a finding which has been confirmed in numerous contemporary studies[13] The fact is that elderly adults with low levels of cholesterol are just as atherosclerotic as those with high levels. That high cholesterol is not a risk factor for CHD has been documented in many studies on a broad range of groups, including women, Canadian men, Swedes, Maoris, elderly people and patients with CHD[14]. IIn a meta-analysis of nineteen studies that included about 68,000 senior citizens that analyzed the relationship between LDL and mortality, those with the highest values lived the longest.[15] Finally, despite claims that statins produce dramatic improvements in CVD outcomes, the effects of statin treatment at a population level is actually quite miniscule. In fact, any beneficial effects of statins are more likely a result of pleiotropic effects, rather than cholesterol lowering[16], because no trial has shown an association between the degree of cholesterol-lowering and the magnitude of beneficial outcomes[13].

Despite the largely disappointing findings from 50 years of cholesterol lower trials, the indictment and conviction of cholesterol as the causal agent in CVD has stood the test of time. In this chapter we have rigorously assessed a broad range of research which has targeted cholesterol reduction with dietary or pharmacological approaches as a means with which to improve cardiovascular health and increase longevity. We have thoroughly evaluated the methodology and findings in this area of research and have reached the conclusion that the grand effort to reduce cholesterol as a strategy to improve health has failed.

The Dietary Trials

It is a fact that an exchange of saturated fat (SFA) with polyunsaturated fatty acids (PUFA) can lower serum cholesterol. This finding has led many researchers to assume that exchanging animal fat for vegetable oil consumption will therefore lower the risk of CHD. Few seem to realize that the reduction of serum cholesterol levels is actually caused by the increased intake of omega-6 PUFA and not by the decrease of the intake of SFA. In accordance, several trials in which a diet rich in SFA was compared with a diet where SFA had been exchanged with food rich in omega-6 PUFA, such as soybean or corn oil, provided findings, which did not support the cholesterol hypothesis.

In the first trial published in 1965 by Rose et al.[17], a diet high in PUFA (corn oil supplementation) produced the goal of a significant reduction of serum cholesterol levels, and yet, resulted in a higher CHD and total mortality in the treatment group. In six similar trials mortality was either higher in the diet group, or no difference was seen between the intervention and control groups[18].

A trial by Dayton et al, which included 800 male war veterans at a nursing home, appeared to have produced a positive result. After seven years a slightly smaller number of those who had consumed the soybean oil diet had died from CHD, but the lower number of CHD deaths was offset by a higher number of cancer deaths. Moreover, although serum cholesterol had been lowered in the treatment group, there was no difference between the degrees of atherosclerosis in the two groups. In fact, those who had consumed the soybeen diet, had more cholesterol in the aorta than those who had administered the nursing home's standard fare. In addition, what is often not mentioned in reviews of this study is that there were significantly more heavy smokers in the control group[19].

The Finnish Mental Hospital Trial is one of the most often cited dietary trials in support of the assertion that there are benefits to reducing saturated fat[20]. About 700 middle-aged male patients were studied at two mental hospitals in Finland. At one of them the patients were given a diet low in saturated fat and cholesterol and high in polyunsaturated fat; at the other hospital they were given the usual hospital diet. Six years later the diets were reversed and the trial continued for another six years. During the trial some of the patients dropped out, and after the first six years the oldest patients in both groups were exchanged with younger patients. Furthermore, there were considerably more smokers, more who had high blood pressure, and more who were treated with drugs in the control groups.

During both periods there were fewer heart events in the diet group, but with one exception the differences were not statistically significant. It is notable that the almost complete absence of significant effects occurred despite the fact that the authors had used a less demanding method to assess significance, the one-tailed t-test. Ultimately, however, how could they know whether the number of heart attacks in the second period was a consequence of the diet the patients had consumed during the first six year period, or whether it was the result of their present diet?

It is abundantly clear that this trial was terribly flawed. It was neither randomised, nor blinded, and what is not widely known is, that it included female patients, as well. In that part of the trial, published four years later[21], there was no benefit at all, although the cholesterol levels in the women were reduced even more than in the men. Nevertheless, the authors' conclusion was that *although the observed changes in CHD incidence fall short in attaining conventional criteria of statistical significance, the results of our trial support the idea that among female populations, as well as male, the use of a diet low in saturated fats and cholesterol and relatively high in polyunsaturated fats, exerts a preventive effect upon coronary heart disease.*

MRFIT. Many researchers thought that an intervention limited to a low-fat diet, alone, was not sufficient to improve CVD outcomes. Therefore several multifactorial trials were performed. One of them was the Multiple Risk Factor Intervention Trial (MRFIT); the largest and probably the most expensive cholesterol-lowering trial[22]. After a routine investigation of more than 360,000 middle-aged men, the researchers selected about 12,000 who were considered especially prone to get a heart attack. The subjects were randomly assigned to two groups of equal size. Those in the treatment group and their families were taught how to avoid cholesterol and saturated fat and increase the intake of polyunsaturated fat and how to quit smoking. High blood pressure was treated energetically, and subjects with weight problems were taught how to reduce calories and get more exercise.

Seven years later blood pressure had been lowered considerably and many had quit smoking. But their cholesterol levels had decreased by only seven per cent and it had decreased in the control group as well, so the difference between the two groups was only two per cent. Other risk factors had changed in the control group as well. The only difference worth mentioning was that significantly more of the control subjects continued to smoke. The outcome of this trial was not impressive; CHD mortality was non-significantly lower in the treatment group (115 vs 124) and total mortality was a little higher (265 vs 260).

With statistical manipulation, the directors of the study improved the appearance of the findings. The participants were divided into smaller groups, and by excluding a subgroup with a particularly poor outcome, the overall result was better. Almost all the other subgroups had fewer fatal heart attacks. Therefore the trial directors concluded that the intervention program might have had a favorable effect for most of the participants. If some of the men had more heart attacks, it was because of the drugs used to lower blood pressure (although in another subgroup treated with such drugs, the outcome was better). It was also obvious that the outcome was favorable for those who had quit smoking. In fact, the change in smoking habits explained the whole difference.

But the investigators claimed that the figures proved the benefit of lowering blood cholesterol. More prudent diet-heart supporters acknowledge that MRFIT was a failure, but they usually add that the failure occurred because a two percentage lowering of blood cholesterol is too small to have any effect. But with this objection diet was declared worthless as a preventive measure, because the subjects in the treatment group had almost halved their intake of cholesterol, they had lowered their intake of saturated fat by more than 25 per cent, and they had eaten 33 per cent more polyunsaturated fat, whereas the diet was practically unchanged in the placebo group[23].

Overall, dietary trials restricting SFA with increased PUFA has been a disappointment to the advocates of the cholesterol hypothesis. This limitation of diet to improve CVD outcomes has provided the impetus to drug trials to more directly target cholesterol reduction. In the next section we have described how this approach, as well, has been a dismal failure.

Drug Trials in the Pre-Statin Era

Before the introduction of the statins, several cholesterol-lowering drugs were tested, all of them with unimpressive results. The following is a review and analysis of a subset of these trials, including an assessment of how their directors misled the public in producing consensus statements on the effectiveness of cholesterol lowering, when indeed the actual findings were anaemic in their outcomes.

The Upjohn trial. One of them, colestipol, a bile-acid sequestering resin, was used in a randomized, placebo-controlled trial, which was directed by Albert E. Dorr from the Department of Biostatistics at the Upjohn Company. This trial included 2278 hypercholesterolemic men and women from 108 clinics in the US. About half of the participants had been diagnosed with CVD and/or diabetes[24]. Clinical information about the participants were telephoned to the staff on Upjohn, who made the random assignment. After up to three years of treatment (no information about the mean duration of the trial was given in the report), where cholesterol was lowered by about 15% in the treatment group, 22 men (4.6%) had died in the placebo group, but only nine (1.6%) in the colestipol group, whereas no difference was seen among the women (no figures were given). The data showed however, that the placebo-group must have included more patients with familial hypercholesterolemia, because triglycerides were significantly lower in that group, and the mortality differed only significantly among men below the age of 50. In that group ten died in the placebo group, but none in the treatment group.

The WHO trial. Colestipol was tested in the WHO trial as well. It included ten thousand middle-aged men with hypercholesterolemia, half of which were treated with colestipol. After five years treatment the number of fatal CHD was the same in each group, but the total number of deaths was significantly higher in the treatment group (128 vs 87)[25].

The Coronary Primary Prevention trial (CPPT). Despite the general failure of cholesterol lowering strategies to improve cardiovascular outcomes, in 1984 the Coronary Primary Prevention Trial (CPPT) was published in JAMA[26]. This trial was praised as the first solid evidence that reducing cholesterol levels with a pharmacological treatment (cholestyramine) could reduce coronary events and mortality[27].

In the CPPT trial[26], middle aged men with cholesterol levels in the top 0.8 % of 480,000 screened subjects were included in the study. Thus, the study was limited to an extreme subset of individuals, which were likely to have had familial hypercholesterolemia. They were treated with either cholestyramine, which lowered their LDL-C levels by about 20%, or a placebo, which produced no significant change. After 7.4 years of treatment, only 30 of 1,906 men in the treatment group (1.6%) and 38 of 1,900 men on placebo (2.0%), had died of CHD; a difference of only 0.4%. In addition, all-cause mortality between the two groups was virtually identical.

These findings should have put an end to the war against cholesterol for two reasons. First, despite the extraordinarily high levels of cholesterol these men were quite healthy; the incidence of coronary events and mortality in this group with hypercholesterolemia was unexpectedly very low. This finding alone is strong evidence against the cholesterol hypothesis. Second, pharmacological reduction of their cholesterol had little effect on outcomes.

One would think that with such strong evidence against cholesterol as a causal agent in heart disease that the directors would have given up their fight to demonize cholesterol. It is surprising that despite the meager findings in the CPPT trial, it was promoted as a pivotal victory. A Time Magazine article stated for example that *Cholesterol is proved deadly ... Lowering cholesterol levels markedly reduces the incidence of fatal heart attacks*. Although the trial was a drug study, the article quoted Basil Rifkind, director of the study, who stated that *the research strongly indicates that the more you lower cholesterol and fat in your diet, the more you reduce your risk of heart disease.*

A consensus conference. Undeterred by the unimpressive findings, the study directors held a consensus conference on cholesterol at the National Institutes of Health[28]. The aim of this conference was to discuss how the results of the CPPT trial should be translated into dietary guidelines for the American people. The conference was headed by Basil Rifkind, who also chose the members of the panel that formulated the final recommendations.

According to the medical investigative reporter Thomas Moore, who participated in the conference[29], there was actually no consensus in the audience. Criticism from the audience was swept under the rug, and some of the critics were cut off by the panel chairman Daniel Steinberg, who cited a lack of time; requests to write a minority report were denied as inconsistent with the conference's goal of a consensus.

As also documented in a recent meta-analysis of the trials performed before the consensus conference[30], the dietary guidelines, according to which foods rich in SFA and cholesterol should be exchanged with food rich in carbohydrates and PUFA, were introduced without any scientific evidence. In spite of that, most other countries soon accepted the flawed dietary guidelines as well. Today there is much evidence that a high intake of carbohydrates and omega-6 PUFAs have many adverse effects on health. In accordance both obesity and type 2 diabetes have increased almost epidemically in many countries after the introduction of the American guidelines.

Ignore the contradictions!

The Miettinen trial. In Finland the results from a multifactorial trial was published one year after the publication of the CPPT trial[31]. It included about 1200 middle-aged, more or less overweight male business executives with high cholesterol and high blood pressure. Half of them were given the same advice as in MRFIT. If their cholesterol was high they were even treated with various cholesterol-lowering drugs, whereas the control group continued as before. Again the risk factors changed satisfactorily, but in spite of that twice as many died in the treatment group as in the control group.

You may probably ask how the medical world reacted to this study. Let us therefore see how often their report became cited by other researchers in subsequent years, and let us compare it with how often the CPPT trial was cited. Both papers dealt with the same subject and were published in the same journal, and no one has questioned the honesty of the experimenters or the quality of the studies; at least not the Finnish one. Reasonably, they should have been cited almost equally often. That the CPPT trial, at least according to its directors, was supportive, and the Miettinen trial was not, is unimportant because the aim of research is to find the truth, whether it supports the current theories or not.

According to Science Citation Index the CPPT trial was cited 109, 121, 202 and 180 times, respectively during the following four years, whereas the Miettinen trial was cited only six, five, three and one time during these four years.

The 2009 WHO/FAO report. In a report from WHO published in cooperation with FAO, 28 experts had been selected to scrutinize the scientific literature about dietary fat[32]. This time the authors had looked at every type of study. In the section of the study on saturated fat Skeaff and Miller declared that *the available evidence from cohort and randomised controlled trials is unsatisfactory and unreliable to make judgements about and substantiate the effects of dietary fat on the risk of developing CHD.*

But in another section Elmadfa and Kornsteiner declared, that *there is convincing evidence that substituting SFA with mainly PUFAs reduces the risk of CHD*, and in the conclusion of the report, no changes were made as regards the dietary recommendations.

It would appear that the twenty-eight authors didn't confer with each other because Skeaff and Miller's figure 12 clearly shows that a high intake of PUFAs is associated with an increased risk of dying from heart disease, whereas figure 8 shows no association with intake of SFA.

The Statin Trials

Despite the absence of evidence that cholesterol reduction, with either diet or drugs, has been effective in improving health outcomes, the last 20-year epoch has been a clear victory for the advocates. We are now in a period in which the dominant approach to CVD treatment is based on the use of statins. The development of these drugs in the 1990's has almost silenced debate and objections. The statins have been praised as miracle drugs and the best anti-atherosclerotic insurance[33], as well as the most powerful inventions to prevent cardiovascular events[34]. The praise for their apparent effectiveness has been near universal, with the latest recommendations by the ACC/AHA that statin treatment would benefit as many as half of all older Americans, as well as children and adolescents with elevated levels of cholesterol[35].

The quandary that the reader is faced with is that statins have generated so much support as the saviour of hearts, and yet skeptics have been vocal in their opposition. We have previously provided a thorough assessment of deception as a tool for statin advocates[36,37]. As an example we have chosen the JUPITER trial to show trial directors' strategy to amplify the miniscule benefits from statin treatment and to minimize the adverse effects. We have also included a section about EXCEL, the first primary-preventive statin trial; a trial which should have stopped all future trials on healthy individuals because already after 48 weeks the number of deaths was almost twice as high in the treatment groups as in the control group.

The JUPITER trial. In this trial, rosuvastatin (Crestor) or placebo was administered to 17,802 healthy people with elevated C-reactive protein and normal cholesterol. The primary outcome was a major cardiovascular event[38]. The trial was stopped after a median follow-up of 1.9 years. The number of subjects with a primary end point was 251 (2.8%) in the control group and 142 (1.6%) in the rosuvastatin group, thus resulting in an absolute risk reduction (ARR) of 1.2 percentage points. The benefit as regards the number of fatal and non-fatal heart attacks was even smaller; 68 (0.76%) versus 31 (0.35%) events, respectively, eg. an ARR of 0.41 percentage points. Thus, less than one half of one per cent of the treated population benefited from rosuvastatin treatment, and 244 people needed to be treated to prevent a single fatal or non-fatal heart attack. Despite this meagre effect, in the media the benefit was stated as "***more than fifty per cent avoided a fatal heart attack***", because 0.41 is 54% of 0.76.

It is also worth noting that the ARR of 0.41 percentage points was the combination of fatal and nonfatal heart attacks. There was little attention paid to the fact that more people had died from a heart attack in the treatment group. Even experienced researchers may have overlooked this finding because the figures were not explicitly stated in the report. One needs to subtract the number of non-fatal CHD from the number of any myocardial infarction to see that there were 11 fatal heart attacks in the treatment group, but only 6 in the control group.

According to a table in the JUPITER report there was no difference between the numbers of serious adverse effects between the two groups. However, in the rosuvastatin group there were 270 new cases of diabetes, but only 216 in the control group (3% vs. 2.4%; p<0.01). Unlike beneficial effects, which the authors amplified by using the relative risk reduction (RRR), the significant effect of new onset diabetes was expressed correctly in the ARR form.

An objective assessment of the JUPITER findings should therefore be conveyed to potential patients in the following manner: *Your chance to avoid a non-fatal heart attack during the next two years is about 97 % without treatment, but you can increase it to about 98% by taking a Crestor every day. However, you will not prolong your life and there is a risk you may develop diabetes, not to mention other serious adverse effect*s.

But in the media the JUPITER findings were presented as very impressive. In an article in Forbes Magazine, John Kastelein, a co-author of the study, proclaimed: *It's spectacular ... We finally have strong data"* that a statin prevents a first heart attack. Shortly afterwards an FDA advisory panel recommended Crestor treatment for people with elevated C-reactive protein levels and normal levels of cholesterol. As a result Crestor became the second most highly prescribed statin in 2015.

A pertinent question is, why did they stop the trial already after 19 months? According to figure 1 in the trial report the mortality curves of the two groups clearly were approaching each other. Had they continued a few months more, they may have crossed each other, meaning that mortality may have become greater in the treatment group. The significant increase of the number of diabetics might also have increased even more if the trial has continued. A relevant reason to stop a trial is of course, if the outcome becomes worse in the treatment group. Better to stop it before such bad things happen. In the EXCEL trial, the first primary-preventive statin trial, the same strategy was followed.

The EXCEL trial was started by Merck two years after the start of 4S, their second-preventive statin trial. It included 8245 healthy people with high cholesterol divided into five groups, four of which received various doses of lovastatin[39]. The trial was ended after 48 weeks. According to a correspondence between Merck and UR the reason was that the aim of the trial was to see if lovastatin would lower cholesterol and to see if the participants tolerated the drug; according to the authors, this was indeed the case.

To plan, develop and initiate a trial including more than 8000 participants from 362 clinical sites takes place at phenomenal cost. Once initiated, the cost of a trial is relatively low and potential benefits of reporting positive effects of treatment come at a minimal cost. It was therefore paradoxical that Merck terminated the trial after only 48 weeks. One wonders, therefore, why they didn't continue the trial? Clearly the costs of continuing that trial would have been minimal compared with the costs starting a new trial. We will provide a logical explanation for its early termination.

With EXCEL, in contrast to almost all other reports from the statin trials, no precise information was provided regarding the number of participants or events in each group. In the placebo group 0.2 per cent died; in the four lovastatin groups the numbers were 0.5, 0.3, 0.6 and 0.5 per cent, respectively. Thus, even if the numbers were small, total mortality was 1.5-4 times higher in the treatment groups after 48 weeks. According to the authors the differences were not statistically significant, but it is easy to calculate, that the difference is close to a p-value of 0.05. Nothing was mentioned about these figures in the abstract.

Stopping the EXCEL trial after 48 weeks had the consequence that it would not be included in any meta-analysis of statin trial outcomes, because all meta-analyses have excluded trials with a duration shorter than one year.

How trial directors have minimized the appearance of adverse effects of statins.

As we have reviewed here and elsewhere[36,37], the magnitude of the benefits of statin treatment is meager, typically in the range of a one to two percentage point reduction in the rate of coronary events and even lower as regards mortality. Nevertheless, at a global level, a reduction of coronary events and death in 2% of the population could make a substantial difference if the statins were harmless. However, the adverse effects of statins are substantial, including cancer, cataracts, diabetes, cognitive impairment, impotency, renal failure and musculoskeletal disorders. Whereas the benefits are routinely reported as relative risk, adverse effects are always expressed in terms of absolute risk or not at all. In the following we have briefly summarized the deceptive strategies used by the trial authors to minimize the appearance of adverse effects. More detailed information is available in our published paper[36].

Cancer. Several statin trials have reported an increase in the incidence of cancer in the treated populations. In three of them the increase was statistically significant. In the CARE trial[40], breast cancer had occurred in 12 (4.2%) of the women in the pravastatin group but in only one (0.34%) in the placebo group. The authors dismissed the significant difference (p=0.002) by stating, that *there is no known potential biologic basis...the totality of evidence suggests that these findings in the CARE trial could be an anomaly.* In the two secondary-preventive trials named PROSPER[41] and SEAS[42], cancer occurred significantly more often as well. The authors of PROSPER downplayed the finding by referring to a meta-analysis of all other pravastatin-trials, which didn't find an excess of cancer, but they did not mention, that on average the participants in PROSPER were 25 years older than those in the other trials. The authors of SEAS classified it as chance, and nothing was mentioned about it in the abstract.

Although the directors of the statin trials typically dismiss a link between statins (or low cholesterol, in general) and cancer, there are well-established mechanisms that can explain a statin-cancer association. For example, it is well established that the lipoproteins participate in the immune system by binding to and inactivating all kinds of microorganisms and their toxic products[43], and there is a well-established role of viruses in cancer development[44]. Several case-control studies of cancer patients and healthy controls have also shown that the cancer patients had been using statins significantly more often[45]. Supporters of statin-treatment typically dismiss these findings by referring to meta-analyses of the statin-trials, which report no evidence of an association of statin treatment to the incidence of cancer. There are serious biases in these meta-analyses, however.

First, almost all statin trials ignore reports of skin cancer. This strategy appears to have begun with the two first simvastatin-trials

4S and HPS[46,47], in which more patients in the treatment groups were diagnosed with non-melanoma skin cancer. Although these figures appeared in the tables, the authors did not mention this finding in the text, possibly because the differences were not statistically significant, but if the data from both trials are combined, the statin-skin cancer association was significant (256/12 454 vs. 208/12 459; $p < 0.028$). It is notable that skin cancer is relatively easy to detect at an early stage of development, and its exclusion from the statin reports has introduced a serious underestimation of the number of cancer.

Second, most statin trials are terminated within 2-5 years. As the latent period between exposure to a carcinogen and the incidence and detection of cancer in humans may be 10 to 20 years or more, the absence of any controlled trials of this duration means that we do not know whether statin treatment will lead to an increased rate of cancer in the coming decades. Concern over the risk of statins as carcinogens is validated by experiments, which have shown that serum concentrations similar to those achieved in human beings can produce cancer in rodents[48].

No significant increase of cancer was seen in a ten-year follow-up of the participants in the 4S trial and the authors therefore concluded that ten years of statin treatment does not induce cancer. Neither does ten years smoking. But in a case-control study of several thousand women there was a doubling of the risk of ductal and lobular breast cancer among those who had used statins for more.than 10 years (odds ratio 2.00; 1.26-3.17)[49].

Myopathy. According to the reports from the statin trials muscular problems occur in less than one per cent of the patients. However, myopathy has only been recorded, if the level of creatine kinase was at least ten times higher than the upper normal level at two successive determinations,

One may wonder if the extraordinarily high threshold for categorizing adverse effects of statins for myopathy is designed to minimize the detection of harm, a strategy which will produce the appearance that statins are harmless, but is inconsistent with the Hippocratic oath whereby the clinician must *first, do no harm.* The fact is that microscopic examinations of muscle tissue from statin-treated patients with muscular symptoms and normal creatine kinase have shown signs of damage[50]. Even patients without overt muscular symptoms may be damaged. In a study of muscle tissue using electron microscopy, the structural integrity of skeletal muscle fibres was compromised in 10 of 14 statin-treated patients without any subjective complaints, compared to one of eight control individuals[51].

According to independent researchers, myopathy is the commonest adverse effect of statins, and is seen more often in women and elderly people. For instance, Sinzinger et al. have reported that muscular weakness and pain occur in one out of four statin-treated patients who exercise regularly[52]. They also noted that seventeen out of twenty-two professional athletes with familial hypercholesterolemia treated with statins stopped because of that particular side effect[53]. Furthermore, in an RCT that included 1016 healthy men and women with high LDL-C, Golomb et al found that after six months statin treatment 40% of the women suffered from exertional fatigue[54].

Another way to minimize the muscular symptoms is to separate them into numerous categories. According to the FDA Adverse Event Reporting System (FAERS), adverse muscular symptoms are recorded in 11 categories (muscle disorder, myopathy, muscle tightness, musculoskeletal stiffness, myalgia, muscular weakness, muscle cramp, muscle enzyme, muscle fatigue, muscle necrosis and muscle spasm). In most of them a low incidence are reported, but taken together the number of myopathy-related events is substantial.

Muscular side effects are not benign phenomena; they may in particular have a deleterious effect on elderly people, because the least expensive and the least risky way to prevent heart disease is regular exercise. Even worse is that severe muscular damage may cause serious renal diseases. In a 6.4 year long follow-up study including 6342 statin-treated "patients" and 6342 non-treated controls corrected for many variables, almost 4 % more in the statin group suffered from acute renal failure, chronic kidney disease, nephritis, nephrosis or renal sclerosis[55].

Neurological effects. Nothing is mentioned about cerebral side effects in the statin trials, although several independent researchers have reported that such symptoms are common. For example, in a meta-analysis of cholesterol lowering trials, Muldoon et al found a statistically significant increase in the number of deaths from accidents, suicide, or violence in the treatment groups[56]. Furthermore, it has been shown by several authors that low cholesterol is a biological marker of major depression and suicidal behavior, whereas high cholesterol is protective[57,58]. In accordance Davison et al. found that the incidence of suicidal ideation among adults with mood disorders was more than 2.5 times greater in those taking statins [59]. Moreover, several studies have shown that low cholesterol is associated with poorer cognition and Alzheimer's disease, and that high cholesterol is protective[60]. For instance, in a study of 143 patients with memory loss or other cognitive problems associated with statin therapy, Evans and Golomb reported that 90% of them improved after discontinuation of their statin treatment[61]. In a study by Padala et al. eighteen older statin-treated subjects with Alzheimer's disease were asked to stop their statin treatment. Twelve weeks later, their performance on several cognition tests had improved significantly and after having started the treatment again, their performance on the tests worsened significantly[62].

There are at least two reasons why such symptoms are ignored in the statin trials. The cerebral symptoms usually do not occur immediately. If they occur in elderly patients several weeks or months after the start of the treatment, both the doctor and the patient may interpret them as symptoms of advancing age. The other reason is that cerebral side effects are classified into many different subgroups. According to FAERS, adverse events from cerebrospinal dysfunctions are classified in 23 separate terms (suicidal attempt, suicidal ideation, suicidal behavior, aphasia, balance disorders, coordination abnormal, amyotrophic lateral sclerosis, amnesia, memory impairment, transient global amnesia, cognitive or confusional state, irritability, paranoia, disorientation, dementia, depression, depressed mood, neuropathy, pain in extremity, Guillain-Barre syndrome, ALS and multiple sclerosis). The incidence of statin-related side effects in the many different subcategories is present at a low rate, but if all of them were to be combined, the total number of adverse events may be substantial.

With the high incidence of neuromuscular adverse effects, it is reasonable to ask why the FDA has not been more forthcoming about informing the public about the well-documented muscle and neurological adverse effects of statins.

About unethical reporting. *Adverse effects from statin treatment are very rare.* This is what Sir Rory Collins, Professor of Medicine and Epidemiology at Oxford told the media in a fierce comment to two papers published in British Medical Journal (BMJ) where the authors claimed that 18%-20% of patients on the cholesterol-lowering drugs suffered adverse events. According to Collins side effects occur in only one in 10,000 people, and he therefore insisted that BMJ should withdraw the papers, but Collins' protest only resulted in a correction of a minor error.

The large difference between the number of side effects according to the trial reports and those reported by independent researchers has led several researcher to ask the trial directors for access to the primary data, but this has always been denied. By this reason new penal EU regulations on clinical trials came into effect in 2004 according to which *essential documents must be archived and be accessible for audit and inspection by regulatory authorities*[63]. It is a striking fact that the benefits recorded in statin trials published since then have become minimal or totally absent[64].

How to cover up that high cholesterol is not a risk factor. Almost everyone "knows" that high cholesterol is a risk factor for heart disease, but as mentioned above, many studies have shown this apparent truism is actually incorrect. The idea was promoted by the Framingham group after their first follow-up of a group of middle-aged inhabitants in the town. However, in the 30-year follow-up of these people they found, that high cholesterol was not a risk factor after the age of 47. In fact, high cholesterol seemed to be beneficial, because, as they wrote: *For each 1 mg/dl drop of cholesterol there was an 11% increase in coronary and total mortality*[65].

With these results in hand why did the authorities not reveal to the public the great value in maintaining high levels of cholesterol with advanced age? Because the findings were ignored, or more directly, the directors misrepresented them entirely, i.e., they lied about the findings. In an extraordinary feat of deception, reminiscent of "doublethink", the highly refined form of deception in George Orwell's novel, *Nineteen Eighty Four*, the 30-year follow-up of the Framingham project is instead used as *support* of the cholesterol hypothesis. Consider for instance the joint statement by the American Heart Association and the National Heart, Lung and Blood Institute in their

153

review entitled The Cholesterol Facts: *The results of the Framingham study indicate that a 1% reduction…..of cholesterol corresponds to a 2% reduction in CHD risk*[66], and here they refer to the opposite result of the 30-year Framingham follow-up study.

One of their strongest arguments is an analysis of the screenees in the WHO trial. The figures from this trial included both the 12,000 participating men, but also the more than 300,000 men who were excluded for various reasons. A large number of studies concerning the follow-up of these people has been published in well-known international medical journals, and these studies are cited again and again as the strongest proof that there is a linear association between blood cholesterol concentrations and the risk of future heart disease.

But these data are not reliable. In a systematic search of the literature on the MRFIT study, Lars Werkö, then director of the Swedish Council on Technology Assessment in Health Care, an independent governmental agency known for its integrity, found 34 papers based on data from MRFIT reporting the relationship between serum cholesterol and mortality[67]. He asked himself whether it really was necessary to publish all these reports, as their results were so similar. *Have the editors really judged the original scientific value of each of these similar articles and deemed them worthy of publication? Or have they been impressed by the status of the research groups that authored these repetitive manuscripts, with the prestigious National Heart, Lung and Blood Institute in the background, and found that they have to succumb to the authorities?*

Worse than being repetitive, the data were inconsistent and of questionable veracity. For instance, the number of screenees varied greatly between the studies, from 316,099 to 361,266. In particular, Werkö was critical of the studies reporting how many had died and why, because it is highly unlikely that all of 361,266 individuals could have been tracked after 6-12 years.

How the cause of death had been established was not reported but we can be rather confident that most of the reported causes were based on death certificates written by general practitioners. Not only is the information from death certificates highly unreliable, but in up to 20% of the reports, death certificates were missing. Yet some of the reports gave a detailed list of diagnoses for almost all deaths.

Furthermore, during the initial screening it came to light that one of the participating centers had falsified its data to increase the number of participants in the trial, possibly in order to obtain more financial support from the National Institutes of Health. This embarrassing matter received little mention in the follow-up reports, nor did the study authors mention the possibility that data falsification could have occurred in other centers as well. Wrote Werkö: *In the many publications regarding the MRFIT screenees, it is obvious that the authors are more interested in the mathematical treatment of large figures than in the quality of these figures or how they were obtained.*

In spite of all these irregularities, the follow-up reports on the MRFIT screenees are still cited as *the most exact database regarding the relation of risk factors to mortality in the healthy male US population.*

Similar methods have been used by others. In an analysis of the statements by three major American consensus committees it appeared that of twelve groups of controversial papers only two of them were quoted correctly, and only in one of the reviews. About half of the papers were ignored. The rest were quoted irrelevantly; or insignificant findings in favour of the hypothesis were inflated; or unsupportive results were quoted as if they were supportive. Furthermore, only one of six randomized cholesterol-lowering trials with a negative outcome were cited and only in one of the reviews, whereas each review cited two, four, and six non-randomized trials with a positive outcome, respectively[68].

Conclusion

The war on cholesterol is reminiscent of the Hans Christian Andersen story of the emperor who had been deceived by swindlers who sold him magnificent clothes, which were invisible to all but the feeble-minded. The king, his advisors and the townspeople were all afraid to admit that the clothes were invisible to them. In this chapter we have served in the role of the child, who stated that the emperor wore no clothes. In like manner, we have spoken out against conformity to the prevailing, but incorrect, view of cholesterol as inherently atherogenic. We have scrutinized the literature to describe how dominant figures in the field of heart disease have, for decades, created the illusion that cholesterol causes heart disease and that the diet and drug-induced reduction of cholesterol is beneficial to cardiovascular outcomes. We have described how advocates of the war on cholesterol have created the illusion that cholesterol is atherogenic by ignoring all conflicting observations from critical and independent scientists, by citing studies incorrectly to make them look supportive of the cholesterol hypothesis, and with the use of deceptive statistics which have distorted and exaggerated trivial findings.

David M. Diamond, PhD*, Uffe Ravnskov, MD, PhD**

* Departments of Psychology and Molecular Pharmacology & Physiology, Center for Preclinical & Clinical Research on PTSD, University of South Florida
ddiamond@usf.edu

** Independent Researcher
ravnskov@tele2.se
www.thincs.org

References

1. Steinberg D. The cholesterol controversy is over. Why did it take so long? Circulation 1989;80:1070-8.

2. Steinberg D. In celebration of the 100th anniversary of the lipid hypothesis of atherosclerosis. J Lipid Res 2013;54:2946-9

3. Pinckney ER, Pinckney C. The Cholesterol Controversy. Sherbourne Press, Los Angeles, 1973.

4. Reiser R. Saturated fat in the diet and serum cholesterol concentration: a critical examination of the literature. Am J Clin Nutr 1973;26:524-55.

5. Reiser R. A commentary on the Rationale of the Diet-Heart Statement of the American Heart Association. Am J Clin Nutr 1984;40:654-8.

6. Stehbens WE. An appraisal of the epidemic rise of coronary heart disease and its decline. Lancet 1987;1:606-11.

7. Stehbens WE. The lipid hypothesis and the role of hemodynamics in atherogenesis. Prog Cardiovasc Dis 1990;33:119-36.

8. Smith RL. Diet, blood cholesterol and coronary heart disease: a critical review of the literature. Vector Enterprises. Vol. 1, 1989; Vol. 2, 1991.

9. Ravnskov U. Cholesterol lowering trials in coronary heart disease: frequency of citation and outcome. BMJ 1992;305:15-9.

10. Gurr MI. Dietary lipids and coronary heart disease: old evidence, new perspective. Prog Lipid Res 1992;31:195-243.

11. Rosenman RH. The questionable roles of the diet and serum cholesterol in the incidence of ischemic heart diseae and its 20th century changes. Homeostasis 1993;34:1-43.

12. Landé KE, Sperry WM. Human atherosclerosis in relation to the cholesterol content of the blood serum. Arch Pathol 1936;22:301–12.

13. Ravnskov U. Is atherosclerosis caused by high cholesterol? QJM 2002;95:397-403.

14. Ravnskov U. The Cholesterol Myths. New Trends Publishing; Washington: 2000

15. Ravnskov U, Diamond DM, Hama R et al. Lack of an association or an inverse association between low-density-lipoprotein cholesterol and mortality in the elderly: a systematic review. BMJ Open 2016;6: e010401. doi:10.1136/ bmjopen-2015-010401

16. Ravnskov U. Implications of 4S evidence on baseline lipid levels. Lancet 1995;346:181

17. Rose GA, Thomson WB, Williams RT. Corn oil in treatment of ischaemic heart disease. BMJ 1965;1:1531-3

18. Ravnskov U. The questionable role of saturated and polyunsaturated fatty acids in cardiovascular disease. J Clin Epidemiol 1998;51:443-60

19. Dayton S, Pearce ML, Hashimoto S, Dixon WJ. Tomiyasu U. A controlled clinical trial of a diet high in unsaturated fat in preventing complications of atherosclerosis. Circulation 1969;40 (Suppl. 2):1-63.

20. Turpeinen O, Karvonen MJ, Pekkarinen M et al. Dietary prevention of coronary heart disease: the Finnish Mental Hospital Study. Int J Epidemiol 1979;8:99-118.

21. Miettinen M, Turpeinen O, Karvonen MJ et al. Dietary prevention of coronary heart disease in women: the Finnish mental hospital study. Int J Epidemiol 1983;12:17-25.

22. Multiple Risk Factor Intervention Trial Research Group. Multiple risk factor intervention trial. Risk factor changes and mortality results.. JAMA 1982;248:1465-77.

23. Gorder DD, Dolecek TA, Coleman GG et al. Dietary intake in the Multiple Risk Factor Intervention Trial (MRFIT): nutrient and food group changes over 6 years. .J Am Diet Assoc. 1986;86:744-51.

24. Dorr AE and others. Colestipol hydrochloride in hypercholesterolemic patients-effect on serum cholesterol and mortality. J Chron Dis 1978;31:5-14.

25. A co-operative trial in the primary prevention of ischaemic heart disease using clofibrate. Report from the Committee of Principal Investigators. Br Heart J 1978;40:1069-118.

26. The Lipid Research Clinics Coronary Primary Prevention Trial results. I. Reduction in incidence of coronary heart disease. JAMA 1984;251:351-64.

27. Steinberg D. The Cholesterol Wars: The skeptics vs the preponderance of evidence. Elsevier 2007.

28. Consensus Conference: Lowering blood cholesterol to prevent heart disease. JAMA 1985;253:2080-6.

29. Moore TJ. Heart Failure, Random House, New York, 1989.

30. Harcombe Z, Baker JS, Cooper SM et al. Evidence from randomised controlled trials did not support the introduction of dietary fat guidelines in 1977 and 1983: a systematic review and meta-analysis. Open Heart. 2015;2:e000196. doi: 10.1136/openhrt-2014-000196.

31. Miettinen TA, Huttunen JK, Naukkarinen V. Multifactorial primary prevention of cardiovascular diseases in middle-aged men. Risk factor changes, incidence, and mortality. JAMA 1985;254:2097-102.

32. Burlingame B, Nishida C, Uauy R, Weisell R. Fats and Fatty Acids in Human Nutrition. Ann Nutr Metab. 2009;55:5-7.

33. Jeger R, Dieterle T. Statins: have we found the Holy Grail? Swiss Med Wkly 2012;142:w13515

34. Roberts WC. The underused miracle drugs: the statin drugs are to atherosclerosis what penicillin was to infectious disease, Am J Cardiol 1996;78:377-8.

35. de Ferranti S, Ludwig DS. Storm over statins--the controversy surrounding pharmacologic treatment of children. N Engl J Med 2008;359:1309-12

36. Diamond DM, Ravnskov U. How statistical deception created the appearance that statins are safe and effective in primary and secondary prevention of cardiovascular disease. Expert Rev Clin Pharmacol. 2015;8:201-10.

37. Diamond DM, Ravnskov U. Additional commentary on deception in statin research. Expert Rev Clin Pharmacol 2015;9:1-2.

38. Ridker PM, Danielson E, Fonseca FAH et al. Rosuvastatin to prevent vascular events in men and women with elevated C-reactive protein. N Engl J Med 2008;359:2195–207.

39. Bradford RH, Shear CL, Chremos AN et al. Expanded clinical evaluation of lovastatin (EXCEL) study results. Arch Intern Med 1991;151:43-9.

40. Sacks FM, Pfeffer MA, Moye LA, Rouleau JL, Rutherford JD, Cole TG, et al. Effect of pravastatin on cardiovascular events in women after myocardial infarction: the cholesterol and recurrent events (CARE) trial. N Engl J Med 1996; 335:1001–9.

41. Shepherd J, Blauw GJ, Murphy MB et al. Pravastatin in elderly individuals at risk of vascular disease (PROSPER): a randomised controlled trial. Lancet 2002; 360:1623–30.

42. Rossebø AB, Pedersen TR, Boman K et al. for the SEAS Investigators. Intensive lipid lowering with simvastatin and ezetimibe in aortic stenosis. N Engl J Med 2008;359:1343-56.

43. Ravnskov U, McCully KS. Vulnerable plaque formation from obstruction of vasa vasorum by homocysteinylated and oxidized lipoprotein aggregates complexed with microbial remnants and LDL autoantibodies. Ann Clin Lab Sci 2009;39:3–16.

44. McLaughlin-Drubin ME, Munger K. Viruses associated with human cancer. Biochim Biophys Acta 2008;1782:127–50.

45. Ravnskov U, McCully KS, Rosch PJ. The statin-low cholesterol-cancer conundrum. QJM 2012;105:383-8.

46. Scandinavian Simvastatin Survival Study Group. Randomised trial of cholesterol lowering in 4444 patients with coronary heart disease: the Scandinavian Simvastatin Survival Study (4S). Lancet 1994;344:1383–9.

47. Heart Protection Study Collaborative Group. MRC/BHF Heart Protection Study of cholesterol lowering with simvas- tatin in 20,536 high-risk individuals: a randomised placebo-controlled trial. Lancet 2002;360:7–22.

48. Newman TB, Hulley SB. Carcinogenicity of lipid-lowering drugs. JAMA 1996;275:55-60.

49. McDougall JA, Malone KE, Daling JR, et al. Long-term statin use and risk of ductal and lobular breast cancer among women 55 to 74 years of age. Cancer Epidemiol Biomarkers Prev 2013;22:1529-37

50. Phillips PS, Haas RH, Bannykh S et al. Statin-associated myopathy with normal creatine kinase levels. Ann Intern Med 2002;137:581-5.

51. Draeger A, Monastyrskaya K, Mohaupt M et al. Statin therapy induces ultrastructural damage in skeletal muscle in patients without myalgia. J Pathol. 2006;210:94-102

52. Sinzinger H, Wolfram R, Peskar BA. Muscular side effects of statins. J Cardiovasc Pharmacol 2002;40:163-71.

53. Sinzinger H, O'Grady J. Professional athletes suffering from familial hypercholesterolaemia rarely tolerate statin treatment because of muscular problems. Br J Clin Pharmacol 2004;57:525-8.

54. Golomb BA, Evans MA, Dimsdale JE et al. Effects of statins on energy and fatigue with exertion: results from a randomized controlled trial. Arch Intern Med 2012;172:1180-2

55. Acharya T, Huang J, Tringali S et al. Statin use and the risk of kidney disease with long-term follow-up (8.4-year study). Am J Cardiol 2016;117:647-55.

56. Muldoon MF, Manuck SB, Matthew HA. Lowering cholesterol concentrations and mortality: a quantitative review of primary prevention trials. BMJ 1990;301:309-14

57. Kim YK, Lee HJ, Kim JY, et al. Low serum cholesterol is correlated to suicidality in a Korean sample. Acta Psychiatr Scand 2002;105:141-8

58. Vilibić M, Jukić V, Pandžić-Sakoman M et al. Association between total serum cholesterol and depression, aggression, and suicidal ideations in war veterans with posttraumatic stress disorder. Croat Med J 2014;55:520-9.

59. Davison KM, Kaplan BJ. Lipophilic statin use and suicidal ideation in a sample of adults with mood disorders. Crisis 2014;35:278-82

60. Hoyer S, Riederer P. Alzheimer disease—no target for statin treatment. Neurochem Res 2007;32:695-706

61. Evans MA, Golomb BA. Statin-associated adverse cognitive effects: survey results from 171 patients. Pharmacotherapy 2009;29:800-11.

62. Padala KP, Padala PR, McNeilly DP et al. The effect of HMG-CoA reductase inhibitors on cognition in patients with Alzheimer's dementia: a prospective withdrawal and rechallenge pilot study. Am J Geriatr Pharmacother 2012;10:296-302

63. Bollapragada SS, Norrie JD, Norman JE. Review of new regulations for the conduct of clinical trials of investigational medicinal products. BJOG 2007;114:917-21

64. Okuyama H, Langsjoen PH, Hamazaki T et al. Statins stimulate atherosclerosis and heart failure: pharmacological mechanisms. Expert Rev Clin Pharmacol 2015;8:189-99. Erratum in: Expert Rev Clin Pharmacol. 2015;8:503-5.

65. Anderson KM, Castelli WP, Levy D. Cholesterol and mortality. 30 years of follow-up from the Framingham Study. JAMA 1987;257:2176-80.

66. LaRosa JC, Hunninghake D, Bush D et al. The cholesterol facts. A summary of the evidence relating dietary fats, serum cholesterol, and coronary heart disease. A joint statement by the American Heart Association and the National Heart, Lung, and Blood Institute. The Task Force on Cholesterol Issues, American Heart Association. Circulation. 1990;81:1721-33.

67. Werkö L. Analysis of the MRFIT screenees: a methodological study. J Intern Med 1995;237:507-18.

68. Ravnskov U. Quotation bias in reviews of the diet-heart idea. J Clin Epidemiol 1995;48:713-9.

Chapter Eight

People with High Cholesterol Live Longer

Tomohito Hamazaki, MD, PhD

Abstract

High blood cholesterol is recognized as a major cause of coronary heart disease (CHD). Although cholesterol levels in Japan are just the average of Western European countries, its CHD mortality is very low compared with those countries. In fact, all-cause mortality in Japan is inversely correlated with LDL-cholesterol levels irrespective of age and sex. The only exception in Japan to this finding is NIPPON DATA80 study (ND80), in which the all-cause mortality of the highest cholesterol group (both sexes combined) was significantly higher than that of the other groups. This phenomenon can be reasonably explained by higher proportions of familial hypercholesterolemia in the ND80 cohort than in the other study cohorts. (Cholesterol is not the cause of CHD in familial hypercholesterolemia though; see the text.) The Cholesterol Guidelines of Japan Atherosclerosis Society (2012) used ND80 results for the most important chart of the Guidelines, which indicated the relationship between 10-year CHD mortality, and sex, age, smoking, blood pressure and cholesterol. However, the unfortunate point is that the number of CHD deaths included in the men's chart was only 18 deaths or so in 10 years; furthermore no mention of statistical significance was made. MEGA Study, the top intervention study with statin in Japan, had serious flaws, and was hardly able to prove any beneficial effects of statin. Cholesterol is a friend; it should not to be feared as dangerous. Neither epidemiological nor intervention studies have been able to prove that cholesterol is the enemy in Japan—*the* country where there has been low CHD mortality from the outset and where anti-cholesterol myth campaigns can be conducted more easily than in any other countries.

Introduction

In Japan, the four leading causes of death are cancer, heart disease, pneumonia, and stroke, in that order [1]. Mortality from ischemic heart disease (IHD)* accounts for about 40% of heart disease, but only 6% of all-cause mortality[1]. If mortality from a certain disease (IHD for instance) could be reduced by two-thirds in any country, it would be an astonishing success. In fact, Japan has succeeded in doing this from the very outset in a sense. As we can see in Fig 1, Japan is lucky enough to enjoy the lowest age-specific mortality from IHD among some 14 countries[2], at roughly one-third of the mean mortality of the other countries. Why is IHD mortality so low in Japan? The major reason is probably that Japanese people regularly eat a lot of fish and have a high intake of α-linolenic acid. So, do they have very low cholesterol levels? Actually they don't. If we look at the cholesterol values of the countries listed on the right in Fig 1, which are the mean values for 2005 through 2009 for both sexes[3], the median cholesterol value of those countries (5.2 mmol/L or 200 mg/dL) is randomly scattered among them. This does not support the notion that cholesterol is an important risk factor for IHD.

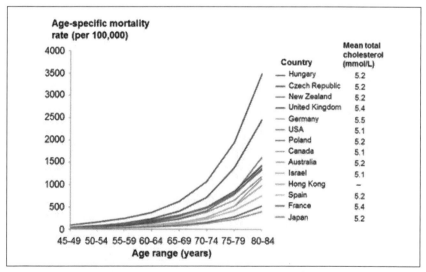

FIGURE 1 **Age-specific mortality rate of ischemic heart disease for 14 countries**

---

* For the sake of simplicity, IHD and CHD are used as they were in the original cited papers but are used interchangeably in this chapter.

The most recent year of available data between 2005 and 2009 is shown[2]. The mean total cholesterol values between 2005 and 2009 were calculated from the table provided by WHO[3].

Moreover, Sekikawa et al[4] reported very interesting trends in blood cholesterol levels and mortality from coronary heart disease (CHD) in the following 8 countries: Australia, Canada, France, Japan, Spain, Sweden, the UK, and USA. Age-adjusted CHD mortality continuously declined between 1980 and 2007 in all these countries. The decline was accompanied by a constant fall in total cholesterol except for in Japan where total cholesterol levels continuously rose. With Fig 1 in mind, is this a Japanese paradox so to speak? In fact, as explained in this chapter, cholesterol issues in Japan are much more than that. Cholesterol levels are a good indicator of longevity irrespective of age and sex. If you look at cholesterol issues in Japan, you will clearly understand what cholesterol is—a friend, not an enemy.

What's important is how many people with familial hypercholesterolemia are in the cohort

Before explaining the issue of cholesterol in Japan, I would like to point out the key to understanding the situation between cholesterol and CHD, namely, the existence of familial hypercholesterolemia (FH). Although many epidemiological studies point to hypercholesterolemia as the cause of CHD, most importantly, mean cholesterol levels do not differ between individuals with heterozygous FH who develop it and those who do not (see Fig 3-A in a previous review[5] for details). Because cholesterol levels and CHD mortality are both much higher in individuals with homozygous FH than in those with heterozygous FH, the similar cholesterol levels seen between individuals with heterozygous FH with CHD and those without CHD cannot be explained by the ceiling effect of cholesterol. Instead, abnormalities of the hemostatic system in FH may explain the high CHD incidence[6]. It is also possible that the LDL receptor defect in FH causes undernutrition of the arteries; through the LDL receptors, LDL particles provide the important nutrients of lipid soluble antioxidants and triglycerides to blood vessels as well as provide the cholesterol necessary for blood vessel repair. At any rate, the association between high cholesterol levels and CHD mortality in Japanese men is most likely due to the presence of individuals with FH in the very high cholesterol groups examined. As for Japanese women, CHD mortality has rarely shown an association with cholesterol levels (the panel for women in Fig 3 is a good example); in the Jichi Medical School Cohort Study, no deaths from myocardial infarction were found at the highest total cholesterol levels (≥6.21 mmol/L or ≥240 mg/dL) in about 7,500 women aged 40-69 years during an average follow-up of 11.9 years[7]—another "Japanese paradox", if you will.

For the association of CHD mortality with cholesterol to be explained by the presence of FH, the slope of the association between cholesterol and CHD mortality would become flatter and flatter as the cohort ages, and there would be fewer and fewer CHD-prone FH participants in the cohort. In fact, this is precisely the case in many epidemiological studies, as Okuyama et al first reported[8] (see also Chapter 3 of our review[5]).

Cholesterol levels and all-cause mortality in Japanese people

Do Japanese people really live longer with higher cholesterol levels irrespective of age and sex? If they do, this must provide the answer to many so-called cholesterol paradoxes and inform us about how to deal with cholesterol.

Let us take a quick look at the largest Japanese epidemiological study on cholesterol undertaken to date. Men and women (N=91,219) aged 40-79 years with no history of stroke or CHD were followed for 10.3 years in the Ibaraki Prefectural Health Study[9]. Figure 2 shows the relationship between all-cause mortality and LDL cholesterol. The hazard ratio (HR) for all-cause mortality was calculated according to LDL cholesterol levels with adjustment for age and many potential confounding factors, and revealed that all-cause mortality was essentially inversely correlated with LDL cholesterol levels in both men and women. The first reaction of well-informed advocates of the cholesterol theory to the findings of this Japanese study would be that this kind of phenomenon can be easily explained by the presence of participants with an as yet subclinical serious disease (e.g., hidden cancer), where some of them who had lower cholesterol levels due to their hidden disease died during the study period (reverse causality). To exclude this possibility of reverse causality, the authors of the Ibaraki Prefectural Health Study re-analyzed the data excluding deaths that occurred within the first 2 years after baseline measurement and, interestingly, found that their initial results were not substantially changed[9].

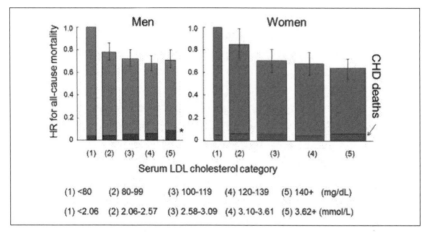

FIGURE 2 **Relationship between serum low density lipoprotein (LDL) cholesterol level and the hazard ratio (HR) for all-cause mortality: Ibaraki Prefectural Health Study[9]**

A total of 30,802 men and 60,417 women were followed for a median 10.3 years. HRs were adjusted for age and many potential confounding factors. Darker colors represent CHD deaths. The height of the bar for CHD deaths is set according to the ratio between the number of CHD deaths and the number of all-cause deaths in the respective groups. The width of each column is proportional to the number of participants in that group. The vertical lines represent 95% confidence intervals. HRs for all-cause mortality for each standard deviation increment of LDL cholesterol were 0.88 (0.85-0.91) for men and 0.90 (0.86-0.93) for women. (Created from the data given in Tables 1 and 2 of reference 9.) *: Significantly different from the reference group (<80 mg/dL) with regard to CHD deaths.

Figure 2 also shows the relationship between LDL cholesterol levels and CHD mortality (indicated by darker colors) according to sex. In men, the HR for CHD mortality was significantly higher than that of the lowest group. However, in women, no differences were observed between any groups. Figure 2 is a good representation of the situation in Japan with regard to cholesterol. This relationship between cholesterol and CHD mortality is not linked to genetic differences between Western and Japanese populations. Japanese emigrants to Hawaii, where Japanese culture is still preserved to a certain degree, were shown to have CHD mortality rates intermediate between those of Japanese men living in Japan and those of Japanese American men living in San Francisco, where the latter group had CHD mortality similar to the general population in San Francisco[10].

Similar results were also found in the Isehara Study, which analyzed the data collected from the annual checkups of residents in Isehara City (population: about 100,000) between 1994 and 2004, with a mean follow-up of 7.1 years[11]. (Since 1982, Japanese citizens aged ≥40 years have been eligible for annual health checkups by law.) The final database for 8,340 men (aged 64±10 years) and 13,591 women (61±12 years) was compiled after applying the following exclusion criteria: death within 1 year of baseline, incomplete lipid data, attended a single check-up only, and serum triglyceride levels beyond the Friedewald equation limits (4.5 mmol/L or 400 mg/dl; 198 men, 126 women). Mean blood LDL cholesterol levels were calculated for individuals from all their available LDL cholesterol values except that at their last checkup. As shown in Fig 3, LDL cholesterol was again found to be a negative risk factor for all-cause mortality.

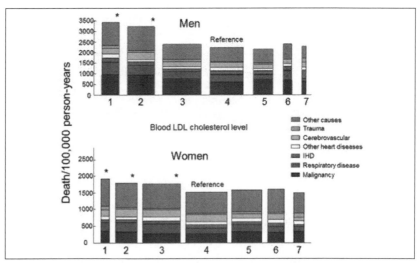

FIGURE 3 **Low density lipoprotein (LDL) cholesterol and mortality in the Isehara Study**[11]

Over 11 years (1994-2004), 8,340 men (aged 64±10 years) and 13,591 women (61±12 years) were followed in Isehara City, Japan. Deaths during the first year of follow-up were excluded. Mean follow-up period was 7.1 years. Cox's proportional hazards regression analysis was employed to calculate age-adjusted relative risks in both men and women. The width of each column is proportional to the number of participants in that group. Cholesterol level of each category is as follows (mg/dL, mmol/L): category 1: <80, <2.1; category 2: 80-99, 2.1-2.5; category 3: 100-119, 2.6-3.0; category 4: 120-139, 3.1-3.5; category 5: 140-159, 3.6-4.0; category 6: 160-179, 4.1-4.6; category 7: ≥180, ≥4.7. *: p<0.001, Cox's proportional hazard regression analysis with Bonferroni adjustment. (Redrawn with permission from the publisher, with slight modifications.)

A very exceptional study: NIPPON DATA80

There is one very exceptional Japanese epidemiological study in which participants with the highest total cholesterol levels had the highest all-cause mortality. This was the National Integrated Project for Prospective Observation of Non-communicable Disease and Its Trends in the Aged, 1980, known as NIPPON DATA80 (ND80)[12] (see black bars in Fig 4). Figure 4 is a carefully redrawn version of the original figure[12] with some important information that I newly added in red. In this study, 9,216 participants were followed for 17.3 years. However, we must exercise extreme caution in interpreting the results. First, let's examine the results of ND80 without combining data from both sexes. Figure 5, which I created from the data given in Table 2 of the same ND80 report[12], shows that neither men nor women had significantly higher all-cause mortality in the higher or highest cholesterol groups at all. In fact, all-cause mortality in the highest cholesterol group was only significantly higher when both sexes were combined, as indicated by the black bars in Fig 4. Moreover, their data were adjusted for serum albumin levels. Because albumin, a good marker for longevity, correlates well with cholesterol level, the adjustment for albumin diminishes the good characteristics of cholesterol. Comparing two figures from the same study (Figs 4 and 5 here), the readers can see how the authors of ND80 exaggerated the risk of high cholesterol levels; they even erased the zero point of the hazard ratio for all-cause mortality. There are more exaggerations: for example, the gray bars are results without deaths due to liver disease (Fig 5), meaning these bars no longer indicate all-cause mortality.

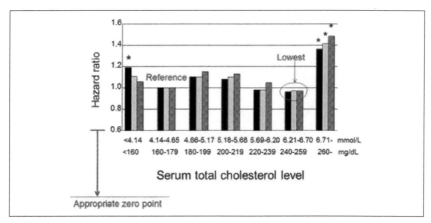

FIGURE 4 Hazard ratio (HR) for all-cause mortality according to serum total cholesterol level: NIPPON DATA80 study, 17.3 years of follow-up[12]

More than 9,000 participants aged ≥30 years were followed for 17.3 years. All data sets (black, gray, and hatched bars) were combined data for both sexes. HRs of all-cause mortality were adjusted for sex, age, serum albumin levels, body mass index, hypertension, diabetes, smoking, and drinking. Black bars: HRs for all-cause mortality without any exclusions. Gray (middle) bars: HRs for all-cause mortality after excluding deaths from liver disease during the entire follow-up period. Hatched (right) bars: HRs for all-cause mortality after further excluding all-cause deaths within the first 5 years of follow-up. Whatever technique the authors of the NIPPON DATA80 might have used to emphasize the risk of hypercholesterolemia, participants in the cholesterol range 6.21-6.70 mmol/L (240-259 mg/dL) show the lowest risk of all-cause mortality. *: p<0.05. (Redrawn with permission from the publisher, with slight modifications.)

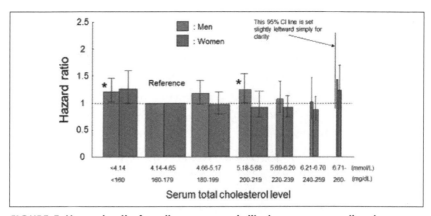

FIGURE 5 Hazard ratio for all-cause mortality by sex according to serum total cholesterol level: the same data from NIPPON DATA80 study[12]

168

So why were the HRs of all-cause mortality slightly high in the highest cholesterol groups of ND80 irrespective of significance in the first place? The answer is very simple: the proportion of participants with FH reported in NIPPON DATA80 is reasonably estimated to be 3-fold higher than that in the general population among male participants and 1.5-fold higher in female participants. (The proportion of FH participants was calculated using the difference between the mean and median cholesterol values in comparison with the general Japanese population[5].) The presence of more FH participants in the ND80 cohort was due to, first, probably a higher proportion of participants with high cholesterol given that the Japanese title of ND80 includes the term "circulatory disease" and, second, the recruitment of ND80 participants from 300 districts across Japan, which made it easy to recruit more FH participants than recruiting them from only one area, especially when the number of participants was large.

Unfortunately, ND80 with its 19-year follow-up[13] served as the basis for the most important charts given in the 2012 guidelines of the Japan Atherosclerosis Society[14]. The charts beautifully show straightforward, positive relationships between 10-year CHD mortality and age, blood pressure (BP), total cholesterol levels, and smoking status, although relationships with age and smoking status only were found in women. Many Japanese physicians follow these 2012 guidelines out of fear of possible malpractice law suits. However, the most unfortunate point is that the number of CHD deaths included in the men's chart was only 35 or so in 19 years, which is very close to 18 deaths in 10 years. How can a chart be drawn indicating absolute CHD mortality in 10 years according to 6 cholesterol categories, 5 BP categories, 3 age categories, and 2 smoking status categories (180 subgroups as a total)? Moreover, the highest risk of CHD mortality in the group with the highest BP, highest cholesterol levels, highest age group, and who were smokers (5-10% in 10 years) was >10 times higher than that in the youngest (40s) group who were non-smokers (<0.5% in 10 years). While this is mathematically possible, we have to question whether there is any clinical or epidemiological importance here, given that no mention of statistical significance was made.

What happens in elderly Japanese people?

When we look at cohorts of elderly people, the proportion of CHD-prone FH participants is very small and negligible, and only beneficial effects of cholesterol are shown in them. Two epidemiological studies with elderly Japanese people have been reported, both of which show that high cholesterol levels are good for longevity.

The first of these studies, the Tokyo Metropolitan Institute of Gerontology Longitudinal Interdisciplinary Study on Aging (TMIG-LISA) Study followed 1,048 Japanese individuals aged 65-85 years living at home in Tokyo or Akita Prefecture for 8 years[15]. As shown in Fig 6, the survival rate was lowest for the lowest quartile of total cholesterol and highest in the highest quartile (without any adjustment). As can be seen from the figure, the relationship between the lowest and highest cholesterol groups does not markedly change with the exclusion of deaths during the first 3 years of the study. The multivariate HR for all-cause mortality for the lowest quartile of total cholesterol was 1.51 compared with the reference (highest quartile) after adjustment for 15 possible confounding factors including grip power and usual walking pace.

The second study of Japanese elderly participants focused on 207 participants only. However, they were all 85 years old at the start, lived in Fukuoka Prefecture, and were followed for 10 years[16]. The mortality rates according to serum total cholesterol levels were 77.4%, 62.5%, and 50% in the bottom, middle, and top tertiles, respectively (Fig 7). A multivariate Cox proportional hazards regression model, with adjustment for sex, smoking, alcohol intake, history of stroke or heart disease, serum albumin concentration, body mass index, and systolic BP, revealed that the total mortality in the bottom tertile was 1.7-fold higher than that in the top tertile. Without albumin adjustment, the difference might have been larger (see above for the discussion on albumin).

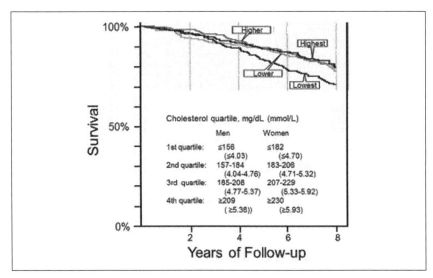

FIGURE 6 Survival curve according to cholesterol quartile in Japanese elderly people: TMIG-LISA Study[15]

A total of 1,048 elderly participants were followed for 8 years. Survival rates are depicted according to cholesterol quartile. No adjustment was performed. The hazard ratio for the 1st quartile was 1.51 compared with that of the 4th quartile after adjustment for 15 factors. (Courtesy of Dr Shoji Shinkai, with slight modifications.)

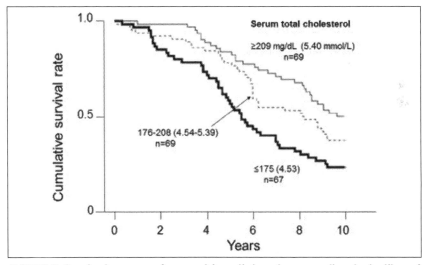

FIGURE 7 Survival curves of very old participants according to tertiles of total cholesterol level: a study in Fukuoka Prefecture[16]

171

Participants all aged 85 in Fukuoka Prefecture were followed for 10 years. Participants in the top and intermediate tertiles of total cholesterol levels survived longer than those in the bottom tertile. See the text for details.

Are statins effective in Japan?

The Management of Elevated Cholesterol in the Primary Prevention Group of Adult Japanese (MEGA) Study is essentially the only statin trial in Japan with a seemingly valid control group (only half-valid, though, as discussed below). It was designed as a prospective randomized, open-labeled, blinded-endpoint (PROBE) study[17]. Because this study is the most important and influential intervention study in Japan, I will discuss it in detail. Men and postmenopausal women weighing ≥40 kg, aged 40-70 years, and with total cholesterol values of 5.69-6.98 mmol/L (220-270 mg/dL) were enrolled between February 1994 and March 1999. Note that this period is of critical importance in understanding the nature of the then diet. Individuals with familial FH or a history of CHD or stroke were excluded. Half of the participants were randomly assigned to the diet alone group and the other half to the diet + pravastatin (10-20 mg/day) group. Follow-up of 5 years was planned.

Unfortunately, this study was seriously flawed. First, randomization seems to have been broken due to a protocol violation: "on the basis of recommendations from the data and safety monitoring committee, the study was continued for an additional 5 years to increase the number of events"[17]. This means that the committee considered there were too few events to obtain significant results at the 5-year mark; so again, Japanese people succeeded in having low CHD mortality from the beginning.

Second is a point that even lay people might have some doubts about (see Fig 9). No CHD cases were observed for more than 1 year starting just before the end of originally planned intervention of 5 years. This looks extremely unnatural. Healthy participants must have been selected in the diet + pravastatin group, intentionally or unintentionally. Actually the numbers of participants in both groups dropped suddenly after 5 years. This study should have reported only the results obtained at the end of the first 5 years.

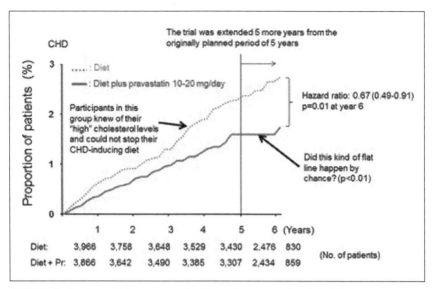

FIGURE 8 **Kaplan-Meier curves for the primary endpoint of first occurrence of coronary heart disease: MEGA Study[17]**

Patients with hypercholesterolemia without any history of CHD or stroke were randomly assigned to the diet or diet + pravastatin group for the mean follow-up period of 5.2 years[17]. CHD was significantly lower in the diet + pravastatin group than in the diet alone group (66 versus 101 events, p=0.01). Besides the flaws described in the text, there are more: the ratio of participants who could not be confirmed to be alive was significantly higher in the pravastatin + diet group than in the diet alone group. Hama et al[18] collected relevant data from papers published on the MEGA Study and from the study's website and also obtained a Japanese version of a slide set on the MEGA Study presented at the American Heart Association Scientific Sessions, 2005. According to the Japanese slides, 13.5% of participants in the pravastatin + diet group compared to 11.9% of participants in the diet alone group could not be confirmed to be alive (odds ratio: 1.16, 1.01-1.33, p=0.031). Also, participants who were diagnosed with cancer within the first 6 months of the study were excluded from the analysis. (Remade with permission from the publisher, with slight modifications.).

Let's look at the results for the first 5 years only. The incidence curve of the diet group is above that of the diet + pravastatin group irrespective of significance. Why is this so? The authors of the study would say with confidence that it was because of statin, but my answer is completely different; it was because of diet. Probably the readers of this chapter have no real experience of the unfortunate reason for this: according to the thinking of that time, the diet recommended for the MEGA Study participants was not nutritionally appropriate for CHD prevention. Butter was replaced with margarine rich in linoleic acid and/or *trans* fatty acids, and fatty fish was avoided because of its high cholesterol content. In fact, as we know now, this diet was CHD *inducing*. The diet + statin group did not likely stick to the diet because they and their doctors knew that their cholesterol levels decreased soon after statin prescription, and thus they thought that the diet were no longer necessary. However, the "diet alone" participants could do nothing except stick to the harmful diet (because it was the only major intervention recommended to them to reduce their risk for CHD) and therefore they had higher incidental CHD than the diet + statin group. This appears to be the major reason for the difference in IHD incidence between the two groups.

Another very important problem with this study was that it was open-label and participating physicians were presumably pro-statin, otherwise they wouldn't have participated in the study. Therefore, the differences in angina and revascularization events between the two participant groups should be discounted. Both of these events were dependent on the physicians' subjective judgment, especially if they viewed those patients who were not receiving the statin to be at higher risk for CHD than those receiving it. If we discount these two events that are open to subjective bias, there would be no difference between the two groups irrespective of significance.

There are some other problems with the study, which are mentioned in the legend to Fig 8. So, even the most important statin-intervention study did not actually prove anything much at all about CHD prevention in Japan.

Conclusions

Cholesterol is in fact a friend; it should not to be feared as dangerous and we should not try to reduce our blood levels of it. Neither epidemiological nor intervention studies have been able to prove that cholesterol is the enemy. This situation is especially clear in Japan— *the* country where there has been low CHD mortality from the outset and where anti-cholesterol myth campaigns can be conducted more easily than in any other countries.

What an irony it is that the first statin was discovered in Japan!

Tomohito Hamazaki, MD, PhD

Professor Emeritus, University of Toyama
Senior Visiting Scientist, RIKEN
Department of Medicine, Toyama Onsen Daini Hospital
hamazakit2016@gmail.com

References

1. Health, Labour and Welfare Statistics Association. Health in Japan: recent vital statistics. J Health Welfare Stat. 2015/2016;62 (No 9 (Suppl)).

2. Finegold JA, Asaria P, Francis DP. Mortality from ischaemic heart disease by country, region, and age: statistics from World Health Organisation and United Nations. Int J Cardiol. 2013;168:934-45.

3. World Health Organization. Mean total cholesterol trends (age-standardized estimate). Data by country. http://appswhoint/gho/data/nodemainA891.

4. Sekikawa A, Miyamoto Y, Miura K, et al. Continuous decline in mortality from coronary heart disease in Japan despite a continuous and marked rise in total cholesterol: Japanese experience after the Seven Countries Study. Int J Epidemiol. 2015;44:1614-24.

5. Hamazaki T, Okuyama H, Ogushi Y, Hama R. Towards a Paradigm Shift in Cholesterol Treatment⬜A Re-Examination of the Cholesterol Issue in Japan. Ann Nutr Metabol 2015;66 (Suppl 4):1-116. Free access: http://www.karger.com/Journal/Issue/266692.

6. Sugrue DD, Trayner I, Thompson GR, et al. Coronary artery disease and haemostatic variables in heterozygous familial hypercholesterolaemia. Br Heart J. 1985;53:265-8.

7. Nago N, Ishikawa S, Goto T, Kayaba K. Low cholesterol is associated with mortality from stroke, heart disease, and cancer: the Jichi Medical School Cohort Study. J Epidemiol. 2011;21:67-74.

8. Okuyama H, Ichikawa Y, Sun Y, Hamazaki T, Lands WE. Association of high total cholesterol with coronary heart disease mortality differs among subject populations--familial hypercholesterolemia as a key concept. World Rev Nutr Diet. 2007;96:19-36.

9. Noda H, Iso H, Irie F, Sairenchi T, Ohtaka E, Ohta H. Gender difference of association between LDL cholesterol concentrations and mortality from coronary heart disease amongst Japanese: the Ibaraki Prefectural Health Study. J Intern Med. 2010;267:576-87.

10. Benfante R. Studies of cardiovascular disease and cause-specific mortality trends in Japanese-American men living in Hawaii and risk factor comparisons with other Japanese populations in the Pacific region: a review. Hum Biol. 1992;64:791-805.

11. Ogushi Y, Kurita Y. Resident cohort study to analyze relations between health check-up results and cause-specific mortality. Mumps (M Technology Association Japan) 2008;24:9-19 (in Japanese).

12. Okamura T, Tanaka H, Miyamatsu N, et al. The relationship between serum total cholesterol and all-cause or cause-specific mortality in a 17.3-year study of a Japanese cohort. Atherosclerosis. 2007;190:216-23.

13. NIPPON DATA80 Research Group. Risk assessment chart for death from cardiovascular disease based on a 19-year follow-up study of a Japanese representative population. Circ J. 2006;70:1249-55.

14. Japan Atherosclerosis Society ed. Japan Atherosclerosis Society (JAS) Guidelines for the prevention of atherosclerotic cardiovascular diseases, 2012. Issued from Japan Atherosclerosis Society, Tokyo. 2012 (in Japanese).

15. Suzuki T, Shibata H. An introduction of the Tokyo Metropolitan Institute of Gerontology Longitudinal Interdisciplinary Study on Aging (TMIG-LISA, 1991-2001). Geriatr Gerontol Int. 2003;3:S1-S4.

16. Takata Y, Ansai T, Soh I, et al. Serum total cholesterol concentration and 10-year mortality in an 85-year-old population. Clin Interv Aging. 2014;9:293-300.

17. Nakamura H, Arakawa K, Itakura H, et al. Primary prevention of cardiovascular disease with pravastatin in Japan (MEGA Study): a prospective randomised controlled trial. Lancet. 2006;368:1155-63.

18. Hama R, Sakaguchi K. Pravastatin (mevalotin) reduces survival rates –a critical examination on MEGA Study– NNH 48: Administration of pravastatin to 48 subjects for 5.3 years reduces one survivor. Informed Prescriber 2006;21:84-6 (in Japanese).

Chapter Nine

A Role for Sulfur Deficiency in Coronary Heart Disease

Stephanie Seneff, PhD

Abstract

Despite decades of research, many questions remain unanswered about the pathogenesis of cardiovascular disease. Why does cardiovascular plaque accumulate only in arteries, and preferentially in arteries supplying the heart? Multiple pathogenic microbial species take up residence in the plaque, yet antibiotic therapy has generally been unsuccessful. Inflammation is now believed to be a critical factor, yet the question of why inflammation occurs itself remains unanswered. Geographical studies show a strong inverse relationship between sunlight availability and heart disease, yet studies on vitamin D supplements have been disappointing. Here, I propose a unifying theory for the etiology of cardiovascular disease, where the atheroma develops to supply cholesterol sulfate to the heart, due to pathologies in the normal supply chain. Sun avoidance and consumption of chemical-laden processed foods are major contributors to the development of coronary atherosclerosis. Appropriate preventive measures include sulfur-containing foods and supplements, organic diet, and sun exposure.

Introduction

Despite many decades of research, atherosclerosis remains a poorly explained phenomenon. The field of cardiovascular disease is in a state of confusion, as doctors continue to focus on high serum cholesterol

177

levels as the main culprit, whereas correlations between cholesterol and ischemia risk are low and insignificant. On the other hand, while factors such as various infective agents and elevated serum homocysteine are correlated with heart disease risk, active treatment of these conditions consistently fails to show benefit. The simple story that is presented to the public is that excess cholesterol accumulates in the blood and lodges in the artery wall, eventually obstructing flow. However, it is striking that the lipid deposits accumulate only in arteries – never in veins. And what is even more striking is that the arteries supplying the heart are the most vulnerable.

In this chapter, all of these seemingly contradictory facts are explained via the theory that heart disease is a condition resulting from deficiencies in the supply of cholesterol sulfate to the vasculature. The atheroma is then viewed as a site where cholesterol sulfate is actively synthesized, and the sulfate is later redistributed to the capillary wall to protect from vascular damage and support the smooth passage of red blood cells. The atheroma is constantly remodelled as its components are repeatedly built up and broken down by metalloproteinases. The deficiency comes about because the enzymes that normally maintain serum levels of cholesterol sulfate are disrupted by environmental toxicants, such as aluminum and glyphosate.

According to this alternative view, the atheroma subserves the heart by providing it with vital nutrients, namely, cholesterol and sulfate. It follows that the cause of heart disease is inadequate supply of cholesterol sulfate to the heart. I will further argue that cholesterol sulfate is normally produced in the skin by keratinocytes, red blood cells, and platelets, catalyzed by sunlight. This theory predicts that sunny climates reduce heart disease risk and that sulfur-rich soil and water derived from basalt rock are protective. Indeed, France and Spain have much lower rates of death from myocardial infarction (MI) than the United Kingdom, and people living on islands enriched with sulfur-containing volcanic basalt rock, such as Japan, Iceland, and Crete, enjoy low MI risk and extended life expectancy.

Early studies on primates showed that a high-fat, high-cholesterol diet fed to monkeys could induce atherosclerosis, but that simultaneous supplementation with sulfur-containing metabolites was protective[1]. Similarly, experiments on rats showed that a diet supplemented with excess cholesterol, cholic acid and vitamin D2 can induce aortic lesions expressing calcification and plaque formation, but such lesions can be completely prevented by simultaneous supplementation with chondroitin sulfate[2]. Children with disorders of cysteine metabolism develop arterial damage at an early age resembling atherosclerosis[3]. The consumption of garlic is inversely correlated with the progression of cardiovascular disease, and this benefit is likely due to the fact that garlic is a rich source of sulfane sulfur[4]. Synthetic hydrogen sulfide donors can remarkably protect mitochondria in endothelial cells from oxidative damage[5]. All of these examples point to the hypothesis that impaired sulfur supply to the vasculature is the key factor in cardiovascular disease.

Cholesterol Sulfate Synthesis in the Skin

Geographical data show an inverse relationship between cardiovascular disease and annual sunlight availability[6]. In a study conducted in the British Isles, 49% of the variance in mortality from coronary heart disease was accounted for by mean annual sunshine hours[7]. However, despite the fact that vitamin D deficiency is associated with cardiovascular disease risk[8], placebo-controlled trials have failed to show any benefit from vitamin D3 supplementation[9].

We suggest that the benefit comes from cholesterol sulfate synthesis instead. In[10], it was proposed that sulfate is produced from reduced sulfur sources in the skin, catalyzed by sunlight. The enzyme that likely carries out this function was identified as endothelial nitric oxide synthase (eNOS), the same enzyme that produces nitric oxide to relax the artery wall. We hypothesize that the overuse of sunscreen has played a dual damaging role not only because sunlight catalysis is suppressed but also because the aluminum in high-SPF sunscreens actively disrupts eNOS' function, due to displacement of the iron in the heme group[11]. eNOS is a cytochrome P450 (CYP) enzyme, and many other environmental chemicals also disrupt CYP enzymes, including mercury[12,13], arsenic[14], cadmium[12], and glyphosate[15,16], the active ingredient in the pervasive herbicide, Roundup.

It is well established that eNOS produces superoxide as well as nitric oxide, but this has always been viewed as a pathology[17]. At the same time, the fact that RBCs contain abundant eNOS has always posed a puzzle to biologists, because nitric oxide would disrupt hemoglobin's ability to transport oxygen[18]. But if the superoxide synthesis by eNOS represents an alternative function to oxidize sulfur, then both of these puzzles are explained. Thiosulfate, derived from hydrogen sulfide gas via oxidation in the mitochondria, may be the primary source of sulfur that is oxidized by eNOS to ultimately yield two sulfate anions[10].

Correlation does not always imply causation, but it would be surprising for causative factors not to be correlated with the disease they cause. Most people assume that elevated serum lipids are a causal factor in coronary artery disease (CAD). Therefore, a plot over time of the hospital discharge rates for hyperlipidemia should be highly correlated with a similar plot for CAD.

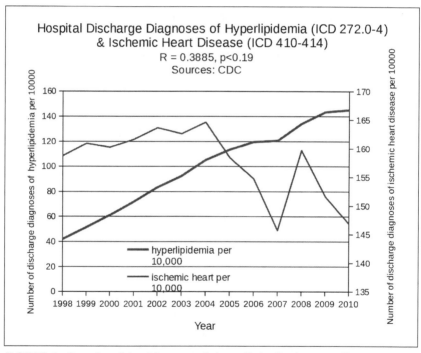

FIGURE 1 **Graph of incidence of hospital discharge diagnoses of hyperlipidemia (ICD 272.0- 4) and ischemic heart disease (ICD 410-414) over time from 1998 to 2010, available from the CDC.**

As Figure 1 shows, this is not the case. The correlation value is 0.39 with an insignificant p-value of 0.19. Yet, tens if not hundreds of millions of people are advised by their doctor to take a statin drug to protect them from CAD because their serum lipid levels are high.

There is a much stronger, highly significant, correlation between hyperlipidemia and glyphosate application to corn and soy crops: R = 0.97, and $p < .000018$, as shown in Figure 2.

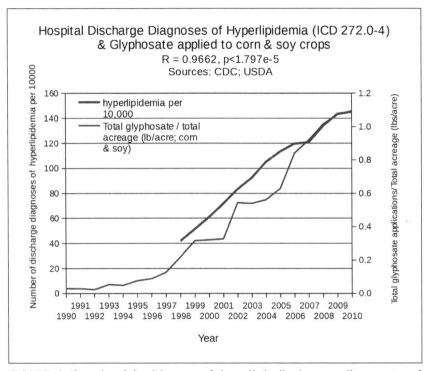

FIGURE 2 Graph of incidence of hospital discharge diagnoses of hyperlipidemia (ICD 272.0- 4), available from the CDC, and the rate of glyphosate application to corn and soy crops, obtained from the US Department of Agriculture.

Glyphosate application rates have steadily increased over time due to the widespread appearance of glyphosate resistant weeds growing among the crops that are increasingly engineered to be glyphosate resistant. Serum lipids have also risen in step with this increase in glyphosate, despite the increase in statin drug prescriptions.

It is not unreasonable to propose that glyphosate is causal in hyperlipidemia. Glyphosate disrupts CYP enzyme activity in the liver[19], and multiple CYP enzymes are needed to produce bile acids[20]. Bile acids contain sulfated oxysterols derived from cholesterol through the action of CYP enzymes, which eventually make their way into chylomicrons that enter the lymph system from the gut and exit into the vascular system in the large veins feeding directly into the heart. Thus, normally, bile is a major source of sulfated sterols to supply the heart.

A rat study assessing the impact of glyphosate, clofibrate and two phenoxyacid herbicides on liver function showed that glyphosate reduced the activity of CYP enzymes in the liver much more than any of the other pesticides investigated[19]. Bile acids normally export a large amount of cholesterol via the digestive system, most of which is reabsorbed via the chylomicron. Impeded bile acid synthesis due to a defective CYP7A1 gene produced neonatal cholestasis and hypercholesterolemia, specifically, elevation in serum LDL, in mice fed a normal chow diet[21].

It is plausible that glyphosate also disrupts eNOS' ability to synthesize sulfate, given that eNOS is also a CYP enzyme. Glyphosate exposure to eNOS in RBCs is expected, as glyphosate export via the kidney requires transit through the vasculature. Disrupted synthesis of cholesterol sulfate, both through the impaired activity of bile acid enzymes and through eNOS dysfunction, will necessitate an increase in the synthesis of LDL particles to transport cholesterol in the unsulfated form, which is hydrophobic.

Furthermore, glyphosate likely disrupts the metabolism of fructose by gut microbes, due to its impairment of the shikimate pathway[22]. This places a huge burden on the liver to metabolize fructose to fat, which then needs to either be stored locally, inducing fatty liver disease, or exported within lipid particles. Fructose is a major factor in non-alcoholic fatty liver disease (NAFLD) and the metabolic syndrome[23]. Fatty liver disease has become an epidemic worldwide[24]. Furthermore, NAFLD is a strong risk factor for cardiovascular disease[25].

The Atheroma Supplies Cholesterol Sulfate

Davidson et al.[26] proposed that RBCs produce cholesterol sulfate while traversing the surface veins, catalyzed by sunlight, and release it to the tissues in the capillaries. This refurbishes both the cholesterol and the sulfate supply to the endothelial wall, maintaining vascular health. Heparan sulfate proteoglycans (HSPGs) in the glycocalyx play many important roles[27], mediating cellular signaling mechanisms and promoting uptake of various nutrients, including LDL clearance by hepatocytes[28]. But perhaps the most important role in the capillary is to maintain a thick layer of gelled water coating the inner surface. This structuring effect on water is due to the kosmotropic properties of sulfate[29]. It provides a near-frictionless surface contact with the RBCs[10], that is further enhanced by the negative charge in both the glycocalyx and the RBC membrane. As the RBC drops off cholesterol sulfate, it also loses negative charge, which means that the venous end has a lower pH than the arterial end. An increase in carbon dioxide content on the venous side enhances this effect, as is extremely apparent immediately following cardiac arrest, when CO_2 accumulates in the veins and the voltage difference between arteries and veins is sharply increased[30]. Thus, an electrical gradient also propels the negatively charged RBC through the capillary. Capillary resistance is the dominant factor in high blood pressure, which can therefore be expected to correlate with an impoverishment in cholesterol sulfate in RBC membranes and heparan sulfate in the capillary wall. Both increased friction at the walls and decreased force from the electromagnetic field contribute to impeded movement of RBCs through the capillary[31].

The glycocalyx is constantly shed and rebuilt in a dynamic process that is promoted by inflammatory agents[32]. Complement and endotoxin both induce glycocalyx shedding through a G-protein coupled receptor response. Such matrix remodelling is especially active during ischemia/reperfusion. Membrane-bound matrix metalloproteinases can detach fragments of the glycocalyx from the artery wall which can then be redistributed to other parts of the vasculature, such as the capillaries, as reenforcements. Thus, it is highly conceivable that the glycocalyx in atherosclerotic regions is a source of raw materials needed to maintain the health of the HSPGs in the capillary glycocalyx.

The atheroma is uniquely suited to the manufacture of cholesterol sulfate by platelets, where the sulfate is supplied by breaking down homocysteine thiolactone, the cholesterol is supplied from the lipid stores in the macrophages, ATP to energize the reaction is supplied by red blood cells, and superoxide, needed to oxidize the sulfur atom in homocysteine, is provided through the inflammatory response[10]. HDL plays a critical role, because platelets will only take up cholesterol from HDL-A1 (the "good" variant), and they will increase their production of cholesterol sulfate 300-fold in the presence of 3'-phosphoadenosine-5'-phosphosulfate (PAPS), a source of transferrable sulfate produced by sulfation of ATP[33]. ApoE plays a significant role as well, as it induces the export of cholesterol from the macrophages into HDL-A1, but it also induces enrichment of sulfate in the HSPGs[34]. This implies that it escorts cholesterol sulfate out of the cell rather than cholesterol. This idea is also supported by the fact that cholesterol sulfate, unlike cholesterol, is water soluble, and therefore readily traverses the cytoplasmic gap between the endothelial reticulum and the plasma membrane. Both homocysteine[35] and gamma-glutamyltransferase (GGT)[36,37] are risks factors for heart disease, and both can be explained because they provide substrate for sulfate synthesis. GGT breaks glutathione down into cysteinylglycine and glutamate, and cysteine from cysteinylglycine can be oxidized to form sulfate[38].

The atheroma harbors various microbial infections, the most significant of which is probably *Chlamydia pneumoniae*[39,40]. While the concept of antibiotic treatment specific to *C. pneumoniae* was enthusiastically embraced, clinical trials have been disappointing[41]. C. pneumoniae are dormant except when internalized into host cells, and, within these cells, they produce a unique form of heparan sulfate, using a set of enzymes that are not found in any other known species[42]. I hypothesize that they play a special role in enhancing the supply of heparan sulfate to the atheroma, and they may be able to do so in the absence of functional CYP enzymes.

A Role for PCSK9

Cholesterol sulfate, along with its close cousin, dehydroepiandrosterone (DHEA) sulfate, is the most common sterol sulfate in the blood[43], and it will readily enter any lipid membrane, including the lipid monolayer of the suspended LDL and HDL particles. I hypothesize that it serves a protective role in preventing oxidative and glycation damage to these particles. The "small dense LDL particles" are the most atherogenic, and they arise because glycation and oxidation prevents the reuptake and recycling by the liver.

Proprotein convertase subtilisin/kexin type 9 (PCSK9) is a proprotein convertase that is synthesized mainly by hepatocytes in the liver. When present in the cytoplasm of hepatocytes, it binds to the LDL receptors and causes them to be metabolized, resulting in reduced liver uptake of spent LDL particles, thus raising serum LDL levels[44]. However, after it is glycosylated and tyrosine-sulfated in the golgi, PCSK9 sulfate is secreted[45], and, once in the serum, it binds to LDL particles[46]. Thus it can be hypothesized that PCSK9 serves a protective role similar to that of cholesterol sulfate in preventing LDL particles from becoming oxidized and glycated, through the structuring effects of sulfate on water. It may also be the case that accumulation of unsulfated PCSK9 in the cytoplasm is an indicator of either sulfate deficiency or impaired sulfotransferase capacity. Statin drugs induce an increase in PCSK9 synthesis[47]. It can be conjectured that reduced supply of cholesterol sulfate necessitates increased supply of tyrosine sulfate to compensate.

It appears then that, when sulfation capacity is impaired in hepatocytes, poorly protected LDL particles accumulate in the serum due to the loss of LDL receptors in the liver. These vulnerable LDL particles are then oxidized and taken up by macrophages in the atheroma, where their contents become substrate for cholesterol sulfate synthesis. There is considerable enthusiasm for a new class of monoclonal antibody drugs that intefere with PCSK9 function on the LDL receptor[44]. A single injection of monoclonal antibodies to PCSK9 resulted in a greater than 60% drop in LDL cholesterol, due to enhanced reuptake by the liver. I predict that these drugs will cause some unexpected consequences both because LDL particles will be more vulnerable to attack by oxidizing and glycating agents, due to loss of protection from PCSK9, and because the liver will try to recycle more cholesterol than it can safely dispose of through the bile acids, which may lead to fatty liver disease. The impaired sulfation capacity that PCSK9 should be signaling will still exist even though there is insufficient PCSK9 to adequately signal the problem.

Cholesterol Sulfate and Leukotrienes

Arachidonic acid (AA), produced by polymorphonuclear cells (PMNLs), is a key stimulating factor in the inflammatory cascade that leads to allergy, asthma and atherosclerosis[48,49]. The first step in this cascade is the conversion of AA to leukotriene A4, mediated by the highly regulated enzyme 5-lipoxygenase (5-LO). The 5-lipoxygenase pathway has been implicated in the pathogenesis of atherosclerosis[50,51]. 5-LO is activated by calcium influx, which induces its binding to the nuclear membrane[52].

Cholesterol sulfate has a profound inhibitory effect on 5-LO, which likely depends on its internalization and trafficking to the endoplasmic reticulum[53]. Membrane fluidity is a key modulator of the activity of 5-LO, and cholesterol decreases the permeability of membranes, thereby decreasing fluidity[54,55,56]. I hypothesize that the sulfate anion provided by cholesterol sulfate mobilizes the cholesterol in the ER, such that it can now populate the nuclear membrane and inhibit the activity of 5-LO. I further hypothesize that the conversion of AA to leukotrienes is a key mechanism by which PMNLs signal cholesterol sulfate deficiency, in order to provoke a system-wide inflammatory response that will restore sulfate supplies to the vasculature, through oxidation of sulfur in homocysteine or cysteinylglycine by superoxide, thereby mobilizing cholesterol.

Chagas Syndrome, Down Syndrome and Statin Drugs: Multiple Pathways to Heart Failure

Deaths from MI have steadily decreased in the industrialized world over the past few decades[57,58], but we are simultaneously experiencing an increasing health care burden in an emerging epidemic in heart failure[59]. In fact, heart failure is the single most frequent cause of hospitalization for those over 65 years old, affecting 5 million Americans as of 2010[60]. I maintain that heart failure is a direct sequela to insufficient supply of cholesterol and sulfate to the heart. Since the atheroma plays a significant role in supplying these nutrients, it can be anticipated that factors that interfere with the healthy function of the atheroma will lead over time to heart failure.

Chagas syndrome is an infectious disease endemic to regions of South America caused by the Tryptanosoma cruzi pathogen[61,62]. Recovered patients are susceptible to premature death by heart failure many decades later. However, they have been noted to be remarkably free of atherosclerosis, although they suffer from frequent small heart attacks[62]. The explanation for this unique profile follows logically from the fact that T. cruzi produces an antigenic molecule that closely mimics cholesterol sulfate[61]. As a result, these patients develop antibodies to cholesterol sulfate, which would render the synthesis of cholesterol sulfate by the atheroma counterproductive, but lead to system-wide deficiencies in cholesterol and sulfate.

Down syndrome (trisomy 21) is associated with a low risk to atherosclerosis[63,64] combined with a premature susceptibility to heart failure[65] and Alzheimer's disease (AD)[66]. A key enzyme present on chromosome 21 is Cu/Zn superoxide dismutase (SOD), which is thus 50% overexpressed in association with Down syndrome[67]. SOD dismutates superoxide to hydrogen peroxide, thus reducing the bioavailability of superoxide for the oxidation of reduced sulfur sources, such as homocysteine thiolactone and cysteinylglycine (derived from glutathione)[36], to form sulfate. Downs patients are susceptible to AD at least 20 to 30 years earlier than is normally expected, and dementia is clinically detected in association with Down syndrome at least 3 times more frequently than in those without trisomy 21[68]. Sulfate deficiency likely plays a significant role in the AD brain, as evidenced by the severe deficiency in sulfatide, the only sulfonated lipid, observed in association with AD[69].

Many have argued that statin drugs produce their pleiotrophic effects through an anti-inflammatory effect[70,71,72], and, further, that other treatments aimed at reducing inflammatory signaling might be effective treatments[73]. I predict that both statin therapy and these other treatments will lead to heart failure. Statins also disrupt G- protein coupled receptor signaling via their suppression of the synthesis of geranylgeranyl pyrophosphate, leading to defective protein prenylation[74], which explains their induction of arterial calcification[75]. Thus, I propose that statin drugs promote heart failure through impairment of cholesterol sulfate synthesis in the atheroma, both by reducing the bioavailability of LDL to the atheroma and by interfering with the inflammatory response. Not surprisingly, low cholesterol is consistently associated with poor survival statistics in heart failure[76,77,78]. In heart failure, total cholesterol levels under 200 mg/dl increase risk of dying by up to 3 fold[76,77]. Fonarow et al. state, provocatively: "Could elevated total cholesterol, which is so firmly established to be deleterious for the development of coronary heart disease and coronary heart disease mortality, actually turn out to be good for patients with chronic HF?"[78], p. 1941.

Does Taurine Replenish Sulfate in MI?

Taurine (aminoethanesulfonic acid) is the only sulfonated amino acid, and its roles in the body are yet to be fully clarified. The highest concentrations of taurine are found in the heart, and taurine represents 50% of the free amino acid pool there[79]. Although some bacteria can utilize taurine as a fuel source[80], it has long been maintained that taurine can not be metabolized by mammalian cells. However, reperfusion injury following coronary bypass surgery is decreased by preoperative infusion of taurine[81], and taurine supplementation improves heart function following MI in rat studies[82].

Taurine clearly plays a critical though poorly understood role in cardiovascular disease. It is stored in large concentrations in the brain, heart and liver, and it is also retained in blood platelets. Acute left ventricular ischemia in the dog as well as whole heart anoxia in the rat heart in vitro resulted in the disappearance of taurine from the left ventricle via leakage into the extracellular fluid[83]. Studies on dogs, cats and humans have demonstrated a direct linear relationship between plasma taurine levels and platelet taurine levels[84,85]. Platelets from taurine deficient cats and humans are more sensitive to clotting stimuli[85]. Early studies in dogs showed that taurine was mainly concentrated in the atria, and ischemia induced a 47% loss of taurine in the left ventricle and a 26% loss in both atria[86].

Human polymorphonuclear leukocytes (PMN) produce myeloperoxidase (MPO) during ischemia/reperfusion injury[87], and elevated MPO is an established risk factor for cardiovascular mortality following angiography[88]. Since MPO often serves as a potent bacteriocidal weapon[89], it potentially links to the infectious theory of heart disease[90,40]. Hypochlorite (HOCl), produced in response to

MPO, avidly oxidizes many sulfhydryl-dependent proteins, leading to platelet activation and endothelial adhesion by neutrophils, and it has been proposed that taurine protects from these damaging effects by reacting with and neutralizing HOCl to form taurine chloramine[91]. As we have seen, taurine is released from the heart during ischemia, and it is not taken up by the platelets[92], so it would be readily available in the serum. However, taurine chloramine activates complement, by producing a hemolytic C5-C9 complex[93]. Complement activation, in turn, promotes an inflammatory response, providing oxidizing agents that could in theory promote the oxidation of sulfur in taurine chloramine.

Thus, a novel way to view taurine is as a potential buffer for sulfate renewal in times of acute deficiency. If sulfate insufficiency is an important factor in heart disease, an important question to ask is: can taurine chloramine become a substrate for sulfate synthesis? After all, it already contains sulfur at a +5 oxidation state, so it only needs to oxidize it from +5 to +6 to produce sulfate. Taurine chloramine is a much more reactive compound than its precursor, taurine.

Taurine is not easily catabolized by mammalian cells[94]. However, 25% of the traced sulfur in supplemental taurine turned up in the urine as sulfate. The hypothesis was put forward that the gut bacteria metabolized the taurine to sulfate. Since taurine chloramine is more reactive, perhaps it can be metabolized to yield free sulfate, with microbial infective agents playing a facilitative role. If so, this would justify both cardiac storage of taurine as a source of sulfate during times of severe deficiency, as well as the presence of microbes in cardiovascular lesions[90,40], and it would lend further credibility to the infectious theory of heart disease.

Taurine offers protection during ischemia/reperfusion, although the mechanism has not yet been worked out[95]. There is a severe loss of taurine from the heart during ischemia that can lead to heart failure if the taurine is not replenished. A World Health Organization population study revealed an inverse association between taurine excretion and ischemic heart disease mortality[96]. Reperfusion causes a burst in oxygen consumption through diversion of the electrons from the electron chain into superoxide production[97,98]. We argue that a key purpose of this superoxide is to oxidize sulfur derived from cysteine or homocysteine from a -2 oxidation state to a +6 oxidation state, producing sulfate from sulfide and consuming two superoxide anions. Several enzymes working in conjunction with the mitochondrial electron chain are involved in oxidizing H_2S to sulfate and thiosulfate[99]. As described in[100], homocysteine thiolactone is converted to sulfate in the presence of superoxide, catalyzed by vitamin A and vitamin C, possibly explaining the positive role of vitamin C in protection from cardiovascular disease[101].

Taurine offers many health benefits to the cardiovascular system[102]. Taurine has been shown to inhibit the osteoblastic differentiation of vascular smooth muscle cells that leads to artery calcification[103]. Taurine showed protection against the loss of mechanical function in rat hearts in both a heart failure and ischemia model[104]. In particular, taurine suppresses the production of superoxide during reperfusion[105]. We propose here that this suppressive effect is achieved mainly due to the fact that it contains sulfur already at a +5 oxidation state, and hence only 1/6 as much superoxide is needed to produce an equivalent amount of sulfate. The fact that taurine is normally inert makes it a great choice for buffering as a precursor to sulfate. However, HOCl is needed to convert it into the more reactive molecule, taurine chloramine, from which sulfate can be derived, with the help of superoxide and perhaps microbial enzymes. Species of Clostridium are able to utilize sulfonate forms of sulfur, such as taurine, as an energy source, and, more generally, it has been confirmed that anaerobic bacteria can convert taurine directly to thiosulfate[80].

Experiments have confirmed that taurine can be broken down to sulfoacetaldehyde by neutrophils, with taurine chloramine as an intermediary, through nonenzymatic hydrolysis catalyzed by hydrogen peroxide[106]. With an adequate source of energy, sulfoacetaldehyde can react with phosphate to produce acetyl phosphate and sulfite. Sulfite can then be oxidized to sulfate via enzymatic action of sulfite oxidase. We propose that this reaction takes place during MI. A China-based study of possible associations between biochemical, diet, and lifestyle factors and cardiovascular disease did not find any relationship with serum cholesterol, but showed a protective effect for molybdenum[107]. This could be explained by the fact that molybdenum is a cofactor for sulfite oxidase.

It is possible that a resonance phenomenon in structured water plays a role. Del Giudice et al.[108] argue that coherent oscillation of almost-free electrons in water molecules within an exclusion zone surrounding a kosmotropic hydrophilic surface can become a source of free electrons for chemical reactions. The water molecules are resonating in tune with an electromagnetic field, and they serve to capture energy within the exclusion zone to excite and mobilize electrons. The Schumann resonance frequency of the earth's geomagnetic field at 7.83 Hz is a possible source. It has been suggested that low frequency (< 10Hz) alpha waves in the brain are influenced by geomagnetic pulsations in the ionosphere ranging from 0.1 to 10 Hz[109]. It has also been argued that encephalopathy is a mechanism to renew sulfate supplies to the brain, by metabolizing taurine to sulfate, using seizures as a source of energy to induce resonance phenomena in the structured water[110]. So, here we are suggesting an analogous mechanism in the heart.

Atrial fibrillation (AFIB) is a frequent occurrence in the context of MI, particularly in the elderly[111]. Frequency analysis of recordings made during AFIB reveal a peak frequency response in the range of 5 to 7 Hz[112,113]. We propose that low frequency energy generated by cardiac arrhythmia, analogous to similar low-frequency stimulation from seizures, may serve as an energy source to create such coherence domain oscillations within the water at the surface of certain cell types within the heart, providing energy needed to produce sulfate from taurine. Clearly, much more research is needed to explore these possibilities.

Cardiovascular Disease Prevention and Treatment

If the ideas proposed here are valid, they suggest some very simple measures that can be taken to decrease the risk of cardiovascular disease. Consuming a strictly organic diet that is rich in sulfur-containing foods and spending significant time outdoors without sunscreen on sunny days are two important lifestyle changes. Many sulfur-containing compounds have been shown to benefit cardiovascular health. Garlic, an excellent source of sulfane sulfur, has been consistently recognized as a healthy supplement[4,114]. α-Lipoic acid is cardioprotective[115], and its benefit may derive from its ability to increase sulfane sulfur levels and rhodanese activity in the heart, liver and kidney[116]. Chondroitin sulfate and glucosamine sulfate reduce the levels of inflammatory markers such as interleukin 1β[117], and this may well be mainly because they are a source of sulfate. The synthetic chemical, AP39, has been shown in rat studies to supply hydrogen sulfide gas to mitochondria and protect them from DNA oxidation damage[5]. It may therefore be a promising future prevention/treatment option for humans. Vanadyl sulfate is cardioprotective[118]. This may be mainly due to its ability to supply sulfate, as its sulfate anion dissociates rapidly in solution. N-acetyl cysteine has shown significant benefit during acute myocardial infarction, through multiple effects including reduction in oxidative stress, more rapid reperfusion, better left ventricular perservation and function, and reduced infarct size[119]. A placebo-controlled experiment on magnesium sulfate supplements during acute myocardial infarction revealed a 24% relative reduction in all-cause mortality and a 25% relative reduction in left ventricular failure in the treatment group[120]. Is it possible that the sulfate rather than the magnesium is the critical beneficial factor? Thus, a broad range of biologically active molecules that have been recognized as being cardioprotective have in common the feature that they supply sulfur to the body.

The Body Electric

While the topic of electricity in the body is beyond the scope of this chapter, I want to leave you with an image of a solar-powered electrical circuit connecting all parts of the body, where the "wires" are the blood vessels. The biosulfates in the glycocalyx play an essential role in maintaining an "exclusion zone" of gelled water lining all the vessel walls, within which electrons are mobilized in the gel and protons at the interface to produce electrical current that powers the muscles and neurons[108,121,122]. Thus, cholesterol sulfate captures sunlight energy in the bound sulfate anion to fuel both mobility and neuronal signaling, just as chlorophyll endows plants with the ability to convert sunlight energy into stored sugars, starches, and fats. Life on the earth's surface has always had access to sunlight as an energy source, and animals and plants have found distinct ways to utilize it.

Sunlight is used by animals to oxidize oxygen to superoxide, and then to oxidize sulfur to sulfate. Cholesterol is the carrier molecule that distributes the sulfate over the vasculature. It too is oxidized by sunlight to form vitamin D, a signaling molecule that communicates to the tissues that all is well. As the negatively charged RBC traverses the capillary, it creates a dynamic electromagnetic signal called the "streaming potential" that oscillates with the rhythm of the heart beat. Endothelial cells respond to this signal by releasing nitric oxide, which relaxes the vessel and promotes flow[123].

Conclusion

In this chapter, I have proposed a hypothesis that explains the complex processes that take place in the atheroma as a mechanism to assure cholesterol sulfate supplies to the heart. Cholesterol sulfate is an important source of sulfate to maintain the RBCs' negative surface charge and to populate the extracellular matrix of the endothelial wall. This results in near frictionless trafficking of RBCs through capillaries. I maintain that the modern lifestyle of sun avoidance and exposure to toxic chemicals through food, sunscreen or other environmental insults results in impaired cholesterol sulfate synthesis in the skin mediated by sunlight. This pathology necessitates a mechanism to store cholesterol in the artery wall to be made readily available for cholesterol sulfate synthesis whenever sulfur sources such as homocysteine or cysteinyl-glycine are available, along with superoxide and ATP as sources of oxygen and energy to fuel the reaction. In an emergency, a myocardial infarction can initiate a programmed response that depletes taurine reserves to restore sulfate supplies. Microbes such as *C. pneumoniae* can assist in replenishing heparan sulfate to the artery wall. I argue that statin therapy interferes with cholesterol sulfate production, leading to increased risk to heart failure, which is now a major contributor to rising health care costs.

If the ideas contained in this chapter are widely embraced, the field of cardiovascular disease treatment will be revolutionized. Patients will be encouraged to spend significant time outdoors on sunny days without sunscreen, and will be encouraged to eat a diet consisting of organic whole foods that are rich in sulfur content. Nutritional supplements that contain sulfur, such as α-lipoic acid, N-acetyl cysteine, garlic extract, chondroitin sulfate, etc., will be prescribed by doctors. Statin drugs will become a thing of the past, because it will be recognized that any benefit they provide in terms of reduced rate of myocardial infarction are completely offset by the serious side effects incurred because of the further depletion of the supply of cholesterol sulfate to the tissues. It will finally be acknowledged that statin therapy is a poor option in heart disease prevention.

Stephanie Seneff, PhD

Senior Research Scientist
Computer Science and Artificial Intelligence Laboratory, MIT
seneff@csail.mit.edu

References

Papers of special note have been highlighted as:

* of interest
** of considerable interest

1. Mann GV. Effects of sulfur compounds on hyper-cholesteremia and growth in cysteine-deficient monkeys. Am J Clin Nutr 1960;8:491-497.

** *This early paper demonstrated a clear protective effect of sulfur-containing metabolites in preventing cardiovascular plaque buildup in monkeys.*

2. Morrison LM, Bajwa GS, Alfin-Slater RB, Ershoff BH. Prevention of vascular lesions by chondroitin sulfate A in the coronary artery and aorta of rats induced by a hypervitaminosis D, cholesterol-containing diet. Atherosclerosis 1972;1(1):105-118.

3. McCully KS. Vascular pathology of homocysteinemia: Implications for the pathogenesis of arteriosclerosis. Am J Pathol 1969;56(1):111-128.

4. Benavides GA, Squadrito GL, Mills RW, Patel HD, Isbell TS, Patel RP, Darley-Usmar VM, Doeller JE, Kraus DW. Hydrogen sulfide mediates the vasoactivity of garlic. PNAS 2007;104(46):17977-17982.

5. Szczesny B, Mo´dis K, Yanagi K, Coletta C, Le Trionnaire S, Perry A, Wood ME, Whiteman M, Szabo C. AP39, a novel mitochondria-targeted hydrogen sulfide donor, stimulates cellular bioenergetics, exerts cytoprotective effects and protects against the loss of mitochondrial DNA integrity in oxidatively stressed endothelial cells in vitro. Nitric Oxide 2014;41:120-30.

6. Grimes DS, Hindle E, Dyer T. Sunlight, cholesterol and coronary heart disease. Q J Med 1996;89:579-589.

** *This paper demonstrates a clear geographical link between sunlight abundance and protection from cardiovascular disease.*

7. MacPherson A, Bacs´o J. Relationship of hair calcium concentration to incidence of coronary heart disease. Science of the Total Environment 2000;255(1-3):11-19.

8. Wang TJ, Pencina MJ, Booth SL, Jacques PF,Ingelsson E, Lanier K, Benjamin EJ, D'Agostino RB, Wolf M, Vasan RS. Vitamin d deficiency and risk of cardiovascular disease. Circulation 2008;117:503-511.

9. Wood AD, Secombes KR, Thies F, Aucott L, Black AJ, Mavroeidi A, Simpson WG, Fraser WD, Reid DM, Macdonald HM. Vitamin D3 supplementation has no effect on conventional cardiovascular risk factors: A parallel-group, double-blind, placebo-controlled RCT. J Clin Endocrinol Metab 2012;97(10):3557-68.

10. Seneff S, Lauritzen A, Davidson R, Lentz-Marino L. Is endothelial nitric oxide synthase a moonlighting protein whose day job is cholesterol sulfate synthesis? Implications for cholesterol transport, diabetes and cardiovascular disease. Entropy 2012;14:2492-2530.

** *This paper explains the theory that sulfate synthesis in the skin by eNOS, catalyzed by sunlight, is critical for the health of the vasculature and the tissues.*

11. Tian Q-Y, Sun D-H, Zhao M-G, Zhang W-H. Inhibition of nitric oxide synthase (NOS) underlies aluminum-induced inhibition of root elongation in Hibiscus moscheutos. New Phytologist 2007;174(2):322-331.

12. Alexidis AN, Rekka EA, Kourounakis PN. Influence of mercury and cadmium intoxication on hepatic microsomal CYP2E and CYP3A subfamilies. Research Communications in Molecular Pathology and Pharmacology 1994;85(1):67-72.

13. Korashy HM, El-Kadi AOS. Modulation of TCDD-mediated induction of cytochrome P450 1A1 by mercury, lead, and copper in human HepG2 cell line. Toxicology in Vitro 2008;22(1):154-158.

14. Anwar-Mohamed A, El-Sherbeni AA, Kim SH, Althurwi HN, Zordoky BN, El-Kadi AO. Acute arsenic toxicity alters cytochrome P450 and soluble epoxide hydrolase and their associated arachidonic acid metabolism in C57Bl/6 mouse heart. Xenobiotica 2012;42(12):1235-47.

15. Samsel A, Seneff S. Glyphosate's suppression of cytochrome P450 enzymes and amino acid biosynthesis by the gut microbiome: Pathways to modern diseases. Entropy 2013;15:1416-1463.

16. Samsel A, Seneff S. Glyphosate, pathways to modern diseases II: Celiac sprue and gluten intolerance. Interdiscip Toxicol 2013;6(4):159-184.

17. Verhaar MC, Westerweel PE, van Zonneveld AJ, Rabelink TJ. Free radical production by dysfunctional eNOS. Heart 2004;90:494-5.

* *This paper demonstrates that eNOS produces superoxide as well as nitric oxide, which is considered to be a dysfunctional response rather than a catalyst for sulfate synthesis in the artery wall.*

18. Kleinbongard P, Schulz R, Rassaf T, Lauer T, Dejam A, Jax T, Kumara I, Gharini P, Kabanova S, O zu¨yaman B, et al. Red blood cells express a functional endothelial nitric oxide synthase. Blood 2006;107:2943-2951.

19. Hietanen E, Linnainmaa K, Vainio H. Effects of phenoxyherbicides and glyphosate on the hepatic and intestinal biotransformation activities in the rat. Acta pharmacol et Toxicol 1983;53:103-112.

This paper demonstrates the disruption of multiple enzymes in rat liver following glyphosate exposure.

20. Lorbek G, Lewinska M, Rozman D. Cytochrome P450s in the synthesis of cholesterol and bile acids – from mouse models to human diseases. FEBS J 2012;279:1516-1533.

21. Erickson SK, Lear SR, Deane S, Dubrac S, Huling SL, Nguyen L, Bollineni JS, Shefer S, Hyogo H, ohen DE, Shneider B, Sehayek E, Ananthanarayanan M, Balasubramaniyan N, Suchy FJ, Batta AK, Salen G. Hypercholesterolemia and changes in lipid and bile acid metabolism in male and female CYP7A1-deficient mice. JLR 2003;44:1001-1009.

This paper shows a direct link between impaired bile acid synthesis in the liver and elevated serum LDL in mice.

22. Samsel A, Seneff S. Glyphosate, pathways to modern diseases IV: cancer and related pathologies. J Biol Phys Chem 2015; 15:121-159.

23. Lim JS, Mietus-Snyder M, Valente A, Schwarz J-M, Lustig RH. The role of fructose in the pathogenesis of NAFLD and the metabolic syndrome. Nature Rev Gastroentero Hepatol 2010;7: 251264.

24. Hassan K, Bhalla V, El Regal ME, A-Kader HH. Nonalcoholic fatty liver disease: A comprehensive review of a growing epidemic. World J Gastroenterol 2014;20(34): 1208212101.

25. Targher, G, Day CP, Bonora E. Risk of cardiovascular disease in patients with nonalcoholic fatty liver disease. N Engl J Med 2010;363:1341-1350.

26. Davidson RM, Seneff S. The initial common pathway of inflammation, disease, and sudden death. Entropy 2012;14:1399-1442.

27. Tumova S, Woods A, Couchman JR. Heparan sulfate proteoglycans on the cell surface: versatile coordinators of cellular functions. The International J Biochem Cell Biol 2000;32(3):269-288.

28. MacArthur JM, Bishop JR, Stanford KI, Wang L, Bensadoun A, Witztum JL, Esko JD. Liver heparan sulfate proteoglycans mediate clearance of triglyceride-rich lipoproteins independently of LDL receptor family members. J Clin Invest 2007;117(1):153-164.

29. Collins KD. Charge density-dependent strength of hydration and biological structure. Biophys J 1997;72:65-76.

30. Grundler W, Weil MH, Rackow EC. Arteriovenous carbon dioxide and pH gradients during cardiac arrest. Circulation 1986;74:1071-1074.

31. Seneff S, Davidson RM, Lauritzen A, Samsel A, Wainwright G A novel hypothesis for atherosclerosis as a cholesterol sulfate deficiency syndrome. Theoretical Biology and Medical Modeling 2015;12:9.

32. Mulivor AW, Lipowsky HH. Inflammation- and ischemia-induced shedding of venular glycocalyx. Am J Physiol Heart Circ Physiol 2004;286:H1672-H1680.

33. Yanai H, Javitt NB, Higashi Y, Fuda H, Strott CA. Expression of cholesterol sulfotransferase (SULT2B1b) in human platelets. Circulation 2004;109(1):92-6.

34. Paka L, Kako Y, Obunike JC, Pillarisetti S. Apolipoprotein E containing high density lipoprotein stimulates endothelial production of heparan sulfate rich in biologically active heparin-like domains: A potential mechanism for the anti-atherogenic actions of vascular apolipoprotein E. J Biol Chem 1999;274:4816-4823.

" This paper links ApoE to both cholesterol and sulfate transport in the atheroma, by explaining how it promotes both cholesterol export from macrophages and sulfate enrichment in the glycocalx.

35. McCully KS. Chemical Pathology of Homocysteine. IV. Excitotoxicity, Oxidative Stress, Endothelial Dysfunction, and Inflammation. Ann Clin Lab Sci 2009;39(3):219-232.

36. Emdin M, Pompella A, Paolicchi A. Gamma-glutamyltransferase, atherosclerosis, and cardiovascular disease: Triggering oxidative stress within the plaque. Circulation 2005;112:2078-2080.

37. Qi X, Xu W, Song H, Xu, M, Ma W, Zhou L. Serum gamma-glutamyl transferase: A novel biomarker for coronary artery disease. Med Sci Monit 2014;20:706-710.

38. Joseph CA, Maroney MJ. Cysteine dioxygenase: Structure and mechanism. Chem Commun 2007;32:3338-3349.

39. Shi Y, Tokunaga O. Chlamydia pneumoniae and multiple infections in the aorta contribute to atherosclerosis. Pathology International 2003;52(12):755-63.

40. Tufano A, Di Capua M, Coppola A, Conca P, Cimino E, Cerbone AM, Di Minno G. The infectious burden in atherothrombosis. Semin Thromb Hemost 2012;38(05):515-523.

41. Neumann F-J. Chlamydia pneumoniae-atherosclerosis link: A sound concept in search for clinical relevance. Circulation 2002;106:2414-2416.

42. Rasmussen-Lathrop SJ, Koshiyama K, Phillips N, Stephens RS. Chlamydia-dependent biosynthesis of a heparan sulphate-like compound in eukaryotic cells. Cellular Microbiology 2000;2(2):137-144.

' This paper explains that C. pneumoniae produce heparan sulfate using a unique set of enzymes not known elsewhere in biological systems.

43. Strott CA, Higashi Y. Cholesterol sulfate in human physiology: what's it all about? J Lipid Res. 2003;44(7):1268-78.

' This is the most comprehensive paper available that describes the various known roles of cholesterol sulfate in human physiology.

44. Seidah NG. Proprotein convertase subtilisin kexin 9 (PCSK9) inhibitors in the treatment of hypercholesterolemia and other pathologies. Curr Pharm Des 2013;19(17):3161-72.

45. Benjannet S, Rhainds D, Hamelin J, Nassoury N, Seidah NG. The proprotein convertase (PC) PCSK9 is inactivated by furin and/or PC56A: functional consequences of natural mutations and post- translational modifications. J Biol Chem 2006;281:30561-30572.

46. Tavori H, Giunzioni I, Linton MF, Fazio S. Loss of plasma proprotein convertase subtilisin/kexin 9 (PCSK9) after lipoprotein apheresis. Circ Res. 2013;113:1290-1295.

47. Mayne J, Dewpura T, Raymond A, Cousins M, Chaplin A, Lahey KA, LaHaye SA, Mbikay M, Ooi TC, Chr'etien M. Plasma PCSK9 levels are significantly modified by statins and fibrates in humans. Lipids in Health and Disease 2008:7:22.

48. Peters-Golden M, Brock TG. 5-Lipoxygenase and FLAP. Prostaglandins Leukotrienes Essent Fatty Acids 2003;69:99-109.

49. Røadmark O. 5-Lipoxygenase-derived leukotrienes: mediators also of atherosclerotic inflammation. Arterioscler Thromb Vasc Biol 2003;23:1140-1142.

50. Hjelte LE, Nilsson A. Arachidonic acid and ischemic heart disease. J Nutr 2005;135(9):2271-2273.

51. Mehrabian M, Allayee H. 5-Lipoxygenase and atherosclerosis. Curr Opin Lipidol 2003;14:447-457.

52. Rouzer CA, Samuelsson B. Reversible, calcium-dependent membrane association of human leukocyte 5-lipoxygenase. Proc Natl Acad Sci USA 1987;84:7393-7397.

53. Aleksandrov DA, Zagryagskaya AN, Pushkareva MA, Bachschmid M, Peters-Golden M, Werz O, Steinhilber D, Sud'ina GF. Cholesterol and its anionic derivatives inhibit 5-lipoxygenase activation in polymorphonuclear leukocytes and MonoMac6 cells. FEBS J 2006;273(3):548-57.

54. Cooper RA. Influence of increased membrane cholesterol on membrane fluidity and cell function in human red blood cells. J Supramol Struct 1978;8(4):413-30.

55. Grunze M, Deuticke B. Changes of membrane permeability due to extensive cholesterol depletion in mammalian erythrocytes. Biochimica et Biophysica Acta (BBA) - Biomembranes 1974;356(1):125-130.

56. Haines TH. Do sterols reduce proton and sodium leaks through lipid bilayers? Progress in Lipid Research 2001;40:299-324.

57. Smolina K, Wright FL, Rayner M, Goldacre MJ. Determinants of the decline in mortality from acute myocardial infarction in England between 2002 and 2010: Linked national database study. BMJ 2012;344:d8059.

58. Allender S, Scarborough P, O'Flaherty M, Capewell S. Patterns of coronary heart disease mortality over the 20th century in England and Wales: Possible plateaus in the rate of decline. BMC Public Health 2008;8:148.

59. Roger VL. The heart failure epidemic. Int J Environ Res Public Health 2010;7:1807-1830.

60. Braunwald, E. Shattuck lecturecardiovascular medicine at the turn of the millennium: triumphs, concerns, and opportunities. N Engl J Med 1997;337:1360-1369.

61. Avila JL, Rojas M, Avila A. Cholesterol sulphate-reactive autoantibodies are specifically increased in chronic chagasic human patients. Clin Exp Immunol 1996;103:40-46.

62. Laranja FS, Dias E, Nobrega G, Miranda A. Chagas' disease: A clinical, epidemiologic, and pathologic study. Circulation 1956;14:1035-1060.

63. Murdoch JC, Rodger JC, Rao SS, Fletcher CD, Dunnigan MG. Down's syndrome: an atheroma-freemodel? Br Med J 1977;2(6081):226-8.

64. Epstein CJ, Avraham KB, Lovett M, Smith S, Elroy-Stein O, Rotman G, Bry C, Groner Y. Transgenic mice with increased Cu/Zn-superoxide dismutase activity: animal model of dosage effects in Down syndrome. Proc Natl Acad Sci U S A 1987;84(22):8044-8.

65. Bittles AH, Bower C, Hussain R, 1,5, Glasson EJ. The four ages of Down syndrome. European Journal of Public Health 2006;17(2):221-225.

66. Lai F, Williams RS. A prospective study of Alzheimer disease in Down syndrome. Arch Neurol. 1989;46(8):849-53.

67. Brooksbank BWL, Balazs R. Superoxide dismutase, glutathione peroxidase and lipoperoxidation in Oown's syndrome fetal brain. Developmental Brain Research 1984;16(1):37-44.

68. Wisniewski KE, Wisniewski HM, Wen GY. Occurrence of neuropathological changes and dementia of Alzheimer's disease in Down's syndrome. Annals of Neurology 1985;17(3);278-282.

69. Han X, M Holtzman D, McKeel DW Jr, Kelley J, Morris JC. Substantial sulfatide deficiency and ceramide elevation in very early Alzheimer's disease: potential role in disease pathogenesis. J Neurochem 2002;82(4):809-18.

70. Davignon J. Beneficial cardiovascular pleiotropic effects of statins. Circulation 2004;109:III-39-III-43.

71. Jasin´ska M, Owczarek J, Orszulak-Michalak D. Statins: a new insight into their mechanisms of action and consequent pleiotropic effects. Pharmacol Rep 2007;59(5):483-99.

72. Weitz-Schmidt G. Statins as anti-inflammatory agents. Trends in Pharmacological Sciences 2002;23(10):482-487.

73. Ridker PM, Lu¨scher TF. Anti-inflammatory therapies for cardiovascular disease. Eur Heart J 2014;35(27):1782-91.

74. Maeda T, Kawane T, Horiuchi N. Statins augment vascular endothelial growth factor expression in osteoblastic cells via inhibition of protein prenylation. Endocrinology 2003;144(2):681-692.

75. Nakazato R, Gransar H, Berman DS, Cheng VY, Lin FY, Achenbach S, Al-Mallah M, Budoff MJ, Cademartiri F, Callister TQ, Chang HJ, Cury RC, Chinnaiyan K, Chow BJ, Delago A, Hadamitzky M, Hausleiter J, Kaufmann P, Maffei E, Raff G, Shaw LJ, Villines TC, Dunning A, Feuchtner G, Kim YJ, Leipsic J, Min JK. Statins use and coronary artery plaque composition: Results from the International Multicenter CONFIRM Registry. Atherosclerosis 2012;225(1):148-153.

76. Horwich TB, Hamilton MA, MacLellan WR, Fonarow GC. Low serum total cholesterol is associated with marked increase in mortality in advanced heart failure. J Card Fail 2002;8:216-24.

77. Rauchhaus M, Clark AL, Doehner W, Davos C, Bolger A, Sharma R, Coats AJ, Anker SD. The relationship between cholesterol and survival in patients with chronic heart failure. J Am Coll Cardiol 2003;42:1933-40.

78. Fonarow GC, Horwich TB. Cholesterol and Mortality in Heart Failure: The Bad Gone Good? J Am Coll Cardiol 2003;42(11):1941-1942.

79. Huxtable RJ. Physiological actions of Taurine. Physiol Rev 1992;72(1):101-63.

80. Denger K, Laue H, Cook AM. Thiosulfate as a metabolic product: the bacterial fermentation of taurine. Arch Microbiol 1997;168(4):297-301.

81. Milei J, Ferreira R, Llesuy S, Forcada P, Covarrubias J, Boveris A. Reduction of reperfusion injury with preoperative rapid intravenous infusion of Taurine during myocardial revascularization. Am Heart J 1992;123(2):339-345.

82. Briet F, Keith M, Leong-Poi H, Kadakia A, Aba-Alkhail K, Giliberto JP, Stewart D, Errett L, David Mazer C: Triple nutrient supplementation improves survival, infarct size and cardiac function following myocardial infarction in rats. Nutr Metab Cardiovasc Dis 2008;18(10):691-9.

83. Crass MF 3rd, Song W, Lombardini JB. Cardiac muscle taurine: effects of acute left ventricular ischemia in the dog and anoxic perfusion of the rat heart. Recent Adv Stud Cardiac Struct Metab 1976;12:259-63.

84. Torres CL, Walker NJ, Rogers QR, Tabliny F. Platelet taurine concentration can be predicted from whole blood taurine concentrations in dogs. J. Nutr 2006;136:2055S-2057S.

85. Hayes KC, Pronczuk A, Addesa AE, Stephan ZF. Taurine modulates platelet aggregation in cats and humans. Am J Clin Nutr 1989;49:12116.

86. Crass MF III, Lombardini JB. Loss of cardiac muscle taurine after acute left ventricular ischemia. Life Sciences 1977;21(7):951-958.

87. Hasegawa T, Malle E, Farhood A, Jaeschke H. Generation of hypochlorite-modified proteins by neutrophils during ischemia-reperfusion injury in rat liver: attenuation by ischemic preconditioning. Am J Physiol Gastrointest Liver Physiol 2005;289:G760-G767.

88. Heslop CL, Frohlich JJ, Hill JS. Myeloperoxidase and C-reactive protein have combined utility for long-term prediction of cardiovascular mortality after coronary angiography. J Am Coll Cardiol 2010;55(11):1102-9.

89. Rosen H, Crowley JR, Heinecke JW. Human neutrophils use the myeloperoxidase-hydrogen peroxide-chloride system to chlorinate but not nitrate bacterial proteins during phagocytosis. J Biol Chem 2002;277:30463-30468.

90. Ravnskov U, McCully KS. Review and Hypothesis: Vulnerable plaque formation from obstruction of vasa vasorum by homocysteinylated and oxidized lipoprotein aggregates complexed with microbial remnants and LDL autoantibodies. Ann Clin Lab Sci 2009;39(1):3-16.

* This paper demonstrates that microbes play a role in cardiovascular disease.

91. McCarty MF. The reported clinical utility of taurine in ischemic disorders may reflect a down-regulation of neutrophil activation and adhesion. Med Hyp 1999;53(4):290-299.

92. Paasonen MK, Penttil a O, Himberg JJ, Solatunturi E. Platelet taurine in patients with arterial hypertension, myocardial failure or infarction. Acta Med Scand Suppl 1980;642:79-84.

93. Vogt W. Complement activation by myeloperoxidase products released from stimulated human polymorphonuclear leukocytes. Immunobiology 1996;195(3):334-346.

94. Sturman JA, Hepner GW, Hofmann AF, Thomas PJ. Metabolism of [35S] taurine in man. J Nutr 1975;105:1206-1214.

95. Schaffer SW, Jong CJ, Ito T, Azuma J. Effect of taurine on ischemia-reperfusion injury. Amino Acids 2014;46:21-30.

96. Yamori Y, Liu L, Ikeda K, Miura A, Mizushima S, Miki T, Nara Y. WHO-Cardiovascular Disease and Alimentary Comprarison (CAR-DIAC) Study Group. Distribution of twenty-four hour urinary taurine excretion and association with ischemic heart disease mortality in 24 populations of 16 countries: Results from the WHO-CARDIAC study. Hypertens Res 2001;24(4):453-7.

97. Chen Q, Moghaddas S, Hoppel CL, Lesnefsky EJ. Ischemic defects in the electron transport chain increase the production of reactive oxygen species from isolated rat heart mitochondria. AJP Cell Physiology 2008;294(2):C460-6.

98. Chen Q, Paillard M, Gomez L, Li H, Hu Y, Lesnefsky EJ. Postconditioning modulates ischemia-damaged mitochondria during reperfusion. J Cardiovasc Pharmacol 2012;59(1):101-8.

99. Stipanuk MH, Ueki I. Dealing with methionine/homocysteine sulfur: cysteine metabolism to taurine and inorganic sulfur. Inherit Metab Dis 2011;34(1):17-32.

100. McCully KS. Chemical pathology of homocysteine. V. Thioretinamide, thioretinaco, and cystathionine synthase function in degenerative diseases. Ann Clin Lab Sci 2011;41(4):300-312.

101. Simon JA. Vitamin C and cardiovascular disease: A review. J Am Coll Nutr 1992;11(2):107-125.

102. Xu Y-J, Arneja AS, Tappia PS, Dhalla NS. The potential health benefits of taurine in cardiovascular disease. Exp Clin Cardiol 2008;13(2):57-65.

103. Liao X-B, Zhou X-M, Li J-M, Yang J-F, Tan Z-P, Hu Z-W, Liu W, Lu Y, Yuan L-Q. Taurine inhibits osteoblastic differentiation of vascular smooth muscle cells via the ERK pathway. Amino Acids 2008;34:525-530.

104. Kramer JH, Chovan JP, Schaffer SW. Effect of taurine on calcium paradox and ischemic heart failure. Am J Physiol 1981;240(2):H238-46.

105. Kingston R, Kelly CJ, Murray P. The therapeutic role of taurine in ischaemia-reperfusion injury. Current Pharmaceutical Design 2004;10(19):2401-2410.

106. Olszowski S, Olszowska E, Kusior D, Szneler E. Sulphoacetaldehyde as a product of taurine chloramine peroxidation at site of inflammation. Amino Acids 2002;22:145153.

107. Guo W, Li JY, King H, Locke FB. Diet and blood nutrient correlations with ischemic heart, hypertensive heart, and stroke mortality in China. Asia Pac J Public Health 1992-1993;6(4):200-9.

108. Del Giudice E, Tedeschi A, Vitiello G, Voeikov V. Coherent structures in liquid water close to hydrophilic surfaces. J Phys: Conf Ser 2013;442:012028.

109. Rusov VD. Can resonant oscillations of the earth ionosphere influence the human brain biorhythm? arXiv:1208.4970 Department of Theoretical and Experimental Nuclear Physics, Odessa National Polytechnic University, Ukraine, 2012.

110. Seneff S, Lauritzen A, Davidson R, Lentz-Marino L. Is encephalopathy a mechanism to renew sulfate in autism? Entropy 2013;15:372-406.

111. Rathore SS, Berger AK, Weinfurt KP, Schulman KA, Oetgen WJ, Gersh BJ, Solomon AJ. Acute myocardial infarction complicated by atrial fibrillation in the elderly prevalence and outcomes. Circulation 2000;101:969-974.

112. Corino VD, Mainardi LT, Stridh M, S ornmo L. Improved time-frequency analysis of atrial fibrillation signals using spectral modeling. IEEE Trans Biomed Eng 2008;55(12):2723-30.

113. Joaqu´ın Rieta J, Alcaraz R. Applications of signal analysis to atrial fibrillation. Chapter 7 in Tong Liu, Ed., Atrial Fibrillation -Mechanisms and Treatment. ISBN 978-953-51-1023-1, February 27, 2013; published under CC BY 3.0 license.

114. Rahman K, Lowe GM Garlic and cardiovascular disease: A critical review. J Nutr 2006;136(3):736S-740S.

115. Wollin SD, Jones PJH. α-Lipoic acid and cardiovascular disease. J Nutr 2003;133(11):3327-3330.

116. Bilska A, Dudek M, Iciek M, Kwiecien´ I, Sokolowska-Jezewicz M, Filipek B, Wlodek L. Biological actions of lipoic acid associated with sulfane sulfur metabolism. Pharmacol Rep 2008;60(2):225-32.

117. Chou MM, Vergnolle N, McDougall JJ, Wallace JL, Marty S, Teskey V, Buret AG. Effects of chondroitin and glucosamine sulfate in a dietary bar formulation on inflammation, interleukin-1β, matrix metalloprotease-9, and cartilage damage in arthritis. Exp Biol Med (Maywood) 2005;230(4):255-262.

118. Bhuiyan MS, Takada Y, Shioda N, Moriguchi S, Kasahara J, Fukunaga K. Cardioprotective effect of vanadyl sulfate on ischemia/reperfusion-induced injury in rat heart in vivo is mediated by activation of protein kinase B and induction of FLICE-inhibitory protein. Cardiovasc Ther 2008;26(1):10-23.

119. Sochman J. N-acetylcysteine in acute cardiology: 10 years later. what do we know and what would we like to know? J Am Coll Cardiol 2002;39(9):1422-1428.

120. Woods KL, Fletcherk S, Roffe C, Haider Y. Intravenous magnesium sulphate in suspected acute myocardial infarction: results of the second Leicester Intravenous Magnesium Intervention Trial (LIMIT-2) The Lancet 1992;339(8809):1553-1558.

121. Pollack, G. Cells, gels and the engines of life: A new, unifying approach to cell function. Ebner and Sons: Seattle WA, USA, 2001.

122. Pollack G. The fourth phase of water: Beyond solid, liquid, ande Vapor. Ebner and Sons: Seattle WA, USA, 2013.

123. Trivedi DP, Hallock KJ, Bergethon PR. Electric fields caused by blood flow modulate vascular endothelial electrophysiology and nitric oxide production. Bioelectromagnetics 2013;34(1):22-30.

** This paper explains how elevated blood pressure and elevated heart rate increase the strength of the streaming potential, produced by the RBCs acting as moving charged particles, promoting blood flow.

Chapter Ten

Stress as Cause of Atherosclerosis:
The Acidity Theory

Carlos E. T. B Monteiro

Abstract

The link between stress and atherosclerosis is well-known with many studies and postulations in this regard. However, there is a general unawareness that stress can induce hyperlactatemia and lactic acidosis, because this relationship has been little discussed in medical science. The influence of adrenaline on lactic acid production was first noticed by Carl Ferdinand Cory in 1925. The heart is an organ of high metabolic activity – that cannot rest as other body muscles, being susceptible to drops in pH during ischemia and hypoxia. The chronic elevated catecholamine release, triggered by sympathetic dominance, may accelerate the myocardial glycolysis leading to significant increase in lactate production. Risk factors for atherosclerosis like hypertension, diabetes, cigarette smoking, stress conditions and high carbohydrate diets are linked to autonomic dysfunction. These risk factors present as well an increased concentration of lactate in plasma. Blood lactate is also associated with carotid atherosclerosis. Plasma lipid abnormalities and myocardial lactate production were significantly associated with subsequent arteriographic progression. The amount of lactate released by the myocardium has been shown to be related to the severity of coronary artery disease. Reduced pH increases the oxidation of low-density lipoprotein that is considered to have a significant role in atherogenesis. According to the acidity theory of atherosclerosis the acidosis evoked by sympathetic dominance or continuous stress leads to changes in shear stress, the final stage in the development of atherosclerotic lesions. The importance of mechanical forces such as those derived from changes in hemodynamic shear stress, as a decisive factor for atherosclerosis, was advocated by Meyer Texon since 1957.

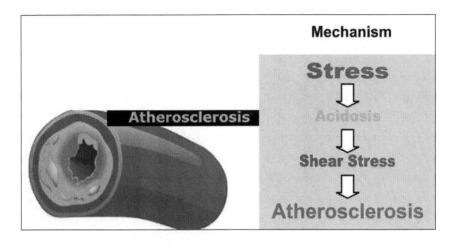

Introduction

In a recent article we presented the history about the acidity theory of atherosclerosis, developed in 2006, addressing its pathophysiology, therapeutics, risk factors and external markers. There I also have wrote about individuals with lower degree or absence of atherosclerosis, and on the reversion or lower progression of atherosclerosis through the use of sympatolytic drugs and by stress reduction approaches[1]. In the current article I extend the discussion about the etiology of the Acidity Theory of Atherosclerosis, aside to present new risk factors and other diseases associated to atherosclerosis, under its point of view. Also, I bring up for discussion the inverse association between cancer and atherosclerosis, confirmed by recent studies.

Our hypothesis

The myogenic theory[2], developed by Dr. Quintiliano H. de Mesquita, from Brazil, became the template for the acidity theory of atherosclerosis. In his point of view the heart disease process involves two distinct pathologies, one for coronary artery disease/atherosclerosis and other for the myocardial disease, what led to his adoption of the terms "coronary-cardiomyopathy" or "coronary-myocardial disease", instead "coronary heart disease" and the term "acute myocardial syndromes" instead "acute coronary syndromes". His reasoning was contrary to the currently accepted thinking which has its cause and effect relationship based in the thrombocentric coronary heart disease model.

Noteworthy is the citation from Dr. George E Burch, a shaper of modern cardiology, which goes strikingly to the point:

"The coronary patient does not die from coronary disease, he dies from myocardial disease." (1972)[3]

Our acidity theory of atherosclerosis fits perfectly well with the myogenic theory of myocardial infarction. The myogenic theory accepts that physical and emotional stresses affect the cardiac muscle dependent on the diseased coronary artery, compromising the myocardial structure. In his book about the myogenic theory from 1979, Dr. Mesquita says: "Thus, the coronary disease contributes to the deterioration of the ventricular segment, constituting areas of myocardial sclerosis or segmental myocardial disease, the possible future site of the myocardial infarction".[4]

Acidity Theory of Atherosclerosis Mechanism

I. Sympathetic dominance by continuous stress plus

II. Deficiency in production of endogenous digitalis-like compounds with alterations of $Na(+)$, $K(+)$-ATPase activity results in:

III. Lowered pH (acidosis) that increases perfusion pressure and provokes effects on contractility of coronary arteries leading to changes in hemodynamic shear stress and atherosclerosis as consequence.

The sequence of events to explain atherogenesis, in the acidity theory concept

Fundamentals

Stress and Acidosis

The heart is an organ of high metabolic activity – that cannot rest as other body muscles, being susceptible to drops in pH during ischemia and hypoxia. The chronic elevated catecholamine release, triggered by sympathetic dominance, may accelerate the myocardial glycolysis leading to significant increase in lactate production. According to a study from 1982 the support for a direct participation of catecholamines in the development and/or maintenance of lactic acidosis includes: 1) the common association of stress and lactic acidosis; 2) the rise in plasma lactate concentration during adrenaline infusion; 3) the precipitation of lactic acidosis by adrenaline intoxication and phaeochromocytoma; and 4) the vasoconstrictor effects of catecholamines leading to tissue anoxia and lactic acid production[5]

The influence of adrenaline on lactic acid production was first noticed by Carl Ferdinand Cory in 1925[6]. Together with his wife Gerty Cory, received a Nobel Prize in 1947 for their discovery of how glycogen– a derivative of glucose – is broken down and resynthesized in the body. John R. Williamson confirmed in 1964 the effects of adrenaline infusion on the increased production of lactate in isolated heart tissue, up to five times the normal production[7].(Note: Lactic acidosis results from increased production of lactate, the final product in the pathway of glucose metabolism. Lactate and lactic acid are not synonymous. Lactic acid is a strong acid which, at physiological pH, is almost completely ionized to lactate)

Hyperlactataemia is common during physiological (exercise) and pathophysiological stress[8*]

Risk factors for atherosclerosis like hypertension[9,10], diabetes[11,12], cigarette smoking[13], stress conditions[14,15] and high carbohydrate diets[16,17] have shown an increased concentration of blood lactic acid or lactate.

---

* Hyperlactatemia is defined as a mild to moderate persistent increase in blood lactate concentration (2-4 mmol/L) without metabolic acidosis, whereas lactic acidosis is characterized by persistently increased blood lactate levels (usually >4-5 mmol/L) in association with metabolic acidosis.

Blood lactate is also associated with carotid atherosclerosis[18].

Lowered pH increases perfusion pressure[19,20,21]. Also, pH changes have profound effects on contractility of coronary arteries[21,22], that may happen through the sodium/potassium pump and K induced relaxation channels[23].

The association of increased lipid levels with abnormal lactate metabolism may provide a useful screening test for the detection of coronary artery disease. It was found that plasma lipid abnormalities and myocardial lactate production were significantly associated with subsequent arteriographic progression. The amount of lactate released by the myocardium has been shown to be related to the severity of coronary artery disease.[24-26]

Additional findings linking lactate/lactic acid and atherosclerosis

1. In advanced plaques the existence of hypoxic areas in the arterial wall – with accumulation of lactic acid in atherosclerotic lesions – seems to be related to a decreased oxygen diffusion capacity and increased oxygen consumption by the foam cells[27]

2. A pathological study has demonstrated that approximately two-thirds of the atherosclerotic plaques show lactate dehydrogenase isoenzyme shifts significantly above the media and intima[28].

3. Macrophages and lymphocytes convert most of their glucose into lactate rather than oxidizing it completely to CO2, and macrophages possess a selective transporter in their plasma membranes for lactic acid. This lactic acid may make the extracelullar space surrounding macrophages acidic in atherosclerotic lesions[29]

4. Lowering pH augments the oxidation of low-density lipoprotein (LDL) by releasing Fe and Cu radicals and decreasing anti-oxidant defense capacity[29,30,31]

5. LDL oxidation occurs not within the interstitial fluid of atherosclerotic lesions but within lysosomes in macrophages in

atherosclerotic lesions. The study also found that this oxidative modification was inhibited by the drug chloroquine, which increases the pH of lysosomes, as oxidation can be promoted by acidic pH[32]

6. In-vitro findings suggest that in areas of atherosclerotic arterial intima, where the extracellular pH is decreased, binding of apolipoprotein B100 containing lipoproteins to proteoglycans and modification of the lipoproteins by acidic enzymes are enhanced. The pH induced amplification of these processes would lead to enhanced extracellular accumulation of lipoproteins and accelerated progression of the disease[33,34]

7. The acidic environment also represents a novel endogenous danger signal alerting the innate immunity. Low pH may thus contribute to inflammation in acidosis-associated pathologies such as atherosclerosis.[35]

Endogenous digitalis like compounds, the sodium potassium pump and cardiac glycosides

There is a postulation that epinephrine (adrenaline) increases lactate formation by a raise in the Na+K+ ATPase activity. This can be inhibited through digitalis or strophanthin/ouabain which are sodium pump inhibitors.[36] The link between adrenaline and increased NA+K+ – ATPase activity is well established.

Endogenous digitalis-like compounds of the cardenolide (digoxin and ouabain / strophanthin) and bufadienolide (Proscillaridin-A and Marinobufagenin) types, isolated from human tissues and body fluids, have similar molecular structure of cardiac glycosides extracted from plants and toad venom[38,39]. Endogenous DLCs are steroidal hormones that are synthesized in, and released from the adrenal gland, whose regulation may be directed by the hypothalamic-pituitary-adrenal (HPA) axis.[40,41]

Endogenous DLCs may serve as effectors of ion-transport activity mediated by their interaction with Na,K-ATPase and thus play a role as a new hormonal axis[37]

Many hormones, including aldosterone, insulin, thyroid hormone and catecholamines regulate not only the expression but also the insertion of Na+, K+-ATPase into the plasma membrane, according to specific physiological needs. The Na+, K+-ATPase which was considered to be the ion transporting pump now appears to have many other unrelated functions, some of which may be regulated by DLCs. In fact DLCs have already been implicated in the regulation of several major physiological parameters including water and salt homeostasis[39]

Perturbation of the endogenous digitalis-like compounds system has been implied in many pathological conditions including cardiac arrhythmias, hypertension, heart failure, cancer and depressive disorders.[39,42] Stress situations may affect the release of endogenous DLCs by the adrenal gland.[41] Also, the extracellular acidification may affect the signaling and transport of endogenous DLCs.[43,44] This raises the possibility that an insufficient production of endogenous DLCs to attend the demand in some medical conditions, like in coronary-myocardial disease, hypothetically can be resolved through the use of cardiac glycosides at low concentration. This is confirmed by clinical studies using digitalis and strophanthin/ouabain drugs with largely positive effects in prevention of acute myocardial syndromes and mortality.[2,45] Low therapeutic doses of digitalis and strophanthin/ouabain drugs have specific sympathoinhibitory response by blocking the overproduction of catecholamine[46,47] that may induce a potent inhibition of glycolysis.[48] We hypothesize that endogenous digitalis-like compounds may have similar action on neurohormonal levels.

Sympatholytic properties from cardiac glycosides (digoxin, digitoxin, ouabain, etc) show positive effects for atherosclerosis including the reduction in plasma levels of total cholesterol, LDL cholesterol and triglycerides. It should take in consideration the fact that stress and other risk factors for atherosclerosis causes the elevation of these elements in blood. Benefic effects of cardiac glycosides are also seen through anti-inflammatory pathways.[49,50,51,52,53,76,95,96,97].

However, inflammation is a result of an injury, not its cause. Incidentally, there are demonstrations about a pivotal role for the sympathetic nervous system and its neurotransmitters in regulating inflammation.[99]

IMPORTANT POINTS:

1. Despite the ongoing advances and recent controversies related to some details[54] of endogenous digitalis-like compounds, our basic reasoning expressed since 2006 about its importance in the acidity theory of atherosclerosis, remains unaffected.[55]

2. Cholesterol is vital for the human body with use in cell membranes, hormones, neurotransmitters, overall nerve function and, among other properties, as a healing agent to repair tissue injuries what occur in atherosclerosis according our concept.[56,57,58] Cholesterol is the major precursor of endogenous digitalis-like compounds.[37] Therefore, the cholesterol lowering by drugs may affect many functions of the body. Incidentally, a study in humans found that statin therapy can be associated with high blood lactate/ pyruvate ratio suggestive of mitochondrial dysfunction.[59] Statins, besides presenting trivial beneficial results in preventing mortality, have many adverse effects, including the promotion of coronary calcification during atheroma[60,61]

Hemodynamic shear stress and atherosclerosis

As the final step in this process the changes in pH may lead to mechanical forces over the coronary blood flow intensifying the damaging action in the development of atherosclerotic lesions.

Atherosclerosis preferentially affects the outer edges of vessel bifurcations. In these predisposed areas, hemodynamic shear stress, the frictional force acting on the endothelial cell surface as a result of blood flow is weaker than in protected regions. Studies have identified hemodynamic shear stress as an important determinant of endothelial function and phenotype[62].

The pulsatile nature of blood pressure and flow creates hemodynamic stimuli in the forms of cyclic stretch and shear stress. The changes in flow patterns can produce potentially deleterious effects on vascular biology. Lowered shear stress and oscillatory shear stress are essential conditions in atherosclerotic lesion size and vulnerability[63,64].

The sympathetic activation with elevation of circulating catecholamine causes coronary vasoconstriction and consequent reduction in blood flow. On the other hand the increased lactate (or decreased blood pH) may evoke vascular smooth muscle relaxation and increase of blood flow. These opposite forces working in sequence - with the sympathetic overdrive leading to metabolic acidosis, in our view, may be reconciled to represent a strong explanation for the occurrence of the resulting abnormal stretching/relaxing of coronary arteries, in different directions, simultaneously, on every heart beat, producing changes in hemodynamic shear stress[65,66,67], leading to atherosclerotic disease.

The most important scientific advances by researchers that paved the way for our acidity theory of atherosclerosis:

1. Walter Holbrook Gaskell demonstrated in 1880 that acid solutions have effects on the contractility of heart tissues and vascular smooth muscle, representing an important mechanism for the local regulation of blood flow during increased metabolic activity.[69]

2. Rudolph Virchow in 1856 described atherosclerosis as "endarteritis deformans" meaning that the atheroma was a product of vascular injury inducing inflammation within the intima of the artery wall, with cholesterol deposit occurring thereafter[70]

3. Carl F Cory in 1925 was the first to observe the influence of adrenaline/epinephrine on lactic acid production.[6]

4. Meyer Texon in 1957 postulated that mechanical forces such as those derived from changes in hemodynamic shear stress could cause atherosclerosis.[71]

[**] The importance in the degree of stretching of an artery, as a mechanical factor for atherosclerosis, is known since the early fifties.[68]

5. Thomas Zsotér et al have demonstrated in 1961 that reduction of blood pH increases blood flow.[18]

6. James P. Henry and Patricia M. Stephens, in 1977, postulated that chronic stress or the constantly heightened sympathetic-adrenomedullary activity might lead to atherosclerosis and cardiovascular disease*.[72]

7. Redford B. Williams, in 1978, postulated that recurrent physiologic actions involving exaggerated heart rate and pressor responses to behavioral stimuli might promote arterial injury via hemodynamic forces such as turbulence and shear stress.[73]

Risk factors for atherosclerosis/coronary artery disease

In a recent article (1) I have presented 24 risk factors for atherosclerosis where the common denominator is the dysregulation of the autonomic nervous system, related to sympathetic dominance, through sympathetic over-activity or withdrawal of the parasympathetic system, with elevation of catecholamine levels. I take this opportunity to add two risk factor linked to autonomic dysfunction, not previously mentioned.

25. **Trans fatty acids:** Trans fatty acids (TFA) consumption are associated with risk of cardiovascular disease. TFA consumption was also linked with abnormal heart rate variability that reflects autonomic dysfunction.[74]

26. **Cold exposure:** In most healthy human subjects, cutaneous application of ice water, the cold pressor test (CPT), increases arterial pressure, heart rate, and vascular resistance. For many years, CPT has been used to evaluate sympathetic neural control of the peripheral and coronary circulations in humans. A recent study has linked sympathetic activation-UCP1 axis and cold-associated hyperlipidemia that contributes to cold-induced accelerated development of atherosclerotic plaques in mice. In order to verify the clinical relevance, the authors conducted a pilot experiment

by recruiting human subjects to their studies. According them this pilot human study further validates the clinical relevance of their mouse studies with the admission of the fact that only a small number of human subjects were recruited at the time, what might lack a sufficient statistical power to justify a definite conclusion[75]

Other diseases associated to atherosclerosis

1. **Osteoporosis:** Studies show a link between osteoporosis and atherosclerosis. One of these reported that hip fracture is two till five times more common in people with cardiovascular disease than in those with no history of this condition. Interesting is that drugs that reduce the elevated production of lactic acid/lactate in the human body like bisphosphonates and beta blockers not only reduced fracture risk in both men and women but also prevented the development of atherosclerosis. It is worth to mention a postulation from 1978, endorsed by other authors, that the body drawn minerals from the bones to neutralize acid and alkaline challenges.[76-78]

2. **Vitamin C deficiency:** Studies using guinea pigs demonstrated that ascorbic acid deficiency produces atherosclerosis. To our knowledge there are no studies directly indicating autonomic dysfunction in this condition. However, it is interesting to note that Vitamin C improves baroreflex sensitivity leading to an inhibition of the sympathetic nervous system. A recent study has demonstrated that intravenous administration of vitamin C reduced cardiovascular adrenergic drive in hypertensive patients. There are also studies showing that intra-periotoneal ascorbic acid greatly inhibits atherosclerosis in guinea pigs. High plasma vitamin C concentrations have been associated with low risk of ischemic heart disease.[68,76,79,80]

3. **Alzheimer's disease:** Pathological, clinical and epidemiological studies indicate that there is an association between Alzheimer's disease (AD) and atherosclerotic disease, through a chronically lowering brain hypoperfusion. Also, current evidence shows that

autonomic dysfunction may be associated with AD. Interesting to note is that the use of sympatholytics (beta-blockers), for the treatment of hypertension resulted in fewer Alzheimer's type brain lesions on autopsy than the use of other hypertensive medications. A recent study confirmed that low cardiac index has been associated with the development of incident dementia and Alzheimer's disease.[81-85]

Inverse association between cancer and atherosclerosis

Recent findings confirm that atherosclerotic lesions are less pronounced in patients suffering from carcinoma than among non-cancerous persons. Interesting to mention is that cancer and atherosclerosis share some risk factors and molecular pathways – acceleration of glycolysis metabolism, therefore increasing lactic acid/lactate concentration in blood and tissues, worsening cancer and atherosclerostic disease. Like in atherosclerosis there are studies indicating that the autonomic dysfunction is the primary cause of cancer[86] On the other hand, some anticancer therapies like chemotherapy, which a recent study found it is related to parasympathetic dysfunction, in addition to promote atherosclerosis show a high risk of cardiovascular morbidity and mortality[87,88,89,90,91]

Also, there are studies investigating the potential impact of cancer and its therapies on coronary artery calcification. A recent paper by the Multi-Ethnic Study of Atherosclerosis trial has demonstrated an increase in the incidence of coronary artery calcification over time in individuals with cancer compared with non-cancer controls.[92]

Some epidemiologic studies suggest a positive association between elevated serum cholesterol level and risk for certain cancer types.[98] As said before I see cholesterol serum elevation as a healing agent to repair tissue injuries, including for cancer

Resting heart rate and all-cause and cardiovascular mortality

Last but not least a recent meta-analysis involving a total of 46 studies with more than a million patients confirms that high resting heart rate is independently associated with increased risk of all-cause and cardiovascular mortality in the general population. Its results suggest the risk is increased by 9% and 8% for every 10 beats/min increment of resting heart rate. According to the authors Higher resting heart rate is a marker of an imbalance between the vagal and the sympathetic tone, and dysfunctional autonomic nervous system, playing a central role in the pathogenesis of numerous adverse health conditions. Also, that a relatively high heart rate has direct detrimental effects on progression of coronary atherosclerosis, on occurrence of myocardial ischemia and ventricular arrhythmias, and on left ventricular function.[93,94]

Notes

A. Our article published at Positive Health Online (1), November 2015, comprises the following matters:

1. The history of the acidity theory of atherosclerosis

2. 24 risk factors where the common denominator is autonomic dysfunction

3. Individuals with lower degree or absence of atherosclerosis

4. Reversion or lower progression of atherosclerosis by sympatholytic drugs and stress reduction strategies

5. External risk markers for atherosclerosis and their relationship with lactic acid or lactate concentration

B. There is additional information on the acidity theory of atherosclerosis that you may find useful in our short (100 pages) and low cost book from 2012[76], which includes our manuscript from 2008[55] Some articles contained in this book: "What causes the elevation of cholesterol levels in blood?", "Hemodynamic shear stress, calcification and atherosclerosis", "The positive impact of humor and negative of stress over the vascular function", etc...

Carlos E. T. B Monteiro

Independent researcher
President at Infarct Combat Project (http://www.infarctcombat.org)
Non-official member of "The International Network of Cholesterol
Skeptics (THINCS – www.thincs.org)
Fellow of the American Institute of Stress (www.stress.org)
Member of the honorary board of Weston A Price Foundation
(www.westonaprice.org/)
secretary@infarctcombat.org

References:

1. Carlos Monteiro, Acidity Theory of Atherosclerosis -- History, Pathophysiology, Therapeutics and Risk Factors – A Mini Review. Positive Health Online, Edition 226, November 2015. Free access at http://goo.gl/AejGAV

2. Carlos Monteiro. **Stress as Cause of Heart Attacks – The Myogenic Theory, Wise Traditions Journal** (Fall edition, 2014) from Weston A. Price Foundation. at http://www.westonaprice.org/modern-diseases/cardiovascular-disease/stress-as-cause-of-heart-attacks/

3. Burch GE and col. Ischemic cardiomyopathy, Am Heart J. 1972 March, 83(3): 340-50

4. Quintiliano H. de Mesquita. Book "Myogenic Theory of Myocardial Infarction", 1979. Summary in English at http://www.infarctcombat.org/LivroTM/parte8.htm

5. Schade DS.1982. The role of catecholamines in metabolic acidosis. Ciba Found Symp;87:235-53

6. Cory CF and Cory GT. The mechanism of epinephrine action IV: The influence of epinephrine on lactic acid production and blood sugar utilization. J Biol Chem 1929, 84: 683 – 698. Full text at http://www.jbc.org/content/84/2/683.full.pdf+html

7. Williamson JR. Metabolic effects of epinephrine in the isolated, perfused rat heart. J Biol Chem 1964, 239: 2721 – 2729 Full text at http://www.jbc.org/content/239/9/2721.full.pdf

8. Mercedes Garcia Alvarez, Paul Marik, Rinaldo Bellomo. Stress hyperlactataemia: present understanding and controversy. The Lancet Diabetes & Endocrinology, November 29, 2013 http:// dx.doi.org/10.1016/S2213- 8587(13)70154-2

9. F. E. Demartini, P. J. Cannon, W. B. Stason, and J. H. Laragh. Lactic Acid Metabolism in Hypertensive Patients. Science 11 June 1965, Vol. 148. no. 3676

10. Juraschek SP, Bower JK, Selvin E, Subash Shantha GP, Hoogeveen RC, Ballantyne

CM, Young JH. Plasma lactate and incident hypertension in the atherosclerosis risk in communities study. Am J Hypertens. 2015 Feb;28(2):216-24.

11. Crawford SO et al, Association of blood lactate with type 2 diabetes: the Atherosclerosis Risk in Communities Carotid MRI Study. International Journal of Epidemiology 2010;1–9

12. Juraschek SP et al. Lactate and Risk of Incident Diabetes in a Case-Cohort of the Atherosclerosis Risk in Communities (ARIC) Study. PLoS ONE 2013, 8(1): e55113. doi:10.1371/journal.pone.0055113

13. Yarlioglues M. Kaya MG et al. Dose-dependent acute effects of passive smoking on left ventricular cardiac function in health volunteers. J Investig Med 2012, Feb; 60 (2): 517-22

14. Sharda S, Gupta SN and Khuteta KP. 1975. Effect on mental stress on inter-mediate carbohydrate-and lipid-metabolism. Indian J Physiol Pharmacol. Apr-Jun;19(2):86-9.

15. Hall JB, Brown DA. 1979. Plasma glucose and lactic acid alterations in response to a stressful exam. Biol Psychol. May;8(3):179-88.

16. Harold T. Edwards, Edward H. Bensley, David B. Dill and Thorne M. Carpenter. 1944. Human Respiratory Quotients in Relation to Alveolar Carbon Diox-ide and Blood Lactic Acid After Ingestion of Glucose, Fructose, or Galactose. Journal of Nutrition Vol. 27 No. 3 March, pp. 241-251. Full free paper at http://jn.nutrition.org/cgi/reprint/27/3/241

17. Hallfrisch J. 1990. Metabolic effects of dietary fructose. FASEB J, Vol 4; Jun: 2652-2660. Full free paper at http://www.fasebj.org/cgi/reprint/4/9/2652.pdf

18. Palamaner G et al. Association of blood lactate with carotid atherosclerosis: The Atherosclerosis Risk in Communities (ARIC) Carotid MRI Study. Atherosclerosis 228 (2013) 249e255.

19. Zsotér T, Bandeman L, Chappel CL. The effect of local pH changes on blood flow in the dog. Am Heart J. 1961;61: 777-782

20. von Ardenne M, Reitnauer PG. 1989. Increase of perfusion pressure at constant perfusion rate caused by low pH values, Biomed Biochim Acta, 48(4):317-23

21. Yasushi Horai et al. 2005. Changes in pH increase perfusion pressure of coronary arteries in the rat. J Pharmacol Sci 97; 400: 407

22. Austin C, Wray S. 2000. Interactions Between Ca2+ and H+ and Functional Consequences in Vascular Smooth Muscle, Mini Review, Circulation Research 86:355.

23. Kim YM et al. 2005. Contribution of Na_-K_ pump and KIR currents to extracellular pH-dependent changes of contractility in rat superior mesenteric artery, Am J Physiol Heart Circ Physiol 289:792-800 Full free paper at http://ajpheart.physiology.org/cgi/reprint/289/2/H792

24. G. Jackson, Lynne Atkinson, M. Clark, B. Crook, P. Armstrong, and S. Oram, Diagnosis of coronary artery disease by estimation of coronary sinus lactate. British Heart Journal, 1978, 40, 979-983 Full free text at http://www.ncbi.nlm.nih.gov/pmc/articles/PMC483520/

25. Bemis CE, Gorlin R, et al. Progression of coronary artery disease: A clinical arteriographic study. Circulation, Vol XLVII, March 1973. Full free text at http://circ.ahajournals.org/content/47/3/455.full.pdf

26. Gertz EW, Wisneski JA, Neese R, Bristow JD, Searle GL, Hanlon JT: Myocardial lactate metabolism: evidence of lactate release during net chemical extraction in man. Circulation 1981, 63: 1273-1279. Full free text at http://circ.ahajournals.org/cgi/reprint/63/6/1273

27. T Bjornheden, M Levin, M Evaldsson, O Wiklund. 1999. Evidence of hypoxic areas within the arterial wall in vivo, Arteriosclerosis, Thrombosis and Vascular Biology; 19:870-876

28. Gown MA, Benditt PE. 1982. Lactate dehydrogenase (LDH) isozymes of human atherosclerotic plaques. Am J Pathol 1982, 107:316-321

29. Leake DS. 1997. Does an acidic pH explain why low density lipoprotein is oxidized in atherosclerotic lesions? Atherosclerosis. Mar 21;129(2):149- 57

30. Morgan J, Leake DS. 1995. Oxidation of low density lipoprotein by iron or copper at acidic pH. J Lipid Res. Dec;36(12):2504- 12. Full free paper at http://www.jlr.org/cgi/reprint/36/12/2504

31. Patterson RA, Leake DS. 1998. Human serum, cysteine and histidine inhibit the oxidation of low density lipoprotein less at acidic pH. FEBS Lett. Sep 4;434(3):317- 21.

32. Wen Y, Leake DS. 2007. Low density Lipoprotein oxidation undergoes within lysosome in cells. Circ .Res. 100;1337-1343. Full free paper at http://circres.ahajournals.org/cgi/content/full/100/9/1337

33. Sneck M, Kovanen PT, Oorni K. 2005. Decrease in pH strongly enhances binding of native, proteolysed, lipolysed, and oxidized low density lipoprotein particles to human aortic proteoglycans, Journal of Biological Chemistry, 280;45: Nov. Full free paper at http://www.jbc.org/cgi/reprint/280/45/37449

34. Oorni K and Kovanen PT. 2006. Enhanced extracellular lipid accumulation in acidic environments. Curr Opin Lipidol 17(5);534-40: Oct

35. Rajamäki K et al. Extracellular acidosis is a novel danger signal alerting innate immunity via the NLRP3 inflammasone. The Journal of Biological Chemistry , 2013; V288: N19:

36. Levy B, Gibot S, Franck P, Cravoisy A, Bollaert PE. Relation between muscle Na+K+ ATPase activity and raised lactate concentrations in septic shock: a prospective study. Lancet 365: 871–75. 2005

37. Hassan M. AM Qazzaz et al. 2004. De Novo Biosynthesis and Radiolabeling of Mammalian Digitalis-Like Factors. Clin Chem. Mar;50(3):612-20. Full free paper at http://www.clinchem.org/cgi/content/full/50/3/612

38. Schoner W. 2002. Endogenous cardiac glycosides, a new class of steroid hormones. Eur J Biochem. 268, 2440-2448, Full free paper at http://www.ejbiochem.org/cgi/content/full/269/10/2440

39. Nesher M, Shpolansky U, Rosen H, Lichtstein D. 2007.The digitalis-like steroid hormones: New mechanisms of action and biological significance. Life Sci. May 15;80(23):2093-107

40. Sophocleus A et al. 2003. Circulating endogenous digitalis-like factors (EDLF) in man is derived from the adrenals and its secretion is ACTH-dependent. J Endocrinol Invest Jul;26(7):668-74

41. Weidemann H et al. 2004. Diverse effects of stress and additional adrenocorticotropic hormone on digitalis-like compounds in normal and nude mice, Journal of Neuroendocrinology, Vol 16, 458-463.

42. Rose AM, Valdes RJ. 1994. Understanding the sodium potassium pump and its relevance to disease, Clin. Chem. 40/9: 1674-1685. Full free paper at http://www.clinchem.org/cgi/reprint/40/9/1674

43. Vasilyev A, Khater K, and Rakowski RF. 2004. Effect of Extracellular pH on Presteady-State and Steady- State Current Mediated by the Na+/K+ Pump,. J Membr Biol. March 15; 198(2):65–76. Full free paper at http://www.pubmedcentral.nih.gov/articlerender.fcgi?artid=1357233

44. Li C, Geering K, Horisberger JD. 2006. The Third Sodium Binding Site of Na,K-ATPase Is Functionally Linked to Acidic pH-Activated Inward Current. Membr Biol. 213(1):1-9

45. Kern B. 1970. Der Myokard-Infarkt. Haug-Verlag, Heidelberg.

46. Gheorghiade M, Adams KF, Colucci WS. Digoxin in the Management of Cardiovascular Disorders. Circulation 2004; 109: 2959-2964

47. Gutman Y, Boonyaviroj P. Naunyn Schmiedebergs. 1977. Mechanism of inhibition of catecholamine release from adrenal medulla by diphenylhydantoin and by low concentration of ouabain (10 (-10) M). Arch Pharmacol Feb;296(3):293-6.

48. Calderón-Montaño J, Burgos-Morón E, Lopez-Lazaro M. The Cardiac Glycosides Digitoxin, Digoxin and Ouabain Induce a Potent Inhibition of Glycolysis in Lung Cancer Cells. WebmedCentral CANCER 2013;4(7):WMC004323

49. Jagielska J. et al. Digitoxin elicits anti-inflammatory and vasoprotective properties in endothelial cells: Therapeutic implications for the treatment of atherosclerosis?, Atherosclerosis 2009 Oct;206(2):390-6

50. Kolkhof P et al. Cardiac glycosides potently inhibits C-reactive protein synthesis in human hepatocytes. Biochem Biophys Res Commun. 2010 Mar 26;394(1): 233-9

51. Ihenetu K et al. Digoxin and digoxin-like immunoreactive factors (DLIF) modulate the release of pro-inflammatory cytokines. Inflamm Res. 2008 Nov. 57(11); 519-23

52. Shah VO, Ferguson J, Hunsaker LA, Deck LM, Vander Jagt DL. Cardiac Glycosides Inhibit LPS-induced Activation of Pro-inflammatory Cytokines in Whole Blood through an NF-κB-dependent Mechanism. International Journal of Applied Research in Natural Products Vol. 4 (1), pp. 11-19, Mar-April 2011

53. Yang Q, Huang W, Jozwik C, Lin Y, Glasman M et al. 2005. Cardiac glycosides inhibit TNF-alpha/NF-kappaB signaling by blocking recruitment of TNF receptor-associated death domain to the TNF receptor. Proc Natl Acad Sci USA Jul 5;102(27):9631-6. Full free paper at http://www.pnas.org/cgi/content/full/102/27/9631

54. Buckalew VM. Endogenous digitalis-like factors: an overview of the history. Frontiers in Endocrinology April 2015, V6; A49:1 at http://journal.frontiersin.org/article/10.3389/fendo.2015.00049/full

55. Carlos ETB Monteiro, Acidic environment evoked by chronic stress: A novel mechanism to explain atherogenesis. Available from Infarct Combat Project, January 28, 2008 at http://www.infarctcombat.org/AcidityTheory.pdf

56. Gordts SC. The Impact of Lipoproteins on Wound Healing: Topical HDL Therapy Corrects Delayed Wound Healing in Apolipoprotein E Deficient Mice. Pharmaceuticals 2014, 7, 419-432; doi:10.3390/ph7040419

57. Cheung MC et al. **Phospholipid transfer protein in human plasma associates with proteins linked to immunity and inflammation.** Biochemistry 2010 Aug 31;49(34):7314-22.

58. Kaunitz H. Cholesterol and repair processes in arteriosclerosis. Lipids. 1978 May;13(5):373-4.

59. See comment in PubMed Commons belowDe Pinieux G et al. Lipid-lowering drugs and mitochondrial function: effects of HMG-CoA reductase inhibitors on serum ubiquinone and blood lactate/pyruvate ratio. Br J Clin Pharmacol. 1996 Sep;42(3):333-7. Full free text at http://www.ncbi.nlm.nih.gov/pmc/articles/PMC2042680/

60. Diamond DM and Ravnskov U. How statistical deception created the appearance that statins are safe and effective in primary and secondary prevention of cardiovascular disease. Expert Rev Clin Pharmacol 2015;8:201–10

61. Puri R et al. Impact of Statins on Serial Coronary Calcification During Atheroma Progression and Regression. J. Am. College of Cardiol.2015;65:1273-8

62. Malek AM, Alper SL, Izumo S. 1999. Hemodynamic shear stress and its role in atherosclerosis JAMA 282: 2035-2042

63. Cheng C et al. 2006. Atherosclerotic lesion size and vulnerability are determined by patterns of fluid shear stress. Circulation 113:2744-2753. Full free paper at at http://circ.ahajournals.org/cgi/content/abstract/113/23/2744

64. Cunningham KS and Gotlieb AI. 2005. The role of shear stress in the pathogenesis of atherosclerosis (Mini review), Laboratory Investigation 85, 9-23, Full free paper at http://www.nature.com/labinvest/journal/v85/n1/full/3700215a.html

65. Press release. 2006. Beyond Lipids: Understanding the Mechanics of Atherosclerosis (press release). UCSD News, July 12. At http://www.jacobsschool.ucsd.edu/news/news_releases/release.sfe?id=554

66. Kaunas R, Usami S, Chien S. 2006 Regulation of stretch-induced JNK activation by stress fiber orientation. Cellular Signalling, Nov;18(11):1924-31 at http://www.ncbi.nlm.nih.gov/pubmed/16581230

67. Haga JH, Li Yi-Shuan J. and Chien S. 2007. Molecular basis of the effects of mechanical stretch on vascular smooth muscle cells, Journal of Biomechanics, 40(5):947-60.

68. GC Williams, An experimental study of the intimal ground substance in atherosclerosis. Can Medical Assoc J, 1953 Jul; 69 (1): 17-22 at http://www.ncbi.nlm.nih.gov/pmc/articles/PMC1822858/

69. Gaskell WH. On the tonicity of the heart and blood vessels. J Physiol 1880;3:48-75

70. Rudolph Virchow. Book "Celular Pathology": as based upon Physiological and Pathological Histology: Twenty lectures delivered in the Pathology Institute of Berlin, 1858

71. Texon M. 1957. A hemodynamic concept of atherosclerosis, with particular reference to coronary occlusion. Arch Intern Med 99:418–427

72. Henry J.P., Stephens P.M.. Stress, Health, and the Social Environment: A Sociobiologic Approach to Medicine. Springer; First edition, Dec 21 1977

73. Williams RB: Psychophysiological process, the coronary prone behavior pattern, and coronary heart disease. In Dembroski TM, Weiss SM, Shields JL, Haynes SG, Feinleib M (eds), Coronary Prone Behavior. New York, Springer, 1978, pp 141-146

74. Soares-Miranda L, Stein PK, Imamura F, et al. Tans-fatty acid consumption and heart rate variability in two separate cohorts of older and younger adults. *Circ Arrhythm Electrophysiol.* 2012 August 1; 5(4): 728–738

75. Mei Dong, Xiaoyan Yang, Sharon Lim, Cold Exposure Promotes Atherosclerotic Plaque Growth and Instability via UCP1-Dependent Lipolysis, Cell Metab. 2013 Jul 2; 18(1): 118–129

76. Book "Acidity Theory of Atherosclerosis – New Evidences" , 2012. It can be found for Kindle readers and in paperback at Amazon.com. The printed edition is also being distributed by Barnes and Noble and other bookstores

77. Yang S et al. Association between beta-blocker use and fracture risk: the Dubbo Osteoporosis Epidemiology Study. Bone. 2011 Mar 1;48(3):451-5

78. Issekutz B Jr. Effect of beta–adrenergic blockade on lactate turnover in exercising dogs. *J Appl Physiol* 1984; 57: 1754–59.

79. Bruno RM et al. Effect of acute administration of vitamin C on muscle sympathetic activity, cardiac sympathovagal balance, and baroreflex sensitivity in hypertensive patients. Am J Clin Nutr, 2012 vol. 96 no. 2 302-308. Full free text at http://ajcn.nutrition.org/content/96/2/302.full

80. Kobylecki CJ et al. Genetically high plasma vitamin C, intake of fruit and vegetables, and risk of ischemic heart disease and all-cause mortality: a Mendelian randomization study. Am J Clin Nutr 2015;101: 1135-43

81. Wendell CR, Waldstein SR, Ferrucci L, O'Brien RJ, Strait JB, Zonderman AB: Carotid atherosclerosis and prospective risk of dementia. Stroke 2012, 43:3319–3324.

82. Dolan H, Crain B, Troncoso J, Resnick SM, Zonderman AB, Obrien RJ: Atherosclerosis, dementia, and Alzheimer disease in the Baltimore Longitudinal Study of Aging cohort. Ann Neurol 2010, 68:231–240.

83. Rebecca H. Affoo, Norine Foley John Rosenbek et al. Swallowing Dysfunction and Autonomic Nervous System Dysfunction in Alzheimer's Disease: A Scoping Review of the Evidence. Journal of the American Geriatrics Society, 2013; Volume 61, Issue 12, pages 2203–2213

84. Peila R, White LR et al. Reducing the risk of dementia: efficacy of long-term treatment of hypertension. Stroke 2006;37:1165–1170. Full free text at http://stroke.ahajournals.org/content/37/5/1165.long

85. Carlos Monteiro, The link between atherosclerosis and Alzheimer's disease. February 7, 2013 at http://aciditytheory.blogspot.com.br/2013/02/atherosclerosis-autonomic-dysfunction.html

86. Carlos Monteiro, Cancer, Atherosclerosis and Sympathetic Dominance. Positive Health Online, Issue 223: July 2015 at http://www.positivehealth.com/article/cancer/cancer-atherosclerosis-and-sympathetic-dominance

87. Sajima T, Tanabe A et al. Impact of platinum-based chemotherapy on the progression of atherosclerosis. Climateric 2011 Feb;14 (1): 31-40

88. Kalabova H, Melichar B et al. Intima-media thickness, myocardial perfusion and laboratory risk factors of atherosclerosis in patients with breast cancer treated with anthracycline-based chemotherapy. Med Oncol 2011 Dec; 28 (4): 1281-7

89. Monsuez JJ, Charniot JC, Vignat N, Artigou JY. Cardiac side-effects of cancer chemotherapy. Int J Cardiol. 2010;144(1):3–15.

90. Senkus E, Jassem J. Cardiovascular effects of systemic cancer treatment. Cancer Treat Rev. 2011;37(4):300–11.

91. Adams SC, Schondorf R, Benoit J, Kilgour RD. Impact of cancer and chemotherapy on autonomic nervous system function and cardiovascular reactivity in young adults with cancer: a case-controlled feasibility study. BMC Cancer. 2015 May 18;15:414. doi: 10.1186/s12885-015-1418-3

92. Whitlock MC et al. Cancer and Its Association With the Development of Coronary Artery Calcification: An Assessment From the Multi-Ethnic Study of Atherosclerosis. J Am Heart Assoc. 2015;4:e002533 at http://jaha.ahajournals.org/content/4/11/e002533.full

93. Dongfeng Zhang, Xiaoli Shen, Xin Qi. Resting heart rate and all-cause and cardiovascular mortality in the general population: a meta-analysis. CMAJ November 23, 2015 at http://www.cmaj.ca/content/early/2015/11/23/cmaj.150535

94. Kim Fox, Jeffrey S. Borer, et al. Resting Heart Rate in Cardiovascular Disease. The Heart Rate Working Group. J Am Coll Cardiol. 2007;50 (9):823-830, at http://content.onlinejacc.org/article.aspx?articleid=1138437

95. Campia I, Gazzano et al. Digoxin and ouabain increase the synthesis of cholesterol in human liver cells. Cell Mol Life Sci. 2009 May;66(9):1580-94

96. Campia I, Sala V, Kopecka J et al. Digoxin and ouabain induce the efflux of cholesterol via liver X receptor signalling and the synthesis of ATP in cardiomyocytes. Biochem J. 2012 Oct 15;447(2):301-11.

97. Shi H, Mao X, Zhong Y et al. Digoxin reduces atherosclerosis in apolipoprotein E-deficient mice. Br J Pharmacol. 2016 Feb 16

98. Omer F. Kuzu, Mohammad A. Noory, and Gavin P. Robertson. The Role of Cholesterol in Cancer. Cancer Res; 76(8) April 15, 2016

99. Georg Pongratz; Rainer H Straub. The Sympathetic Nervous Response in Inflammation. Arthritis Res Ther. 2014;16(504) Full paper at http://www.ncbi.nlm.nih.gov/pmc/articles/PMC4396833/

Chapter Eleven

The Role of Infections, Lipoproteins and
Hyperhomocysteinemia in the Pathogenesis of
Vulnerable Atherosclerotic Plaques.

Uffe Ravnskov, MD, PhD, Kilmer S. McCully, MD

Abstract

Although cholesterol-lowering drugs have long been the main pharmacological therapy for prevention of cardiovascular disease (CVD), numerous observations contradict the view that elevated low-density lipoprotein cholesterol (LDL-C) is a causative factor in the pathogenesis of atherosclerosis. Inflammation and oxidized LDL (ox-LDL) have been identified as potent risk factors for CVD, but the origin of these factors is unclear. Our concept is that the vulnerable plaque is a micro-abscess created by obstruction of vasa vasorum by aggregates of microbes and lipoproteins, exacerbated by homocysteinylation of LDL, endothelial dysfunction and impaired erythrocyte deformability. Obstruction of vasa vasorum by lipoprotein aggregates containing microorganisms leads to ischemia of arterial wall, intramural cell death, rupture of capillaries with haemorrhage, and escape of microorganisms into the intima, leading to inflammation and creation of the vulnerable plaque. This explanation resolves the many observations that contradict the cholesterol hypothesis and implicates inflammation and ox-LDL as secondary phenomena in the origin of atherosclerosis.

Clinical contradictions to the cholesterol hypothesis

Numerous observations are incompatible with the hypothesis that either elevated total blood cholesterol (tC) or elevated low-density lipoprotein cholesterol (LDL-C) is a causal factor in CVD:

1. No study of unselected individuals has shown an association between tC or LDL-C and the degree of atherosclerosis[1].

2. Almost all studies have shown that elevated tC and/or LDL-C do not predict CVD in women, nor do they predict CVD in elderly people, although the large majority of cardiovascular deaths occur in people older than 65 years of age[2].

3. Low tC and low LDL-C are risk factors for coronary heart disease in Russians[3] and in patients with rheumatoid arthritis[4].

4. No cholesterol-lowering trial has shown exposure-response, namely an association between the degree of cholesterol lowering and the clinical or roentgenological outcome[2].

5. Recent studies have shown that tC and LDL-C are lower than normal in patients with acute myocardial infarction, and in one study, mortality increased when cholesterol was lowered further[5,6].

6. A recent systematic review showed that LDL-cholesterol in 68 094 elderly people is not associated with or in most cases inversely associated with mortality.[91]

Pathophysiological contradictions to the cholesterol hypothesis

A high level of LDL-C in the blood is said to produce endothelial dysfunction or damage, which allows the migration of LDL-C and monocytes into the arterial wall. According to this view, LDL-C is modified by oxidation, and ox-LDL-C is phagocytized by monocytes or macrophages, a process that converts them to foam cells. These processes are considered as the cause of inflammation in the arterial wall[7]. However, several observations contradict these assumptions:

1. The concept that high LDL-C causes endothelial dysfunction is unlikely because there is no association between the concentration

of LDL-C in the blood and the degree of endothelial dysfunction[8].

2. It is unlikely that endothelial dysfunction leads to influx of LDL-C, because in patients with hyperhomocysteinemia caused by inborn errors of methionine metabolism no lipids are observed in the arterial wall even though there is pronounced endothelial damage[9,10].

3. If inflammation in the arterial wall were the causative factor in atherogenesis, anti-inflammatory treatment should have beneficial effects. However, almost all trials with anti-inflammatory drugs have resulted in increased cardiovascular mortality[11].

4. If the current view of the causative role of LDL-C in atherogenesis were true, both inflammation and the deposits of lipids should occur close to the endothelium, but these changes are found predominately in the adventitia[12-14].

The role of vasa vasorum

In experiments with rabbits Booth et al[15] produced foam cell formation, deposition of extracellular lipid and smooth muscle cell infiltration into the arterial sub-endothelium without any damage of the endothelium by positioning a hollow silastic collar around the carotid artery. Such changes have also been produced by ligating the vasa vasorum of the femoral artery in minipigs[16]. As vasa vasorum are functional end-arteries[17], and as similar findings are seen in early human atherosclerosis, these investigators concluded that atherosclerosis might be initiated by occlusion of vasa vasorum.

Therefore, the crucial question concerns which factors are able to occlude the vasa vasorum. Simanonok suggested that occlusion of the vasa vasorum results from impaired erythrocyte deformability[18]. Stiffened erythrocytes are less able to traverse smaller capillaries and arterioles, and impaired erythrocyte deformability is observed in diabetes, hypertension, smoking, obesity, lack of physical fitness, psycho-emotional stress, advanced age, peripheral arterial disease, acute myocardial infarction and stroke[18].

Another cause of impaired blood flow may be hyperhomocysteinemia, because a high level of homocysteine in the blood causes endothelial dysfunction and a narrowing of the capillaries and arterioles[9,19].

For many years infectious diseases have been known to be associated with CVD. Today at least 100 published reviews discuss this phenomenon, but almost all investigators believe infections to be secondary to CVD. We suggest that infectious microbes are primary participants in the pathogenesis of vulnerable plaques[20,21]. According to our hypothesis, complexes composed of microorganisms and lipoproteins, enlarged by homocysteinylated LDL aggregates and autoantibodies against homocysteinylated LDL or oxidized LDL, obstruct blood flow through capillaries and arterioles. This effect may be most pronounced in vasa vasorum of the arteries because of high extracapillary pressure[20,21]. Our hypothesis explains the ischemia and hypoxia of the arterial wall observed within the macrophage-rich center of the atherosclerotic lesions[22] and is based on the little known, but well documented role of the lipoproteins in the immune system.

The innate lipoprotein immune system

Previously most authorities considered the serum factor anti-streptolysin-S to be an antibody because of its ability to neutralize streptolysin-S, a streptococcal hemolysin toxin. However, in 1939 Todd et al showed that, contrary to the normal reaction of antibodies, the anti-streptolysin-S titer fell below normal values in patients with rheumatic fever at the peak of the clinical symptoms[23]. Subsequently, several research groups demonstrated that antistreptolysin-S is identical with the lipoproteins[20]. In animals HDL has the main protective effect against infectious microbes and their toxins, but in humans all lipoproteins are protective[20]. Human HDL and LDL are able to bind to and neutralize not only streptolysin-S but also many types of bacteria and viruses and their toxic products[20,24]. In agreement with these observations, lipoproteins are found to disappear from the general circulation during infections[25]. Moreover, low LDL is associated with respiratory and gastrointestinal diseases[26], most of which have an infectious origin. Moreover, the increased risk of hospital admission because of an infectious disease is associated with low serum cholesterol[27]. Furthermore, before 1900 persons with familial hypercholesterolemia lived longer than people without this condition, probably because of the protective effect of LDL against the commonest cause of death at that time, infectious diseases[28].

Many studies have shown that the lipoproteins adhere to all kinds of microorganisms, producing aggregation[29,30]. The size of these aggregates may increase in the presence of hyperhomocysteinemia, because the cyclic anhydride of homocysteine, homocysteine thiolactone, reacts with the free amino groups of apoB protein of LDL, causing aggregation of LDL[31,32]. There is also evidence that homocysteinylation of LDL may alter the antigenic properties of LDL, leading to autoantibody formation[33-35]. Reaction with these autoantibodies may further increase the size of the LDL-microbial aggregates.

The vulnerable plaque is a micro-abscess

Aggregates of homocysteinylated lipoproteins with microorganisms may obstruct blood flow within the vasa vasorum, causing ischemia and hypoxia of the arterial wall[20]. This obstruction may lead to intramural cell death, vasa vasorum may rupture causing haemorrhage, and the LDL aggregates with their content of microbial products may enter the arterial wall and cause inflammation. If the immune system is functioning optimally, inflammation and reparatory processes convert the necrotic arterial tissue into a fibrous plaque. If the immune system is sub-optimal, the necrotic arterial wall containing lipoprotein aggregates and micro-organisms may rupture into the intima, creating a micro-abscess, the vulnerable plaque. It has been shown that almost all arterial thrombi are associated with vulnerable plaques. Some thrombi are precipitated by rupture of a vulnerable plaque[36], but in other cases the thrombus is located adjacent to a superficial erosion of a proteoglycan-rich plaque without rupture[37].

In agreement with the conclusion that the vulnerable plaque is a micro-abscess, its temperature is higher than that of the surrounding tissue[38]. Furthermore, fragments from more than 50 different bacterial and virus species[39-42] and even live bacteria[43-46] have been demonstrated in atherosclerotic arteries, but not a single one was found in normal arterial tissue. The concept that vulnerable plaques are loaded with microorganisms is also supported by the finding that about 20 % of patients with acute myocardial infarction complicated by cardiogenic shock have bacteraemia and sepsis[47].

Our concept is that the atherosclerotic, calcified plaques are the healed scars resulting from infections within the arterial wall. We agree with the American pathologist Hans Kaunits, who in a review published almost 40 years ago concluded: "It may perhaps be profitable to pay more attention to speculations that the initiating factor is an infectious agent....In a wide variety of pathological conditions, cholesterol forms a large part of the lesion. This is true in scars, tubercles, gummata, old fibroids, thrombi, cholesteatomata, where it forms a complicated tissue in combination with calcium, fibrin, collagen, and other substances"[48].

Foam cells and atherogenesis

The presence of foam cells is a frequent finding in atherosclerotic arteries. According to the currently prevailing hypothesis, foam cells are created by macrophages which phagocytize oxidized cholesterol by interaction with the scavenger receptor. However, in vitro experiments have shown that lipopolysaccharides (LPS) from several of the pathogens which are most frequently reported in human atheromas are able to convert macrophages to foam cells in the presence of human LDL[49-51].

Macrophages phagocytize lipoprotein aggregates by phagocytosis and destroy the microorganisms by oxidation with reactive oxygen radicals[20]. It is therefore much more likely that the presence of oxidized cholesterol in the artery wall and in the circulation is the result of a normal oxidative process of the innate immune defence system. Therefore, our conclusion is that cholesterol is not oxidized in the interstitium but is oxidized inside the macrophages together with the microorganisms and their toxic products.

Intimal fatty streaks of the aorta and peripheral arteries are composed of aggregated foam cells located close to the arterial endothelium. Probably these foam cells are destined to enter the circulation, and their presence is a normal phenomenon in healthy people. This is the only credible explanation, since aortic and arterial fatty streaks are present even in the fetus and in early childhood[53,54], presumably reflecting a normal and reversible response to infections.

Evidence for infections as a causative factor in atherosclerosis and CVD

Numerous observations and experiments suggest that infections are not secondary to CVD but are primary factors in the pathogenesis[55,56]. For instance, influenza epidemics are associated with an increase of CVD mortality[57,58]. About a third of patients with acute myocardial infarction or stroke have had an infection during the preceding month[59]. Bacteraemia[60,61], HIV[62,63], serological markers of infection[64,65] and periodontal infections[66,67] are risk factors for CVD. Furthermore, infected children who die from an infectious disease have narrowing of the coronary arteries[68], and those who survive have thickening of the carotid intima-media[69].

Animal experiments support microorganisms as pathogenic factors in atherosclerosis

The strongest argument for causality is experimental creation of atherosclerosis by the suspected factor, and several such experiments with infectious microorganisms have been successful. Atherosclerosis has been produced or accelerated in chickens by infection with Marek's disease herpesvirus[70] and in mice by infection with *Chlamydia pneumoniae*, *Mycoplasma pneumonia* and *Porphyromonas gingivalis*[71,72]. Evidence of early atherosclerosis has also been produced both in normocholesterolemic and in hypercholesterolemic minipigs by infection with *Chlamydia pneumoniae*, alone or together with influenza virus[73]. In accordance with our hypothesis vascular damage and endothelial dysfunction in this experiment were most prominent in the co-infected pigs and less pronounced in the hypercholesterolemic pigs.

Prevention and treatment of atherosclerosis

According to our concept of the pathogenesis of atherosclerosis, the war against CVD should concentrate on counteracting infectious diseases, improving immune function, and eliminating factors that obstruct the blood flow within the vasa vasorum.

For many years treatment with cholesterol-lowering statin drugs has been the standard therapy for prevention of CVD. As the lipoproteins protect against infections, it may seem contradictory that cholesterol lowering with statin drugs is protective against CVD. However, no statin trial has shown an association between the degree of cholesterol lowering and outcome[1], and the beneficial effect of statin drugs must therefore depend on other effects. It is likely that statin treatment would be more beneficial if it did not lower cholesterol.

Many authors claim that statin treatment lowers the risk of infectious diseases. However, in these studies the investigators have compared statin-treated patients with non-treated control individuals from the general population. These studies contain a serious bias because of the fact that low cholesterol levels predispose to infectious diseases. Most statin-treated patients have lived most of their lives with high cholesterol levels, whereas many of the untreated controls may have lived their lives with low cholesterol levels. Furthermore, many patients discontinue statin therapy because of unacceptable side effects. It is therefore impossible to know, whether the better outcome of the statin treated patients is caused by their high cholesterol, or by statin treatment. The lack of anti-infectious efficacy of statin therapy has been documented in various ways. For instance, Becker et al have shown that statin treatment of stroke patients increases their risk of infection[74]. In a study of patients with fever by de Saint Martin et al., a significantly larger number of those who were on statin treatment was admitted to intensive care units, compared with non-users (p=0.009)[75].

Prevention of cardiovascular disease by antibiotics has been largely unsuccessful, apparently contradicting our hypothesis. However, in most of these trials patients have received a single antibiotic, and most of them have been of relatively short duration[76]. Since a large number of different microorganisms has been identified in atherosclerotic arteries, use of a single antibiotic is unlikely to be beneficial. Moreover, viral agents, such as *Herpesvirus* or *Cytomegalovirus*, which have also been implicated in atherogenesis, are generally resistant to antibiotics.

In a trial by Paakkanen et al. of 144 patients with acute coronary syndromes, the participants were randomly divided to receive a three-month treatment of clarithromycin or placebo and were followed for an average of 404 days (138-924 days). The outcome of this trial documented a decrease in major adverse coronary and cerebrovascular events (19 % vs 40 % events), and the benefit was most pronounced among those with complement component C4B deficiencies[77].

Antibiotics may be useful in treatment of acute myocardial infarction. As bacteraemia and sepsis are common findings in life-threatening cases, we suggest that a blood culture should be obtained in patients with acute coronary syndrome. If the blood culture is positive, we anticipate that the course of the disease may be improved with an appropriate antibiotic.

Vaccination may also be useful. In a meta-analysis of 11 cohort studies Vlachopoulos et al found that pneumococcal vaccination was associated with a decreased risk of cardiovascular events and mortality in elderly people, in particular among those with high cardiovascular risk[78]. Furthermore, several observational and case-control studies[79] and two randomized trials[80,81] have shown that influenza vaccination protects against CVD.

Periodontal disease is a risk factor for CVD, and Piconi et al. have documented that treatment of patients with periodontal disease had a better angiographic outcome than observed in any statin trial[82]. Furthermore, according to a nationwide population study, tooth scaling is associated with a decreased risk for future cardiovascular events[83].

Infectious diseases are associated with dyslipidemia, reflecting a metabolic response to infections[84,85]. Thus the dyslipidemia associated with atherosclerosis may be attributed to the metabolic response to infection. Young adults with dyslipidemia are associated with an increased coronary artery calcium score later in life[86]. A probable interpretation of this observation is that increased arterial calcification is attributable to healed and calcified atherosclerotic plaques as a result of spontaneously resolved infections. Consequently, prevention and treatment of atherosclerosis is more likely to be accomplished by prevention and elimination of infections than treatment of dyslipidemia, a secondary metabolic response to infections[87].

An apparent contradiction to our hypothesis is that a lowering of blood homocysteine levels by high dose folate, pyridoxal, and cobalamin has generally been ineffective in preventing adverse vascular events[88]. However, the assay for plasma homocysteine determines the quantity of homocysteine bound to plasma proteins by disulphide bonds, but neither homocystine disulphide nor protein-bound homocysteine has been reported to react with the amino groups of LDL to cause aggregation[31]. This effect is only created by homocysteine thiolactone[32]. Although several of the B vitamin secondary prevention trials significantly lowered plasma homocysteine levels[89], none of these trials utilized an assay for plasma homocysteine thiolactone, the only molecular species of homocysteine which causes LDL aggregation[31,32]. Future trials are needed to study the effect of B vitamin intervention and other homocysteine-lowering protocols on prevention of vascular disease by utilizing an assay for plasma homocysteine thiolactone[90], the reactive molecular form of homocysteine that causes aggregation of LDL, leading to obstruction of vasa vasorum and creation of vulnerable plaques[20].

Summary

Our concept is that microbial infection, hyperhomocysteinemia, aggregated lipoproteins, and endothelial dysfunction are major factors in the pathogenesis of atherosclerosis. That elevated LDL-C is the main cause of CVD dominates the view of the worldwide scientific community, although hundreds of observational and experimental studies fail to satisfy most of Bradford Hill's criteria for causality. A major problem is that almost all investigators and medical journals in this field are economically dependent on the drug companies. In recent years there has been increased scepticism among medical scientists concerning the supposed benefits from statin treatment. Our hypothesis may hopefully increase the interest of the medical profession in more effective methods of prevention and treatment of CVD.

Uffe Ravnskov, MD*, PhD, Kilmer S. McCully, MD**

* Independent Investigator

** Associate Clinical Professor of Pathology, Harvard Medical School
VA Boston Healthcare System
Harvard Medical School

References

1. Ravnskov U. Is atherosclerosis caused by high cholesterol? QJM 2002; 95:397-403.

2. Ravnskov U. High cholesterol may protect against infections and atherosclerosis. QJM 2003; 96:927-34

3. Shestov DB, Deev AD, Klimov AN et al. Increased risk of coronary heart disease death in men with low total and low-density-lipoprotein cholesterol in the Russian Lipid Research Clinics prevalence follow-up study. Circulation 1993; 88:846-53.

4. Myasoedova E, Crowson CS, Kremers HM et al. Lipid paradox in rheumatoid arthritis: the impact of serum lipid measures and systemic inflammation on the risk of cardiovascular disease. Ann Rheum Dis 2011; 70:482-7.

5. Sachdeva A, Cannon CP, Deedwania PC et al. Lipid levels in patients hospitalized with coronary artery disease: an analysis of 136,905 hospitalizations in Get With The Guidelines. Amer Heart J 2009; 157:111-7.

6. Al-Mallah MH, Hatahet H, Cavalcante JL, Khanal S. Low admission LDL-cholesterol is associated with increased 3-year all-cause mortality in patients with non ST segment elevation myocardial infarction. Cardiol J 2009; 16:227-33.

7. Hansson GK. Inflammation, atherosclerosis, and coronary artery disease. New Eng J Med 2005; 352:1685-95.

8. Reis SE, Holubkov R, Conrad-Smith AJ et al. Coronary microvascular dysfunction is highly prevalent in women with chest pain in the absence of coronary artery disease: results from the NHLBI WISE study Amer Heart J 2001; 141:735-41.

9. McCully KS Vascular pathology of homocysteinemia: implications for the pathogenesis of arteriosclerosis. Amer J Pathol 1969; 56:111-28.

10. McCully KS. Hyperhomocysteinemia and arteriosclerosis: historical perspectives . Clin Chem Lab Med 2005; 43:980-86.

11. Trelle S, Reichenbach S, Wandel S et al. Cardiovascular safety of non-steroidal anti-inflammatory drugs: network meta-analysis.. BMJ 2011; 342: c7086 doi:10.1136/bmj.c7086

12. Higuchi ML, Gutierrez PS, Bezerra HG, et al. Comparison between adventitial and intimal inflammation of ruptured and nonruptured atherosclerotic plaques in human coronary arteries Arq Bras Cardiol 2002; 79:20–4. 5.

13. Maiellaro K, Taylor WR. The role of the adventitia in vascular inflammation Cardiovasc Res 2007; 75:640–8.

14. Subbotin VM. Neovascularization of coronary tunica intima (DIT) is the cause of coronary atherosclerosis. Lipoproteins invade coronary intima via neovascularization from adventitial vasa vasorum, but not from the arterial lumen: a hypothesis. Theor Biol Med Model 2012; 9: 11-32

15. Booth RF, Martin JF, Honey AC et al. Rapid development of atherosclerotic lesions in the rabbit carotid artery induced by perivascular manipulation Atherosclerosis. 1989; 76: 257-68.

16. Barker SGE, Talbert A, Cottam S et al. Arterial intimal hyperplasia after occlusion of the adventitial vasa vasorum in the pig. Arterioscler Thromb 1993; 13: 70-7

17. Gössl M, Malyar NM, Rosol M et al. Impact of coronary vasa vasorum functional structure on coronary vessel wall perfusion distribution. Am J Physiol Heart Circ Physiol 2003; 285:H2019–26.

18. Simanonok JP. Non-Ischemic Hypoxia of the Arterial Wall is a Primary Cause of Atherosclerosis. Med Hypotheses 1996; 46:155-61

19. McCully KS. Chemical Pathology of Homocysteine. IV. Excitotoxicity, Oxidative Stress, Endothelial Dysfunction, and Inflammation. Ann Clin Lab Sci 2009; 39:219-232.

20. Ravnskov U, McCully KS. Vulnerable plaque formation from obstruction of vasa vasorum by homocysteinylated and oxidized lipoprotein aggregates complexed with microbial remnants and LDL autoantibodies. Ann Clin Lab Sci 2009; 39:3-16.

21. Ravnskov U, McCully KS. Infections may be causal in the pathogenesis of atherosclerosis Amer J Med Sci. 2012; 344:391-4.

22. Sluimer JC, Gasc JM, van Wanroij JL, et al. Hypoxia, hypoxia-inducible transcription factor, and macrophages in human atherosclerotic plaques are correlated with intraplaque angiogenesis. Am Coll Cardiol 2008; 51: 1258–65.

23. Todd EW, Coburn AF, Hill AB. Antistreptolysin S titres in rheumatic fever. Lancet 1939;2:1213-1217.

24. Han R. Plasma lipoproteins are important components of the immune system. Microbiol Immunol 2010; 54: 246-53.

25. Sammalkorpi K, Valtonen V, Koerttula Y et al. Changes in serum lipoprotein pattern induced by acute infections Metabolism 1988;37:859-65.

26. Jacobs D, Blackburn H, Higgins M et al. Report of the Conference on Low Blood Cholesterol: Mortality Associations. Circulation 1992; 86: 1046-60..

27. Iribarren C, Jacobs DR Jr, Sidney S et al. Cohort study of serum total cholesterol and in-hospital incidence of infectious diseases. Epidemiol Infect 1998; 121: 335–47

28. Sijbrands EJ, Westendorp RG, Defesche JC et al. Mortality over two centuries in large pedigree with familial hypercholesterolaemia: family tree mortality study Brit Med J 2001; 322: 1019-23.

29. Van Amersfoort ES, Van Berkel TJC, Kuiper J. Receptors, mediators, and mechanisms involved in bacterial sepsis and septic shock Clin Microbiol Rev 2003; 16: 379-414.

30. Khovidhunkit W, Kim MS, Memon RA et al. Effects of infection and inflammation on lipid and lipoprotein metabolism: mechanisms and consequences to the host J Lipid Res 2004; 45: 1169-96.

31. Vidal M, Sainte-Marie J, Philippot J, Bienvenue A. Thiolation of low-density lipoproteins and their interactions with L2C leukemic lymphocytes. Biochimie 1986; 68: 723-30.

32. Naruszewicz M, Mirkiewicz E, Olszewski AJ, McCully KS. Thiolation of low-density lipoprotein by homocysteine thiolactone causes increased aggregation and altered interaction with cultured macrophages. Nutr Metab Cardiovasc Dis 1994; 4: 70-7.

33. Ferguson E, Parthasarathy S, Joseph J, Kalyanaraman B. Generation and initial characterization of a novel polyclonal antibody directed against homocysteine thiolactone-modified low density lipoprotein. J Lipid Res 1998; 39: 925-33.

34. Undas A, Jankowski M, Twardowska M et al. Antibodies to N-homocysteinylated albumin as a marker for early-onset coronary artery disease in men Thromb Haemost 2005; 93: 346-50.

35. Yang X, Gao Y, Zhou J et al. Plasma homocysteine thiolactone adducts associated with risk of coronary heart disease Clin Chim Acta 2006; 364: 230-4.

36. Falk E. Plaque rupture with severe pre-existing stenosis precipitating coronary thrombosis. Characteristics of coronary atherosclerotic plaques underlying fatal occlusive thrombi. Br Heart J 1983; 50: 127-34,

37. Farb A, Burke AP, Tang AL et al. Coronary plaque erosion without rupture into a lipid core. A frequent cause of coronary thrombosis in sudden coronary death. Circulation. 1996; 93: 1354-63.

38. Madjid M, Naghavi M, Malik BA et al. Thermal detection of vulnerable plaque Amer J Cardiol 2002; 90: 36L-9L.

39. Ott SJ, El Mokhtari NE, Musfeldt M et al. Detection of diverse bacterial signatures in atherosclerotic lesions of patients with coronary heart disease. Circulation 2006; 113: 929-37.

40. Melnick JL, Petrie BL, Dreesman GR et al. Cytomegalovirus antigen within human arterial smooth muscle cells. Lancet 1983; 2: 644-7.

41. Pampou SY, Gnedoy SN, Bystrevskaya VB et al. Cytomegalovirus genome and the immediate-early antigen in cells of different layers of human aorta Virchows Arch 2000; 436: 539-52.

42. Shi Y, Tokunaga O. Chlamydia pneumoniae and multiple infections in the aorta contribute to atherosclerosis. Pathol Int 2002; 52: 755-63.

43. Ramirez JA Isolation of Chlamydia pneumoniae from the coronary artery of a patient with coronary atherosclerosis. The Chlamydia pneumoniae/Atherosclerosis Study Group. Ann Intern Med. 1996; 125:979-82.

44. Jackson LA, Campbell LA, Kuo CC et al. Isolation of Chlamydia pneumoniae from a carotid endarterectomy specimen J Infect Dis 1997; 176: 292-5.

45. Mosorin M, Surcel HM, Laurila A et al. Detection of Chlamydia pneumoniae-reactive T lymphocytes in human atherosclerotic plaques of carotid artery. Arterioscler Thromb Vasc Biol 2000; 20: 1061-7.

46. Lanter BB, Sauer K, Davies DG. Bacteria present in carotid arterial plaques are found as biofilm deposits which may contribute to enhanced risk of plaque rupture MBio 2014; 5:e01206-14. doi: 10.1128/mBio.01206-14.

47. Kohsaka S, Menon V, Lowe AM et al. Systemic inflammatory response syndrome after acute myocardial infarction complicated by cardiogenic shock. Arch Intern Med 2005; 165:1643-50.

48. Kaunitz H. Cholesterol and repair processes in arteriosclerosis. Lipids 1978;13:373-4..

49. Kalayoglu MV, Indrawati, Morrison RP et al. Chlamydial virulence determinants in atherogenesis: the role of chlamydial lipopolysaccharide and heat shock protein 60 in macrophage-lipoprotein interactions. J Infect Dis 2000; 181Suppl 3:S483-9.

50. Qi M, Miyakawa H, Kuramitsu HK. Porphyromonas gingivalis induces murine macrophage foam cell formation Microb Pathog 2003; 35:259-67

51. Nicolaou G, Goodall AH, Erridge C. Diverse bacteria promote macrophage foam cell formation via toll-like receptor-dependent lipid body biosynthesis. J Atheroscler Thromb 2012; 19:137–48.

52. Wen Y, Leake DS. Low density lipoprotein undergoes oxidation within lysosomes in cells. Circ Res. 2007; 100:1337-43

53. Leistikow EA. Is coronary artery disease initiated perinatally? Semin Thromb Hemost. 1998; 24:139-43.

54. Stary HC. Evolution and progression of atherosclerotic lesions in coronary arteries of children and young adults. Arteriosclerosis 1989;9(1 Suppl):I19-32.

55. Rosenfeld ME, Campbell LA. Pathogens and atherosclerosis: update on the potential contribution of multiple infectious organisms to the pathogenesis of atherosclerosis. Thromb Haemost. 2011; 106:858-67.

56. Kozarov E. Bacterial invasion of vascular cell types: vascular infectology and atherogenesis. Future Cardiol. 2012; 8:123-38.

57. Madjid M, Miller CC, Zarubaev VV et al. Influenza epidemics and acute respiratory disease activity are associated with a surge in autopsy-confirmed coronary heart disease death: results from 8 years of autopsies in 34,892 subjects. Eur Heart J 2007; 28:1205-10.

58. Warren-Gash C, Smeeth L, Hayward AC. Influenza as a trigger for acute myocardial infarction or death from cardiovascular disease: a systematic review. Lancet Infect Dis 2009; 9:601–10.

59. Smeeth L, Thomas SL, Hall AJ et al. Risk of myocardial infarction and stroke after acute infection or vaccination. New Eng J Med 2004;351:2611-8.

60. Valtonen V, Kuikka A, Syrjanen J. Thrombo-embolic complications in bacteremic infections Eur Heart J 1993;14 Suppl K:20-3.

61. Dalager-Pedersen M, Søgaard M, Schønheyder HC et al. Risk for myocardial infarction and stroke after community-acquired bacteremia: a 20-year population-based cohort study. Circulation. 2014; 129:1387-96.

62. Gibellini D, Borderi M, Clò A et al. HIV-related mechanisms in atherosclerosis and cardiovascular diseases J Cardiovasc Med (Hagerstown). 2013; 14:780-90.

63. Idris NS, Grobbee DE, Burgner D et al. Cardiovascular manifestations of HIV infection in children Eur J Prev Cardiol. 2015;22:1452-61.

64. Espinola-Klein C, Rupprecht HJ, Blankenberg S et al. Impact of infectious burden on progression of carotid atherosclerosis Stroke 2002; 33:2581-6.

65. Goyal P, Kalek SC, Chaudhry R et al. Association of common chronic infections with coronary artery disease in patients without any conventional risk factors Indian J Med Res. 2007 Feb;125:129-36.

66. Chapple IL. Time to take periodontitis seriously. BMJ. 2014 doi: 10.1136/bmj.g26

67. Nguyen CM, Kim JW, Quan VH et al. Periodontal associations in cardiovascular diseases: The latest evidence and understanding J Oral Biol Craniofac Res 2015; 5:203-6.

68. Pesonen E. Infection and intimal thickening: evidence from coronary arteries in children. Eur Heart J 1994;15 Suppl C:57- 61.

69. Liuba P, Persson J, Luoma J et al. Acute infections in children are accompanied by oxidative modification of LDL and decrease of HDL cholesterol, and are followed by thickening of carotid intima-media Eur Heart J 2003; 24:515-21.

70. Fabricant CG, Fabricant J, Litrenta MM, et al. Virus-induced atherosclerosis J Exp Med 1978; 148:335–40.

71. Damy SB, Higuchi ML, Timenetsky J, et al. Mycoplasma pneumoniae and/or Chlamydophila pneumoniae inoculation causing different aggravations in cholesterol-induced atherosclerosis in apoE KO male mice BMC Microbiol 2009; 9:194–201.

72. Lalla E, Lamster IB, Hofmann MA et al. Oral infection with a periodontal pathogen accelerates early atherosclerosis in apolipoprotein E-null mice. Arterioscler. Thromb Vasc Biol 2003; 23:1405–11.

73. Birck MM, Pesonen E, Odermarsky M, et al. Infection-induced coronary dysfunction and systemic inflammation in piglets are dampened in hypercholesterolemic milieu. Amer J Physiol Heart Circ Physiol 2011; 300:H1595–601.

74. Becker K, Tanzi P, Kalil A et al. Early statin use is associated with increased risk of infection after stroke. J Stroke Cerebrovasc Dis 2013; 22:66-71.

75. de Saint Martin L, Tandé D, Goetghebeur D et al. Statin use does not affect the outcome of acute infection: a prospective cohort study Presse Med 2010; 39:e52-7

76. Rosenfeld ME, Campbell LA. Pathogens and atherosclerosis: update on the potential contribution of multiple infectious organisms to the pathogenesis of atherosclerosis Thromb Haemost 2011;106:858-67.

77. Paakkanen R, Palikhe A, Seppänen M et al. Beneficial effect of clarithromycin in patients with acute coronary syndrome and complement C4 deficiencies Scand Cardiovasc J. 2009; 43:395-401

78. Vlachopoulos CV, Terentes-Printzios DG, Aznaouridis KA et al. Association between pneumococcal vaccination and cardiovascular outcomes: a systematic review and meta-analysis of cohort studies. Eur J Prev Cardiol 2014 pii: 2047487314549512.

79. Madjid M, Awan I, Ali M, et al. Influenza and atherosclerosis: vaccination for cardiovascular disease prevention Expert Opin Biol Ther 2005; 5:91–6.

80. Gurfinkel EP, de la Fuente RL. Two-year follow-up of the FLU Vaccination Acute Coronary Syndromes (FLUVACS) Registry. Tex Heart Inst J 2004; 31:28-32.

81. Phrommintikul A, Kuanprasert S, Wongcharoen W et al. Influenza vaccination reduces cardiovascular events in patients with acute coronary syndrome. Eur Heart J 2011; 32:1730-5.

82. Piconi S, Trabattoni D, Luraghi C, et al. Treatment of periodontal disease results in improvements in endothelial dysfunction and reduction of the carotid intima-media thickness FASEB J 2009; 23:1196–204.

83. Chen ZY, Chiang CH, Huang CC et al. The association of tooth scaling and decreased cardiovascular disease: a nationwide population-based study Am J Med 2012; 125:568-75.

84. Apostolou F, Gazi IF, Kostoula A et al. Persistence of an atherogenic profile after treatment of acute infection with Brucella. J Lipid Res 2009; 50: 2532-2539.

85. Gidding SS, Stone NJ, Bookstein LC et al. Month-to-month variability of lipids, lipoproteins, and apolipoproteins and the impact of acute infections in adolescents. J Pediatr 1998; 133: 242-246.

86. Pletcher MJ, Bibbins-Domingo K, Liu K et al. Nonoptimal lipids commonly present in young adults and coronary calcium score later in life: the CARDIA (Coronary Artery Risk Development in Young Adults) study. Ann Int Med 2010; 153: 137-146.

87. McCully KS. Homocysteine metabolism, atherosclerosis, and diseases of aging. Compr Physiol 2016; 6: 471-505.

88. Huang T, Chen Y, Yang B, Yang J, Wahlqvist ML, Li D. Meta-analysis of B vitamin supplementation on plasma homocysteine, cardiovascular and all-cause mortality. Clin Nutr 2012; 31: 448-454.

89. McCully KS. Homocysteine, vitamins, and vascular disease prevention. Amer J Clin Nutr 2007; 86(suppl): 1563S-1568S.

90. Jakubowski H. The determination of homocysteine thiolactone in biological samples. Anal Biochem 2002; 308: 112-119.

91. Ravnskov U, Diamond DM, Hama R et al. Lack of an association or an inverse association between low-density-lipoprotein and mortality in the elderly: a systematic review. BMJ Open 2016;6:e010401. doi:10.1136/bmjopen-2015-010401

Chapter Twelve

Cardiovascular Disease is Primarily Due to Blood Clotting*

Malcolm Kendrick, MD

Abstract

This chapter proposes that atherosclerotic plaques, the underlying cause of cardiovascular disease (heart attacks and strokes) are caused by two main processes. First, damage to the lining of larger arteries (the endothelium), followed by blood clotting. These clots are then incorporated into the arterial wall where, if the damage is rapidly repeated, or the blood clots formed are larger/more difficult to break down, the clot will turn into an atherosclerotic plaque. Therefore, factors that can damage the endothelium e.g. smoking, stress, high blood sugar levels, areas of turbulent flow will increase the risk of CVD. In addition, pro-coagulant factors will increase the risk of CVD e.g. air pollution, high fibrinogen levels, heat, cold, type II diabetes, stress, steroid use.

This hypothesis explains why plaques never form in veins, or in pulmonary blood vessels – where endothelial cells are under far less biomechanical strain. It also explains how statins reduce CVD risk. Statins increase nitric oxide synthesis, which protects the endothelium, and is the single most potent anticoagulant agent n nature. This hypothesis also explains how LDL can (in some situations increase CVD risk), as LDL stimulates platelet aggregation (the first step in clot formation). On the other hand, HDL has potent anti-coagulant

---

* I have only used references where I have stated something that is highly controversial, little known, or difficult to find easily e.g. data on haemophilia. Everything else can be rapidly be confirmed by using Google or Pubmed http://www.ncbi.nlm.nih.gov/pubmed

properties. This 'clotting' hypothesis of CVD can be used to explain all of the factors known to cause, or protect against, CVD.

Introduction

Over one hundred and sixty years ago Karl von Rokitansky studied the narrowings and thickenings found in human arteries (atherosclerotic plaques) and decided that they looked almost exactly like blood clots. He therefore proposed that they were, in fact, blood clots – in various different stages of 'repair'.

His scientific rival, Rudolf Virchow, studying the same phenomenon, had noted that these plaques contained a high percentage of cholesterol. Based on this single observation, he conjectured that this cholesterol must have been absorbed into the artery walls, from the bloodstream, creating further inflammation and thickenings.

This was the first time that the 'cholesterol hypothesis' had been proposed. Unfortunately, Virchow won the scientific argument with Rokitansky, at which point the cholesterol hypothesis became the bed rock of all future thinking about cardiovascular disease. Even if most researchers have no idea where the original idea came from.

Had Rokitansky won the debate, the direction of research into heart disease would, I believe, have gone in the correct direction. We would have realized that LDL/cholesterol has a very minor and relatively unimportant role in creating atherosclerotic plaques; a role that relates to the down-stream function of lipoproteins within blood clotting. We would long ago have fully understood the underlying mechanism of cardiovascular disease, and our management of it would be far in advance of where it is today.

In this Chapter I will lay out the 'blood clotting' hypothesis in as concise a form as possible. I will look at the process itself, and then establish how it fits with the various risk factors for cardiovascular disease that have been identified. For the sake of simplicity, I will call this hypothesis the 'atherothrombotic hypothesis', although this term has been used before to describe related phenomena, and is not fully accurate in this case.

The complexity of the atherothrombotic process

Before starting, I should state that much of what is described here should be defined as normal and healthy. For example, damage to the innermost layer of the artery, the endothelium, leads to blood clotting. Indeed, the process of clot formation (thrombosis) is a completely healthy physiological phenomenon. It protects us from death each and every day. Without the ability of blood to clot, the smallest scratch could be fatal. One small cut and we would just slowly bleed to death. People with haemophilia, for example, have serious health problems due to bleeding heavily into joints and suchlike.

On the other hand, if we clot too readily, if we are in a 'hypercoagulable' state, this too is far from healthy. People with an increased propensity of blood clotting are far more likely to die from strokes and heart attacks and pulmonary emboli and suchlike. It does not take much, one way or another for the blood clotting system to go wrong. So we are not talking about black and white, on or off, we are looking at a dynamic system that can tip one way or another – causing problems in either direction.

For example, there are two forms of stroke. Haemorrhagic and ischaemic. A haemorrhagic stroke occurs when a blood vessel in the brain bursts and blood enters the brain tissue, destroying parts of it. An ischaemic stroke occurs when a blood clot blocks an artery in the brain, stopping blood flow, preventing oxygenation and causing brain tissue to die.

These are clinically indistinguishable, unless you do a brain scan. One type of stroke is caused by excess bleeding, the other caused by a blood clot. If you try to treat a haemorrhagic stroke with an anti-coagulant, the patient will most likely die. If you try to treat an ischaemic stroke with an anti-coagulant the patient will most likely live.

In addition, it would be true to say that the coagulation system has more feedback loops and complexity than any other in the body. For every ten factors that are trying to get the blood to clot, there are another ten trying to ensure that it does not, or that the clotting process is stopped in its tracks. All is a constant balance, a highly dynamic system – some might say perhaps even chaotic.

It does not take too much to flip the system one way or another. The analogy of a butterfly fluttering its wings in the rain forest and causing a hurricane half way around the world could be appropriate, in that apparently very small and insignificant changes in one part of the clotting system can lead to a major breakdown elsewhere. Often in ways that can seem counter-intuitive.

The idea of chaos theory is further appropriate here in that agents that may appear almost exactly the same can create very different effects. Some anticoagulant drugs decrease the risk of heart disease, whilst others have no effect on the risk of heart disease, or may even increase the risk. Other anticoagulants can decrease the risk of stroke, without affecting heart disease. Simple, it is not.

At the risk of bringing in too much jargon too early, there are also long-term abnormalities e.g. antiphospholipid syndrome, Factor V Leiden and raised Lp(a). These lead to an increased tendency to blood clotting, and an increased risk of cardiovascular disease. In addition, there are temporary factors at work, that that make the blood hypercoagulable (more likely to clot) e.g. stress, smoking, use of steroids, dehydration, hyper/hypothermia and infections. All of these raise CVD risk, but sometimes for only a period of days, hours, or even minutes.

So, when you are looking at blood clotting and blood clotting abnormalities it is difficult to be absolute. A causes B, X leads to Y. But A may only cause B, so long as D and E are present and not Q and V. However, the general theme here is straightforward. Factors that stimulate, or accelerate blood clotting, or interfere with the correct repair of blood clots, will generally increase the risk of cardiovascular disease CVD.

What are the players in the game?

The endothelium

The endothelium is the single layer of cells that lines all blood vessels. These cells are flat, and thin, and join together at their boundaries with no gaps between. A bit like floor tiles, perhaps, although far more flexible and most certainly far more biological active. An important point to note here is that endothelial cells act as a barrier to anything in the blood stream leaking into the wall of the artery itself.

However, having just said this, as blood vessels become smaller and narrower, the endothelial cells develop holes in them known as fenestrations. This does allow various substances to leak out of the blood into the tissues and organs underneath. Were this not the case, few nutrients could get out of the blood, which would somewhat defeat the point of blood circulation.

For the purposes of this discussion we are not interested in the fenestrated form of endothelium lining smaller blood vessels, arterioles, venules and the like, because of the significantly different structure that is present. This form of endothelium does not act as a barrier and, more critically, it does not lie over tissues that contain powerful blood clotting activators. In short, we are looking at the congruent endothelium lining the larger blood vessels.

Whilst it is known that endothelial cells have a vast array different functions, I am restricting myself to looking at three. The first of which is that they produce nitric oxide (NO). Nitric oxide has two major functions. It is the most powerful anti-coagulant agent in the body. It also stimulates the smooth muscle within larger blood vessels to relax. This opens these arteries up, allowing increased blood flow.

This is why most agents used to treat angina are nitrates. The first of them to be identified was glyceryl trinitrate (GTN). The benefits of GTN was first noted by those working in dynamite factories, where men stirring the nitro-glycerin mixture found that their angina disappeared as they did so. Nitro-glycerin was turned into GTN tablets, and renamed. GTN is still used to stop angina attacks which occur when the blood vessels supplying the heart narrow, reducing oxygen supply, and causing heart muscle pain. GTN opens up the arteries, improves blood supply, and stops the pain.

If endothelial cells are 'stressed' or damaged, they produce far less NO. This has two important effects. First, the level of 'anticoagulant' falls, and the blood vessels constrict, raising pressure and turbulent flow over the endothelium. This makes if far more likely that clots will form.

Another important function of endothelial cells, is that they prevent contact between the blood and the inner arterial wall. This is critical because, lying within the arterial wall, is a high concentration of tissue factor (TF). This is the most powerful single clotting factor that exists. It triggers the 'extrinsic' clotting cascade and, essentially, overpowers all feedback systems, until the damage and tissue factor are both covered over.

Clearly this makes sense. If an arterial wall is damaged through trauma, the blood needs to clot very quickly, and directly on the site of the damage, to plug the hole. Therefore, this is where the primary agent for blood clotting lies. Which means that if endothelial cells are damaged, or stripped off, a thrombus will form very quickly over the area of the damage – triggered by tissue factor.

At which point a final essential characteristic of endothelial cells comes into play. Something that requires a bit more explanation, via a slight detour. If we look at skin cells, which grow upwards from the stratum basale, they gradually become thinner, before turning into the stratum corneum (outer surface of the skin). They then flake off and are replaced from underneath.

However, endothelial cells do not move upwards from within the arterial wall. There is no underlying stratum of endothelial cells that grow towards the surface. So, where do the replacement cells come from? The answer is that they are produced in the bone marrow in the form of endothelial progenitor cells (EPCs), which then circulate in the bloodstream.

Which means that if endothelial cells die (for whatever reason) or are stripped off, they are replaced by EPCs from above – if that is the correct way to think of it. EPCs, when they detect an area of endothelial damage, (inevitably already covered by a thrombus), stick to it, mature and form a new layer of endothelium on top of the thrombus.

In this way something very significant just happened. The thrombus now lies underneath the endothelial layer (within the artery wall itself). This actually answers the question from Virchow that Rokitansky could not answer. Namely, how can a blood clot form within the artery wall? Answer, it cannot, the blood clot is created on an area of damaged, or missing endothelial cells, then the endothelium re-grows on top of it.

Once again, from a physiological perspective, this makes perfect sense. If you damage your skin it will bleed, then a clot will form over the area of damage. The skin will then re-grow under the hardened clot (scab), once the skin has repaired underneath, the scab will simply fall off. However, if this happened in an artery wall, the clot/scab that fell off would travel down the artery until it narrows. At which point it would jam, potentially blocking the artery completely. If the thrombus/scab travelled into the brain it would cause a stroke, potentially fatal. So thrombi that form over areas of arterial damage must be resorbed into the artery wall itself.

A final point to mention here is that EPCs do not necessarily become mature endothelial cells. They can also go down another developmental pathway to become monocytes (a form of white blood cell involved in the immune system). These monocytes can further mature into macrophages. Another white blood cell type. Macrophages attack bacteria and viruses and also any other 'alien' tissue that they find.

Macrophages are the 'clear up' cells of the immune system. Interestingly. in order to clear up the waste, macrophages first use NO to 'oxidize' the alien material. This oxidized material is then engulfed by the macrophage which transports it to lymph glands where it is broken down and, eventually, removed from the body.

In summary, the endothelium is a critical player in the health of the cardiovascular system, primarily through NO synthesis. When healthy, the endothelium is also protective against blood coagulation, by separating the blood from the TF found in the deeper arterial wall. If clots do form, EPCs play a further critical role in covering up the clot, and then clearing up the 'damage' by transforming themselves into blood cells. Yes, it is all very clever.

The clotting/coagulation system

This is, as previously mentioned, an enormously complicated system with many, many, different players involved, along with many feedback systems. At the risk of oversimplifying, for the purposes of this discussion we can divide the coagulation system into the extrinsic clotting system and the intrinsic clotting system.

When we are talking about CVD it is primarily the extrinsic clotting system that is more important than the intrinsic clotting system. In general, significant clots will not form without activation of the extrinsic system. [Of course, it is completely artificial to try to separate these systems in this way, as they share many of the clotting factors and overlap all over the place. But for the sake of simplicity I shall talk about intrinsic and extrinsic as though they were different processes].

As with everything, however, there are exceptions to this rule i.e. situations where you have a healthy and intact endothelium and major clots can still form due to activation of the intrinsic clotting system. There are two main clinical situations where this happens:

- Deep vein thrombosis (DVT)

- Atrial fibrillation causing clots to form within the heart

If a patient lies immobile in a bed, in a plaster cast, there is a high risk that the blood can become virtually stationary within a vein. At which point the intrinsic clotting system can activate. This will start a blood clot forming within a vein (blood flow is too rapid and turbulent for this ever to happen in an artery). This is the basic mechanism behind a DVT.

Such clots are relatively weakly stuck together, in comparison to clots formed by the extrinsic pathway. Which means that a section of them, or the whole thing, can break off and travel up into the heart, then travel through the heart into the lungs where it can get stuck as the blood vessels narrow. This causes a pulmonary embolism (PE), which can often be fatal. [If the clot gets stuck in the heart this is inevitably fatal].

The way to protect against this is to use an anticoagulant that blocks some of the clotting factors of the intrinsic clotting system. The most common of these drugs would be warfarin, another would be low molecular weight heparin (LMWH). Many patients in hospital who are bed bound, for one reason or another, are given LMWH as prophylaxis against DVT and PE, until they get back on their feet. You cannot give heparin long term as toxicity builds up.

Warfarin has another major use, in Atrial Fibrillation. Atrial Fibrillation (AF) is a condition whereby the atria (upper chambers in the heart) do not contract in a regular fashion, instead they 'fibrillate', whereby they twitch very fast and in an irregular rhythm. When the atria fibrillate (for whatever reason), small blood clots can form within the chambers of the atria themselves. These can break free, then travel out of the heart and into the rest of the body, where they will get stuck. Most commonly, these clots travel up into the brain where they cause strokes. Thus, people with AF are given warfarin to prevent strokes.

This treatment is highly effective. However, although warfarin, LMWH and other new oral anticoagulation agents (NOACs) can prevent DVTs, PE, and one specific form of stroke, they have little benefit on atherosclerotic plaque formation, or death from heart disease/CHD.

In fact, some studies have shown that warfarin can accelerate plaque development – whilst reducing the risk of MIs (slightly):

'The present study demonstrates that VKA (warfarin) treatment is associated with accelerated calcification of atherosclerotic plaques in humans.' http://www. ncbi.nlm.nih.gov/pmc/articles/PMC3430691/

But there may be other things going on here as well. I only include this fact to emphasize that we are looking at highly complex systems, where the apparently obvious answer is unlikely to be correct. As H.L. Mencken famously said *'For every complex problem there is an answer that is clear, simple, and wrong.'*

In summary, although the intrinsic clotting system – which is mainly responsible for DVT, PE and a specific type of strokes in AF - is an important cause of death from certain forms of, what can be called, cardiovascular disease. It does not have much of a part to play in CVD due to plaque growth and development.

To understand heart attacks and ischaemic strokes we need to look more closely at clots created by the extrinsic system. This system, as mentioned before, is primarily triggered by injury to the endothelium. Perhaps the most concise description of how this works is from Wikipedia

'Coagulation begins almost instantly after an injury to the blood vessel has damaged the endothelium lining the vessel. Exposure of blood to the space under the endothelium initiates two processes: changes in **platelets,** *and the exposure of subendothelial* **tissue factor** *to plasma Factor VII, which ultimately leads to fibrin formation. Platelets immediately form a plug at the site of injury; this is called primary hemostasis. Secondary hemostasis occurs simultaneously: Additional coagulation factors or clotting factors beyond Factor VII respond in a complex cascade to form fibrin strands, which strengthen the platelet plug.'* https:// en.wikipedia.org/wiki/Coagulation

The main players in the initial thrombus formation are platelets (small 'sticky' cells that clump together to form a plug). After platelets have clumped together, fibrinogen acts to bind the thrombus together. Fibrinogen is a small strand of protein which, when many of them are stuck together, end-to-end, form fibrin. Fibrin is a bit like fishing line.

Long, thin, and very strong. It tangles itself around the developing thrombus, binding it together very strongly.

However, at this point it should be emphasized that thrombus contain almost every substance found in the bloodstream. They are not just made up of platelets and fibrin. Once a thrombus gets going everything is either dragged in, or plays a part in thrombus development: platelets, clotting factors, thrombin, white blood cells, red blood cells, lipoproteins, including LDL-C (aka 'bad' cholesterol). Indeed, if you choose to investigate it, you find connections between almost everything found in blood, and the process of coagulation. For example, platelets and LDL-C.

'Platelets and lipoproteins are intimately involved in the pathogenesis of a wide variety of disease including atherosclerosis, thrombosis, and coronary heart disease. Evidence accumulated over the years suggests the possibility of a direct relationship between plasma lipoproteins and the hemostatic function of platelets. A number of studies demonstrated that native LDL enhanced the platelet sensitivity to stimulation and induced platelet activation.' Yashika Gupta, V. Mallika* and D.K. Srivastava: 'INTERACTION OF LDL AND PLATELETS IN ISCHAEMIC AND ISCHAEMIC RISK SUBJECTS' Indian Journal of Clinical Biochemistry, 2005, 20 (1) 97 – 92

In short LDL-C (which is what we call 'bad' cholesterol, in another confusing and scientifically illiterate fashion) makes platelets more 'sticky' and thus thrombi more likely to form. So, here we can see a possible connection between LDL and increased risk of coagulation and thus, of course, CVD.

The enormous complexity of the clotting system is further revealed when we look at High Density Lipoproteins (HDL) a.k.a. 'good' cholesterol. It is widely accepted that HDL is protective against death from CVD. It is generally believed that this protection comes through the process of reverse cholesterol transport i.e. HDL sucks cholesterol out of plaques. [Which I do not believe]

However, this is probably not how HDL works. It has other important and potent effects on blood coagulation:

'Furthermore, HDL stimulates the endothelial production of nitric oxide and prostacyclin, which are potent inhibitors of platelet activation. Thus, HDL's antithrombotic actions are multiple and therefore, raising HDL may be an

important therapeutic strategy to reduce the risk of arterial and venous thrombosis.' http://www.ncbi.nlm.nih.gov/pubmed/24891399

Even red blood cells (RBCs) get in on the act. They appear to have little active role to play in the initial stages of blood clotting, but when a clot gets going RBCs are dragged, in and once this has happened they have a hugely important role in helping the clot to contract and stabilize. They aggregate within the 'core' of a clot, change their structure to polyhedrons and, essentially, work alongside fibrin to prevent the clot breaking apart. http://www.uphs.upenn.edu/news/News_Releases/2014/01/weisel/

RBCs have more recently been found to be a critical component of atherosclerotic plaques where they also seem to have an important role in accelerating plaque formation:

'In summary, potentially the erythrocyte (Red Blood Cell) is a new player in atheromatous lesion formation. The red cell membrane hides constituents that are lipid rich, can bind to macrophage scavenger receptors, and are associated with risk factors for atherosclerotic disease. The hypothesis that red cell membranes contribute to atheroma formation in coronary arteries is challenging.' http://www.ncbi.nlm.nih.gov/pmc/articles/PMC1767211/

In fact, red blood cell membranes are, possibly, the only structure in the human body that can become cholesterol crystals (so much cholesterol do they contain). When Virchow saw cholesterol in plaques what he was looking at, almost certainly, was cholesterol crystals. These have little to do with LDL-C, or any other form of lipoprotein. Their genesis is from RBC membranes.

'The view that apoptotic macrophages (dead macrophages) are the predominant source of cholesterol in progressive (atherosclerotic) lesions is being challenged as new lines of evidence suggest erythrocyte membranes contribute to a significant amount of free cholesterol in plaques.' https://www.researchgate.net/publication/5958670_Free_cholesterol_in_atherosclerotic_plaques_Where_does_it_come_from

Hopefully, at this point, things have not become too unstructured, or confusing. I wished to give the sense of the immense complexity of the systems operating here. Heart disease, or ischaemic heart disease or cardiovascular disease is not, and never was, the case of finding a few 'risk factors' that could explain everything. It is a dynamic and interconnected process. You cannot understand it, bit by bit, in a reductionist fashion. Knowing how each 'factor' works, tells you little about the entire system. It is like trying to describe a football match by accurately describing the pitch and the individual players, without watching the match.

At this point, before attempting to pull everything back into a coherent structure, I will provide one more example of how almost impossibly clever human clotting physiology is, and how many actors there are.

Lp(a)

Lp(a) is the shortened version of Lipoprotein (a). It has long been recognised in certain populations to have a role in increasing the risk of heart disease. Lp(a) is a form of lipoprotein. Interestingly it has exactly the same structure as LDL. The thing that we try to lower with statins and suchlike. Lp(a) could more accurately be called LDL(a). For that is what it actually is.

The only difference between LDL and Lp(a) is that Lp(a) has a different, and complex protein, attached to it, called apolipoprotein (a). This interesting thing about this protein is that it has exactly the same chemical structure as plasminogen. Plasminogen, not mentioned before, is an enzyme. It becomes incorporated into clots as they form. If it is activated, it cuts apart the strands of fibrin and helps to break the clot apart. Plasminogen, in turn, is activated by Tissue Plasminogen Activator (tPA). tPAcan be made artificially and is one of the original 'clotbusters' used in the acute treatment of strokes and heart attacks.

However, apolipoprotein (a) cannot be activated by tPA, because it is folded in a different fashion to plasminogen, which means that tPA simply bounces off. Thus thrombi containing a lot of Lp(a) are highly resistant to being broken down.

Why would the body produce such a thing? What could possibly be its purpose? The answer is that Lp(a) is found in animals that cannot synthesize vitamin C such as: great apes, fruit bats, hedgehogs and, of course, humans. Animals that cannot produce vitamin C are at risk of scurvy. The primary problem in scurvy is that connective tissue cannot be properly formed. Connective tissue supports small blood vessels (capillaries) and so they start to bleed profusely.

When this happens Lp(a), to put its action into its simplest fashion, acts as glue to plug the cracks in the capillaries and stop the bleeding. Thus, Lp(a) protects against some of the most serious effects of scurvy, because a clot that contains a lot of Lp(a) is completely resistant to plasminogen. Thus, once formed, such clots are very difficult to remove.

Of course collagen, and other connective tissue is also present in larger arteries and veins, so cracks can also develop here. Based on this knowledge, a researcher called Matthias Rath made the conjecture that vitamin C supplementation could protect against CVD by ensuring that the blood vessels were kept healthy, and did not have any cracks. No cracks, no activation of Lp(a) and thus far fewer clots forming.

Rath convinced Linus Pauling (the double Nobel prize winner) that this hypothesis was correct and Pauling spent the later years of his life promoting Vitamin C as a cure for heart disease and strokes – and many other things. For which he was widely ridiculed by the medical establishment.

The most interesting fact here is that having a high Lp(a) will not be a risk factor for heart disease in those with healthy endothelial cells and good supportive collagen – and other connective tissue. However, once the endothelium comes under attack (for whatever reason) a high Lp(a) level may well accelerate plaque formation. Which may explain why Lp(a) is a risk factor in some populations, and not others.

Plaques are clots

Whilst I have talked quite a lot about clotting and the endothelium and suchlike I have not yet outlined the overall process of atherosclerotic plaque development and growth. The underlying atherothrombosis hypothesis is that plaques are, simply, blood clots in various stages of repair (as outlined by Rokitansky).

This hypothesis is strongly supported by looking more closely at the structure of plaques. Here are two extracts from a paper in the *American*

Heart Journal called: *'A Definition of Advanced Types of Atherosclerotic Lesions and a Histological Classification of Atherosclerosis.'*

'The architecture of some multilayered fibroatheromas could also be explained by repeated disruptions of the lesion surface, hematomas, and thrombotic deposits. Organization (fibrosis) of hematomas and thrombi could be followed by renewed accumulation of macrophage foam cells and extracellular lipid between the newly formed fibrotic layer and the endothelial surface...

...The fissures and hematomas that underlie thrombotic deposits in many cases may recur, and small thrombi may reform many times. Repeated incorporation of small recurrent hematomas and thrombi into a lesion over months or years contributes to gradual narrowing of the arterial lumen. Some thrombi continue to enlarge and occlude the lumen of a medium-sized artery within hours or days.'
http://circ.ahajournals.org/content/92/5/1355.full

Simplifying the language here, what the *American Heart Journal* paper is saying is that a significant number of plaques effectively have the appearance of tree rings. With layer upon layer building up, one on top of the other. The only possible explanation for such a structure is for blood clots to have formed repeatedly, over the same spot. Of course, not all plaques look like this. I would conjecture that, attack by macrophages and other healing processes, turns many plaques into an amorphous mass with no particular structure. So the evidence of repeated thrombus formation is lost.

Another important point that I want to bring in here is covered by the last part of the second quote: *'Some thrombi continue to enlarge and occlude the lumen of a medium-sized artery within hours or days.'* What this is saying is that the final event in coronary artery disease, the complete blockage of a coronary artery, represents exactly the same process as caused the atherosclerotic plaque to develop and grow in the first place. Namely, thrombus forming over an area of artery wall damage. The final event is the same as all the other events.

Currently with the lipid, or cholesterol hypothesis we require two, essentially, unrelated physiological processes to take place. First LDL-C is absorbed into the artery wall causing inflammation, plaque development and growth. Once the plaque has reached a certain size, or becomes 'vulnerable' it can rupture leading to the final event.

A large blood clot forming over the plaque, blocking an artery and causing a heart attack. Or (if the clot forms in the arteries in the neck – carotid arteries), breaking off and travelling into the brain where it causes a stroke.

Two different processes with two sets of different causal 'factors?' Of course this might be true, but if we are looking at one disease, atherosclerotic plaque development, growth and final blockage, it is much more likely that it is actually caused by a single process, rather than two.

Returning to the actual process of plaque development and growth. The first step in the process is that endothelial cells become damaged, die, or are simply stripped off. At which point a blood clot forms over the area, stimulated primarily by the exposure of the blood to TF. Once the clot has stopped growing it is covered by EPCs, which form a new layer of endothelium over the top of the clot. The clot now lies within the artery wall where it is attacked by monocytes and macrophages. This breaks it down, and clear it away. This is normal, and healthy, and is probably happening all the time in most people.

However, problems start where this sequence happens at an increased frequency, over the same area. At which point, the repair processes become overwhelmed, and the plaque effectively starts to grow within the artery wall. When this starts to happen macrophages, working away to clear up the damage, become overwhelmed by the detritus, bloat up into foam cells – and can no longer function. Many of them then die, releasing the gunk of half-digested lipoproteins, red blood cell membranes, Lp(a), fibrin strands back into the plaque. This gunk is often referred to as the 'lipid core', although it contains far, far, more than lipid.

Adding to the problem, the endothelium lying on top of plaque tends to be less healthy than normal endothelium, it produces less NO etc. Which adds to the likelihood of repeated thrombus formation at the same point, although, until a reaches a significant size, it does not actually cause any narrowing of the artery. Under normal blood pressure the plaque is pushed outwards, causing a swelling of the artery wall, but no narrowing of the lumen.

The end game in this process is when the thin fibrous cap overlying the plaque ruptures, exposing the contents to the bloodstream. The contents are all highly thrombogenic, stimulating rapid blood clot formation which can fully block the artery. This causes a myocardial inflation, or heart attack.

Alternatively, plaque rupture leads to a clot forming on top of an atherosclerotic plaque in an artery in the neck. This will then break off and travel the brain where it gets stuck, causing an ischaemic stroke. And that is pretty much the atherothrombotic hypothesis.

Arteries and veins

Perhaps the strongest single piece of evidence in support of this hypothesis is that atherosclerotic plaques never form in veins (although there are a couple of exceptions to this, which I will explain later). Veins and arteries are bathed by exactly the same substances in the blood. The LDL-C level is exactly the same, for example, so why does not LDL-C becomes absorbed into vein walls, leading to plaques?

Arteries and veins also have exactly the same basic structure. Endothelium lies over smooth muscle with a deeper layer of connective tissue (the adventitia) beneath. Veins are thinner than arteries, as they have to deal with a much lower blood pressure, but otherwise they are identical. So why, in an otherwise healthy person, do plaques never, ever, develop in veins, or in any blood vessels in the lungs (veins or arteries). A fact that cannot be explained by the cholesterol hypothesis.

The answer is, of course, simple. Veins are exposed to far less biomechanical stress. The pressure in veins is far lower, the blood flow is less turbulent, and so the endothelium is far less 'stressed.' Indeed, the main areas where plaques develop in arteries, are at bifurcations (where one artery splits off another one) and in the heart, where the coronary arteries are exposed to the compression of the heart, every second of every minute and every hour of every day.

In short, in places where blood pressure is high, flow is turbulent, and the artery is under constant physical stress, the endothelium is far more likely to die, or be stripped off, and clots are far more likely to form. This level of endothelial 'stress' is not present in veins, so clots don't start here in the first place. Atherosclerotic plaques do not develop in the lungs either, where the blood pressure is far lower than in the arteries in the rest of the body. As with everything, there are exceptions to these rules:

- When veins are used in coronary artery bypass grafts

- When there is higher than normal blood pressure in the lungs (pulmonary hypertension)

'Our understanding of plaque instability may be extended to vein graft atherosclerosis, which appears to represent the end of a continuum of plaque instability. Compared with plaque in native coronary arteries, vein graft atheroma is more diffuse and vulnerable to rupture, and the consequences of plaque rupture in vein grafts seem to be associated with almost certain thrombotic occlusion within 7 to 12 years after surgery.' http://www.onlinepcd.com/article/S0033-0620(02)70017-0/abstract

As can be seen from this, if you take a vein from somewhere else in the body and use it in the heart as a bypass for a blocked artery (Coronary Artery Bypass Graft [CABG]), it is exposed to far higher blood pressure than it is designed for. In general CABGs last only a few years before becoming completely blocked by a large atherosclerotic plaque.

Atherosclerosis in pulmonary arteries/veins in far less common than atherosclerosis in veins used as bypass grafts, even when there is pulmonary hypertension (high blood pressure in the lungs). Probably because, even in pulmonary hypertension the blood pressure never gets as high as in the larger arteries in the rest of the body. But it can happen, as outlined in this case history. '*Primary pulmonary arteries atherosclerosis: discovering an unusual cause of death in forensic practice*':

'In the literature, there are few studies on atherosclerosis in the pulmonary artery in human beings and no cases similar to the one presented has been reported until now. The aim of the study is to describe a particularly unusual case of primary severe pulmonary atherosclerosis, in a 40-year old man...

Case presentation*: The patient had marked atherosclerosis in the pulmonary trunk and its branches, probably caused by a series of hemodynamic and endothelial changes, subsequent to the pulmonary hypertension.' Rom J Leg Med [20] 177-180 [2012]*

As can be seen from these examples, if you raise the blood pressure in a blood vessel that does not normally, ever, develop atherosclerosis, then atherosclerosis will develop. That is simple cause and effect. And the mechanism underlying it appears very straightforward. Increased biomechanical stress, damaging endothelial cells leading to repeated thrombus formation.

From this it seems clear that endothelial damage is the key event for the entire process. With a healthy and intact endothelial layer, none of the other processes, e.g. thrombus formation can occur to cause a plaque to start, and develop. And the single most important cause of endothelial damage is biomechanical stress. Without that, nothing happens. Which is why veins, and blood vessels in the lungs, never become atherosclerotic.

The next steps

If we assume that, in everyone, endothelium is being damaged in areas of high biomechanical stress, what makes the difference between plaques developing and growing, and nothing happening? Or, to put this another way. What are the possible 'causes' of CVD.

Using broad brush strokes, we can split the causes into three main system. Those that occur at:

- Initiation

- Development

- Repair

Initiation

By initiation I mean those factors – on top of biomechanical stress - that will increase endothelial damage, or make endothelial damage worse when it occurs.

One of the most extreme example of a factor that induces endothelial damage is Kawasaki's disease.

'Kawasaki disease (KD) is a systemic vasculitis of childhood with widespread vascular endothelial damage in the acute stage. Long-term complications, such as myocardial infarction and death, are recognized.' http://www.ncbi.nlm.nih.gov/pubmed/8901658

In Kawasaki's there is significant, if short term, endothelial damage. It is associated with a far higher death rate from CVD, and heart attacks can occur in very young children in some cases as young as three. However these are often due to ruptured aneurysms, normally thought to be a late stage manifestation of atherosclerosis, rather than classic blockage due to thrombus formation.

Another 'inflammatory' condition that damages endothelial cells is Systemic Lupus Erythematosus (SLE). Young women with SLE have a fifty-five fold (relative) increase in the risk of dying of heart disease. To put that in another way, that is a 5,500% increase in risk. http://www.ncbi.nlm.nih.gov/pubmed?term=9048514

The main reason for this risk is almost certainly due to significant damage to the endothelial cells – as outlined in a paper called *Imbalance between Endothelial Damage and Repair: A Gateway to Cardiovascular Disease in Systemic Lupus Erythematosus.'* [Sorry, there is a lot of jargon here, but two points are being made. In SLE there is a whole series of 'factors' that can, and do, damage the endothelium]:

'....endothelial dysfunction, one of the earliest steps of atherogenesis, has been demonstrated to occur in lupus patients even when they are naïve for cardiovascular disease. Currently known "endothelium-toxic" factors including type 1 interferon, proinflammatory cytokines, inflammatory cells, immune complexes, costimulatory molecules, neutrophils extracellular traps, lupus-related autoantibodies, oxidative stress, and dyslipidemia, coupled with the aberrant functions of the endothelial progenitor cells (EPC) which are crucial to vascular repair, likely tip the balance towards endothelial dysfunction and propensity to develop cardiovascular disease in lupus patients.' http://www.hindawi.com/journals/bmri/2014/178721/

This paper also mentions another key point – which is somewhat jumping ahead here. Namely that in SLE there is severe dysfunction of EPC function. This doubles the problem. Not only are mature endothelial cells under attack from many different toxins, the repair cells (EPCs) do not work properly.

Of course, Kawasaki's and SLE could be considered extreme conditions, with extreme effects on endothelial cells. They also create a short term increase in the risk of death from CVD. As does, incidentally, rheumatoid arthritis where, once again, we see significant endothelial damage/vasculitis, and a very high risk of CVD.

However, there are many other factors that can 'damage' the endothelium to a lesser degree [I am not referencing this list. I simply suggest going to Google and typing in endothelial damage followed by, any of the factors listed below]:

- Raised blood sugar levels/diabetes

- Cortisol (a key stress hormone)

- Cigarette smoking

- Air pollution

- Raised insulin levels

- High homocysteine levels

- Low levels of vitamin D

- Cocaine use

- etc.

In fact, this is a very simple game to play. If you can find any factor that increases endothelial damage, you will find that it is associated with an increased risk of CVD. Perhaps not the same increased risk in all populations with each factor. Equally, although all of factors listed above damage the endothelium, they do so to very different degrees. And so the increased risk can vary a few percentage points, in the case of air pollution, to 5,500% with SLE.

Development

Once endothelial damage has occurred, and a thrombus has been created, there are related factors that can become involved to build bigger and potentially more damaging blood clots. Very large clots can, of course, completely block arteries, and they can be fatal very early on in the disease process. There have even been cases of people dying of heart attacks, and strokes, due to a single large blood clot in an artery – with no underlying plaque at all. This is relatively uncommon, but far from unknown.

In general, however, the final clotting event takes place where there is a relatively large plaque that has already formed. And plaques can take years, even decades, to do so. Clot upon clot, repair upon repair and then, a major and fatal thrombosis. This would be the 'normal' sequence of events.

Whilst the development of plaques is primarily dependent on repeated endothelial damage, other factors can exacerbate the formation of bigger and more difficult to repair clots. For example, raised blood clotting factors such as: fibrinogen, antiphospholipid syndrome, factor V Leiden, raised Lp(a). With any of these blood clotting abnormalities you are more likely to die from CVD

If we look at, say, antiphospholipid syndrome (APS) a.k.a. Hughes syndrome. This is an autoimmune disease, in which 'antiphospholipid antibodies' react against proteins that bind to plasma membranes. It is more common in women than in men. The exact cause is not known, but the main abnormality is activation of the clotting system. with thrombosis and vascular disease.

'A major cause of morbidity and mortality in the context of the APS is the occurrence of thrombotic events, which may affect any arterial or venous vascular bed. Manifestations are common in these patients: deep vein thrombosis, pulmonary thromboembolism, stroke, transient ischemic attack, and coronary artery disease.' http://www.hindawi.com/journals/jir/2014/621270/

The treatment is lifelong anticoagulation. Unfortunately, this is normally started after someone has had a major CV event, and is subsequently found to have APS.

If we look purely at heart disease (CHD), perhaps the most important single clotting factor here is fibrinogen. In the Scottish Heart Study it was found that a high fibrinogen levels can increase the risk of CHD by over 300%.

'Fibrinogen is a strong predictor of coronary heart disease, fatal or non-fatal, new or recurrent, and of death from an unspecified cause, for both men and

women…. Comparing the two extreme fifths, the hazard ratios for coronary death are 3.01 and 3.42, and for all-cause mortality are 2.59 and 2.20, for men and women respectively.' http://www.ncbi.nlm.nih.gov/pubmed/9503176

Both APS and raised fibrinogen represent long-term/chronic risk factors (although fibrinogen can also be more transiently raised in stress, anxiety, smoking and depression). However, factors that raise blood clotting risk in the short term also increase CVD risk. For example, bacterial infection. It has long been known that bacterial infection greatly raises the short term risk of death from CVD. This is almost certainly due to the fact that bacteria can stimulate blood clotting directly.

'It has long been known that blood often coagulates during sepsis or bacterial infections, but this has generally been regarded as a host's immune and inflammatory response. It also has been known that bacteria can activate factors that precede coagulation, but it had not previously been known that bacteria can pass the coagulation threshold and cause blood clots to form. Once they form, the clots can grow and propagate. Although this may help prevent the dissemination of the bacteria through the host, it often leads to serious vascular damage due to blocked and injured blood vessels.' http://www.sciencedaily.com/ releases/2008/11/081102154519.htm

Just to look at one other factor, cocaine use. This both damages the endothelium and stimulates the entire blood clotting system.

'Our results demonstrated that chronic cocaine consumption alters several functions of the endothelium towards a pro-thrombotic condition and that some of those functions remain abnormal even after short-term drug withdrawal. These observations support the notion that endothelial dysfunction may play a key role in the pathogenesis of ischemic vascular disease observed in cocaine abusers.' http:// www.ncbi.nlm.nih.gov/pubmed/21601240

'In addition to systemic and coronary vascular changes, cocaine has been found to cause alterations in platelet function and coagulation, with multiple cases reported of acute coronary artery thrombosis after cocaine use.' http://www.ncbi. nlm.nih.gov/pmc/articles/PMC3228621/

Once again, it would be possible to go on, outlining factors that are thombophilic (stimulate blood clotting) that also increase the risk of CVD. There are many of them, but the general point is straightforward. Any factor that increases the risk of blood clotting is likely to cause CVD. Either chronic plaque growth, or acute episodes of blood clotting.

On the other hand, we can look at a couple of conditions that reduce blood clotting, and protect against CVD.

Two of the most common would be Haemophilia and Von Willebrand disease. Both are genetic conditions where there is a lack of various clotting factors, and an increased risk of bleeding. This can obviously bring other health problems, but both have clear benefits in CVD.

'In a survey among all haemophilia patients in The Netherlands, the Standardised Mortality Ratio (SMR) for cardiovascular mortality was 0.2.' doi:10.1160/TH10-07-0460 Thromb Haemost 2011; 105: 274–278

A standardised mortality ratio of 0.2 means that the risk of dying is 20% that of the surrounding population. Another way to frame this is that haemophilia represents a fivefold reduction in risk of dying of CVD. Since synthetic clotting factors have been made available, the reduction in risk of CVD has attenuated.

In Von Willebrand Disease there is a significant reduction in the clotting factor known as Von Willebrand factor (VWF)). This stimulates platelet adhesion, a key process in the creation of thrombi. Patients with this condition have a greatly reduced risk of both stroke and death from heart attacks. Around a fifty per cent reduction in total CVD risk. http://www.ncbi.nlm.nih.gov/pubmed/23506463

Repair

After endothelial damage has occurred, and a blood clot has formed, the next stage is repair. This is normally achieved through a combination of EPCs covering over the thrombus, followed by a clear up operation, primarily coordinated by monocytes and macrophages. Therefore, anything that interferes with this will most likely increase the risk of CVD.

There are a number of conditions that reduce the production of EPCs. Probably the most important of these is age. As people get older the synthesis of EPCs in the bone marrow reduces. Which could well explain why CVD kills far more older people than younger people, with the death rate accelerating in an almost logarithmic progression.

Other things that damage EPC production are chronic kidney disease (CKD). This is associated with a greatly increased risk of CVD.

'Most data available support the notion that EPC numbers and function are reduced in CKD patients, and this altered EPC biology may contribute to the high cardiovascular burden of CKD patients due to compromised reparative processes in the vascular system.' http://ndt.oxfordjournals.org/content/25/2/341.full

Obstructive sleep apnoea (OSA) is another condition where EPC production is impaired. OSA is a condition where people, basically, stop breathing at night for periods of time. It is quite common, and it is associated with an increased risk of CVD.

'In most studies (in OSA), a reduction in circulating EPCs has emerged. The possible mechanisms underlying the decrease in the number or function of EPCs include prolonged inflammation response, oxidative stress, increased sympathetic activation, physiological adaptive responses of tissue to hypoxia, reduced EPC mobilization, EPC apoptosis, and functional impairment in untreated OSA.' http:// www.ncbi.nlm.nih.gov/pmc/articles/PMC3804572/

As before, if a factor can be identified that damages the normal EPC development, or function, there will be an increased risk of CVD.

Obviously, there are many other aspects to 'repair' when it comes to plaques. Perhaps the most important is the healthy and efficient functioning of monocytes and macrophages. Both of these white blood cells have a crucial function in clearing up damaged tissue, bacteria, viruses and the like. The macrophage primarily by invagination. A process by which the macrophage will first oxidize the material – often to kill it – it then grows around the material to pinch it off, then ingest it.

Putting it very simply, macrophages eat the plaque and remove it. Macrophages and monocytes work closely in unison to achieve this – macrophages develop from monocytes.

So, anything that can interfere with the effective functioning of monocytes and macrophages will mean that the clear up process does not work so well and the plaque will grow faster. In fact, within large plaques you will often find large bloated macrophages, called 'foam cells' which have lost the ability to digest anything more, or even move. Some of these macrophages simply split apart, and die.

'Macrophage apoptosis (death) is an important feature of atherosclerotic plaque development. Research directed at understanding the functional consequences of macrophage death in atherosclerosis has revealed opposing roles for apoptosis in atherosclerotic plaque progression. In early lesions, macrophage apoptosis limits lesion cellularity and suppresses plaque progression. In advanced lesions, macrophages apoptosis promotes the development of the necrotic core, a key factor in rendering plaques vulnerable to disruption and in acute lumenal thrombosis (a heart attack).'

Again, things are not completely straightforward. At a certain, early, stage of plaque development macrophage death can protect from plaque growth. Later on, it can be very damaging.

Does the atherothrombotic theory fit the facts?

Clearly, any scientific hypothesis should fit with observed facts, and should not be contradicted by them. Contradiction, or confirmation, is notoriously difficult to achieve in absolute terms in medicine, as there are often so many variables in play (known and unknown).

For example, the cholesterol hypothesis is currently the most widely accepted hypothesis about heart disease. Namely that LDL-C, when the level is high, is absorbed into the arterial wall, causing inflammation and plaques. This hypothesis appeared to have been very strongly supported by the fact that statins – which lower LDL-C – also reduce the risk of CVD. Many people feel that this evidence was, in fact, overwhelming proof of the cholesterol hypothesis. (Even if other LDL-C lowering agents have not shown any benefit).

However, it is more likely that statins actually operate in a complete different way. It has been found, in many studies, that statins promote NO synthesis in endothelial cells, they also increase EPC production and function:

'Statins are potent drugs with a variety of cardiovascular protective effects which appear to occur independent of cholesterol reduction. The vasculoprotective effects

of statins might be due to their direct effect on endothelial cells leading to improved nitric oxide (NO) bioavailability....The functional improvement and increased homing capacity of endothelial progenitor cells induced by statin treatment might reverse impaired functional regeneration capacities seen in patients with risk factors for coronary artery disease or documented active coronary artery disease.'
http://www.ncbi.nlm.nih.gov/pubmed/15238818

Indeed, the effects of statins, when viewed in a different way, support the atherothrombotic hypothesis of CVD more powerfully than the cholesterol hypothesis.

In fact, every pharmaceutical agent found to significantly reduce the risk of CVD either protects the endothelium, reduces the propensity of blood clotting or improves EPC production or function. A non-exhaustive list would be:

- Aspirin

- Clopidogrel

- Warfarin

- Statins

- Ace-inhibitors

- tPA

On the other hand, drugs that increase blood coagulation increase the risk of CVD. For example:

- Steroids/corticosteroids

- Non-steroidal anti-inflammatory drugs (NSAIDs)

- Proton Pump Inhibitors (PPIs) – they reduce NO synthesis in endothelial cells

- Avastin (a cancer drug)

Avastin is particularly interesting, in terms of this discussion, in that it inhibits a substance known as Vascular Endothelial Growth Factor (VEGF). Endothelial progenitor cell production is stimulated by vascular endothelial growth factor-A (VEGF-A) http://www.ncbi.nlm.nih.gov/pubmed/24022223

VEGF also stimulates endothelial cell maturation, and function and NO synthesis. So, it should come as no surprise to find that Avastin increases the development of atherosclerotic plaques, and also increases the risk of heart disease.

'Systemic VEGF inhibition disrupts endothelial homeostasis and accelerates atherogenesis, suggesting that these events contribute to the clinical cardiovascular adverse events of VEGF-inhibiting therapies.' http://www.ncbi.nlm.nih.gov/pubmed/23561917

Moving away from the effects of drugs. Does the atherothrombotic hypothesis fit observations of various diseases? As previously mentioned diseases that create endothelial damage also increase the risk of CVD, e.g. SLE, Rheumatoid arthritis and Kawasaki's. Diseases that increase blood coagulation also increase the risk of CVD e.g. Hughes disease and Factor V Leiden. Diseases that damage EPC production increase the risk of CVD e.g. Chronic Kidney Disease and many forms of cancer.

However, probably the most important disease – in terms of sheer numbers – is type II diabetes. It has been observed that type II diabetes increases the risk of death from CVD by a factor of three, in men, and a factor of five, in women.

As you might expect, people with type II diabetes have significant endothelial dysfunction. This may not be due to the raised blood sugar levels themselves:

'Both insulin resistance and endothelial dysfunction appear to precede the development of overt hyperglycemia in patients with type 2 diabetes. Therefore, in patients with diabetes or insulin resistance, endothelial dysfunction may be a critical early target for preventing atherosclerosis and cardiovascular disease.' http://www.ncbi.nlm.nih.gov/pmc/articles/PMC2350146/

However, endothelial function is a key abnormality in type II diabetes and, in part, explains the raised risk of CVD. But of course, type II diabetes also creates a pro-thrombotic state with many different clotting factors raised, and there is a significant reduction in EPC numbers. So, type II diabetes creates all of the factors needed to increase CVD risk.

Finally, to look at stress. This is a vast subject which I will not look at in any great detail here. I will split stress into acute and chronic. Acute stress can be physical, or psychological. Chronic stress tends to be psychological.

In both case the 'flight of fight' system is activated. This has a wide range of different effects. Raised blood pressure, increased heart rate, diversion of blood supply from the GI tract to muscles. Raised blood sugar levels. All physiological systems are affected on one way or another. It should come as no surprise to find that in a situation of acute psychological, or physical stress, the blood becomes hypercoagulable.

'Stress-induced activation of the sympathoadrenal medullary system activates both the coagulation and fibrinolysis system resulting in net hypercoagulability. The evolutionary interpretation of this physiology is that stress-hypercoagulability protects a healthy organism from excess bleeding should injury occur in fight-or-flight situations.' http://www.ncbi.nlm.nih.gov/pmc/articles/PMC4386736/

So, it should be no surprise to find that acute psychological stress often immediately precedes heart attacks (myocardial infarction)

'Observational studies have found repeatedly that patients report excessive anger, anxiety, sadness, grief, or acute stress immediately prior to onset of MI, and recent meta-analyses summarizing these findings reported strong associations between MI occurrence and many of these acute emotions.' http://www.ncbi.nlm.nih.gov/pmc/articles/PMC3549526/

This should not be surprising and, in fact, with the widely accepted knowledge that the final event in a heart attack is the sudden development of a blood clot, that blocks a coronary artery. In fact, this observation fits with both the cholesterol hypothesis and the atherothrombotic hypothesis.

Acute physical stress can also induce blood clotting, and an increase risk of heart attacks. As can getting up in the morning. A time when stress hormones increase blood coagulation.

'Myocardial infarction occurs most often in the early morning hours, perhaps partly because of the increase in catecholamine-induced platelet aggregation and increased serum concentrations of plasminogen activator inhibitor-1 (PAI-1) that occur after awakening.' http://emedicine.medscape.com/article/155919-clinical

Indeed, there is no dispute that acute physical and/or psychological stress are very important triggers for heart attacks and strokes.

Malcolm Kendrick, MD

General Practitioner in the UK
Independent Researcher
www.drmalcolmkendrick.org

Chapter Thirteen

Statins and Cancer: Cause or Cure?

Paul J. Rosch, MD, Luca Mascitelli, MD, Mark R. Goldstein, MD

Abstract

Statins have been referred to as "miracle drugs" because they not only prevent coronary heart disease, but may also reduce the risk of unrelated diseases like Alzheimer's and cancer, despite evidence that the reverse might occur. Any alleged benefits are usually attributed to diverse immunomodulatory, anti-inflammatory, anticoagulant and other pleiotropic effects of statins. Interfering with cellular cholesterol synthesis could theoretically play a role in some malignancies; *in vitro* studies have shown statins to exhibit anti-proliferative properties mediated by a statin induced reduction in mevalonate and downstream geranylgeranylated proteins. However, statins have other pleiotropic immunomodulatory actions that might promote existing cancer. Possible explanations for these conflicting views will be discussed, as well as the difficulty in proving any cause-effect relationship. Importantly, only well-designed prospective trials, free of industry sponsorship, will determine if statins cause or cure cancer

Are Statins Panaceas Or Poisons?

Opinions about statin efficacy and safety tend to be polarized because of the difficulty in obtaining accurate information on the incidence and prevalence of adverse side effects.

Symptoms like increasing forgetfulness, fatigue and inability to concentrate are often attributed to getting older. The incidence of prostate and other cancers also increase with age.[1,2]. In addition, many statin patients, particularly the elderly, frequently take multiple

271

medications that might increase or decrease susceptibility to side effects such as cancer. Adverse side effects of drugs are frequently minimized or concealed in drug company sponsored clinical trials[3,4]. Adverse drug side effects are frequently minimized or ignored in drug company sponsored clinical trials[3,4] and cancer may not surface until decades after a statin has been approved[5]. Symptoms are not recognized as side effects. In one study, almost 4% of all hospitalizations were due to adverse drug reactions that were not recognized by the attending physicians at the time of admission[6]. When patients inquire about the possibility that a statin is causing their problem, physicians often deny or dismiss this as being very unlikely or impossible, even when there is no other plausible explanation[7]. This would be more apt to occur with cancer since publications can be cited to support their opinion.

Studies that do show a likely causal relationship (or are critical of statins and the theory that cholesterol causes coronary disease) are difficult to publish because medical journals do not want to lose their lucrative profits from drug company reprints and advertisements[8]. Studies sponsored by the pharmaceutical industry are also more likely to be published in higher impact factor journals than are studies without industry funding[9]. Only a very small percentage of statin side effects are reported to MedWatch, the FDA Adverse Event Reporting System (FAERS). The majority comes from pharmaceutical companies because regulations mandate this and there are costly penalties for noncompliance. Reporting by health care professionals and consumers is voluntary and only 27 states require hospitals to notify their health departments of adverse drug side effects. There are numerous other criticisms of the current reporting system[10,11]. Side effects shown to be due to statins are not reported by physicians to avoid lawsuits and unfavorable publicity.

Numerous studies from around the world confirm the association between low cholesterol and the subsequent increased risk of various cancers[12-22]. As previously noted, all statins are carcinogenic in laboratory animals but whether this is a direct effect or related to cholesterol lowering is not clear[23]. Because of this and other disabling side effects, many people consider statins to be poisons that should be avoided at any cost. At the other end of the spectrum, enthusiasts believe that statins are so safe they should be added to the water supply like fluoride or given to everyone 50 or older[24].

Are Statins The Holy Grail For Cancer?

That was the title of an editorial by Mayo Clinic authorities[25] who cited meta-analyses and observational studies showing that statin use was associated with reduced risk of prostate, hepatocellular and esophageal cancer[26-29]. How these benefits are achieved is not clear, but it is suggested that in addition to lowering cholesterol, statins may exert antineoplastic effects through blockage of mevalonate and other pathways, or proapoptotic, antiangiogenic, and immunomodulatory effects that prevent cancer growth[30,31].

Support comes from a *New England Journal of Medicine* article that studied the relationship between statin use prior to cancer diagnosis and cancer-related mortality in the entire Danish population from 1995-2009 in adults over the age of 40. It found that statins were associated with a 15% reduction in cancer and all cause mortality in 13 malignancies, as well as improved survival in the four most frequent cancers; lung, colorectal, prostate and breast[32]. The authors also cited evidence that interference with cellular cholesterol synthesis may inhibition cancer growth and metastasis[30,31,33,34]. In addition, statins have been linked to inhibiting key cellular functions and proliferation in cancer cells with resulting antiproliferative effects due to inhibition of key cellular functions in cancer cells[31,35]. Other studies also imply that in addition to prevention, statins can be used to treat cancer of the prostate[36,37], breast[38,39] and kidney[40,41]. It has been suggested that this may also be due to blockage of the mevalonate pathway since mevalonate has been shown to promote the growth of neoplastic and preneoplastic cells[42].

However, a closer look at the study[32] suggests that higher baseline cholesterol levels might actually improve survival in patients with cancer. Baseline total cholesterol concentration of statin-treated populations is often higher than those of the general population[43]. On the other hand, low plasma levels of low-density lipoprotein cholesterol have been shown to be robustly associated with an increased risk of future cancer[44]. Moreover, in a long-term follow-up study, moderate total serum cholesterol was found to have a protective effect on 40-year cancer mortality[45], and an analysis of large statin randomized controlled trials demonstrated an inverse association between on-treatment low-density lipoprotein cholesterol levels and incident cancer[46]. Of note, in the Danish study[32], the absence of a dose–response relationship for statins and cancer-related mortality, accompanied by an increase in cardiovascular mortality in statin-treated patients, clearly suggests that statin use selected the healthy statin user or unselected the unhealthy cancer patients with low cholesterol.

However, the National Cancer Institute (NCI) Fact Sheet indicates that it is funding a study to determine whether lovastatin can reverse precancerous changes in atypical or dysplastic nevi to prevent them from progressing to melanoma skin cancers[47]. It also states that "Two large cardiovascular clinical trials have demonstrated a significant reduction in skin cancer among patients taking lipid-lowering drugs" and "various human trials and preclinical studies suggest that statins may have chemopreventive activity against skin cancer". No references are provided to support this, and it is possible that statins are contributing to the current epidemic of nonmelanoma skin cancers[48]. The agency is also funding a study on colorectal cancer based on a report that statins can reduce risk of this by 47%[49], despite numerous large-scale studies showing no such effect[50-52].

Immunomodulatory action of statins

In vitro studies have shown statins to exhibit anti-proliferative, pro-apoptotic, anti-invasive and radio-sensitization properties mediated by a statin induced reduction in mevalonate and downstream geranylgeranylated proteins[53,54]. These pleiotropic effects of statins might actually prevent the initiation and promotion of cancer. However, statins have other pleiotropic actions that might promote existing cancer. For example, the short-term beneficial effect of statin therapy after cardiac transplantation has been attributed to a statin induced reduction in natural killer (NK) cell cytotoxicity[55]. However, a chronic attenuation of NK cell function will decrease the innate cell-mediated immune response to tumor cells[56]. It is known that statin therapy increases circulating bone marrow derived endothelial progenitor cells (EPCs) with enhanced functional activity[57]. Although EPCs might augment the neovascularisation of ischemic tissue and wounds, they might promote tumor growth by supporting angiogenesis[58,59]. Not surprisingly, the levels of circulating EPCs correlate directly with the stage of invasive breast cancer, and circulating EPCs are significantly higher in stages III and IV when compared with stages I and II breast cancer patients[60]. Likewise, circulating EPC levels are much higher in patients with aggressive compared with less aggressive non-Hodgkin's lymphoma[61]. Recently, statins have been shown to increase the numbers and functionality of peripheral regulatory T-cells (Tregs), in vivo, by inducing the transcription factor forkhead box P3[62].

Among the various mechanisms involved in cancer development, mounting evidence has found that the dysfunction of the immune system may exert an important role. In a malignant environment, immune system homeostasis and control of self-tolerance are significantly altered. Tregs are immunosuppressive cells implicated in autoimmune diseases and malignant processes. They have suppressive functions against the autologous immune reaction, which in turn exerts a fundamental role in the immunosurveillance of malignant tumors. In fact, enhanced Treg numbers and functionality might impair the host anti-tumor immune response[63]. Additionally, Tregs have been shown to promote the induction of alternatively activated monocytes/macrophages, which contribute to hampered anti-tumor immunity[64]. Compared with normal controls, peripheral Treg numbers are increased significantly in cancer patients[65]. In numerous solid tumor types, the accumulation of Tregs predict a reduction in patient survival[66]. In animal models, depletions of Tregs have resulted in total tumor rejection[67].

Therefore, even though the aforementioned immunosuppressive effects of statins might be beneficial in reducing inflammatory cells in arterial walls and promoting plaque stability, they might be detrimental by suppressing antitumor immune responses resulting in microscopic foci of tumor cells escaping dormancy and proliferating[66].

Indeed, it appears that statins increase the risk of cancer in the elderly, who are more likely to harbor cancer cells because of their advanced age and associated immunosenescence[68]. This was evident in several statin trials. In the Prospective Study of Pravastatin in the Elderly at Risk (PROSPER), cancer incidence was increased significantly in subjects randomized to pravastatin over the 3.2-year study period[69]. The mean age at trial entry was 75 years, and the decrease in cardiovascular disease mortality was offset by an equal increase in cancer mortality, resulting in unchanged overall mortality. The post hoc analysis of the Long-Term Intervention with Pravastatin in Ischemic Disease (LIPID) study demonstrated a significant increased cancer incidence in elderly subjects (65–75 years) randomized to pravastatin over the 6-year trial[70]. Furthermore, a secondary analysis of the Treating to New Targets study demonstrated that subjects randomized to atorvastatin 80 mg daily exhibited a trend towards increased death compared to those randomized to atorvastatin 10 mg daily; the increase in death was largely from cancer[71]. It is certainly plausible that the immunomodulatory effect of statins explains the increase in cancer seen in elderly subjects exposed to statin therapy, and there may be a dose–response relationship.

Notably, immunosuppression represents an emerging risk factor for nonmelanoma skin cancer (NMSC). In fact, immunosuppressive treatments seem to act as a catalyst for skin carcinogenesis as they increase the frequency, number, and aggressiveness of such tumors. Recently, the characteristics of specific components of the immune system associated with the development of NMSC among organ transplant recipients have been highlighted[72]. It was reported that kidney transplant recipients with previous NMSC had a higher number of Tregs present in the peripheral circulation than recipients without NMSC. In addition, there was an overrepresentation of Tregs within NMSC removed from kidney transplant recipients compared with matched NMSC from patients who were not taking immunosuppressive treatments. Furthermore, during prospective follow-up, in the select group of transplant recipients who had previous NMSC and therefore were at high risk for new NMSC development, it was found that a high number of Tregs and low number of NK cells improved the accuracy of predicting a more than a six fold increased risk for developing a new NMSC. Disturbingly, the immunomodulatory pleiotropic actions of statins resemble the immune phenotype, which predicts risk for post-transplantation NMSC. Data from randomized trials with statins are revealing. A systematic review found moderate evidence of an increased incidence of NMSC (median risk ratio 1.6, range 1.2–2.2) with statin drugs[73]. Specifically, in the first 2 simvastatin trials, the Scandinavian Simvastatin Survival Study (4S)[74], and the Heart Protection Study (HPS)[75], NMSC was observed more often in the treatment groups.

In the 4S, there were 13 NMSC in the statin group (0.6%) and six (0.3%) in the placebo group[74]. In the HPS, in simvastatin-allocated participants there were 243 NMSC (2.4%) vs. 202 (2.0%) in placebo-allocated individuals[75]. The difference is statistically significant if the results from both studies are combined (in simvastatin groups, 256 of the 12,490 participants; and in control groups, 208 of the 12,490 participants; P = 0.028). After publication of the four trials included in the review[73], NMSC have been excluded in all reports from subsequent statin trials for unknown reasons. Furthermore, an observational study from Finland has shown a standardized incidence ratio (SIR) for Merkel cell carcinoma (MCC) of 1.94 in ages 60–74 and a SIR of 3.16 in ages<60 years among statin users compared to statin nonusers, implying that statin therapy might be increasing the risk of MCC in atypically younger individuals[76]. A similar phenomenon was noted in patients with immunocompromising states[77,78]. Of note, MCC is a rare and aggressive neuroendocrine skin cancer associated with immunosuppression and a novel polyomavirus; its incidence has increased several fold in Denmark since the mid-1980s corresponding to the introduction and increasing use of statins in clinical practice[79].

Also women may be particularly sensible to the immunomodulatory action of statins. Among women randomized to pravastatin (mean age: 59 years) in the Cholesterol and Recurrent Events (CARE) study, a 5-year prospective randomized secondary prevention trial, breast cancer was significantly increased[80]. Breast cancer occurred in 1 patient of 290 in the placebo group and 12 patients of 286 in the pravastatin group (P<0.002) over the trial duration, and some of the cancers were recurrences. This was not reported in other prospective statin trials, but it is of concern since there are observational data suggesting an increase in breast cancer of 28% among elderly women on statin therapy > three years[81]. It has been recently reported that higher 3-hydroxy-3-methylglutaryl-coenzyme-A reductase (HMG-CoAR) expression in breast cancer cells, in vivo, is associated with a less aggressive phenotype[82]. Therefore, the inhibition of HMG-CoAR by statins might increase the aggressiveness of breast cancer. Additionally, statins have been found to activate PI- 3K and ERK1/2 signaling pathways,[83,84] which could promote the invasive growth of ductal carcinoma in situ[85]. These data are particularly disturbing since the prevalence of microscopic breast cancer at autopsy has been reported to be 39% among women 40–49 years dying without clinically diagnosed cancer[86]. A population-based case–control study of long-term (≥10 years) statin use among postmenopausal woman showed a two-fold risk of developing both invasive ductal and lobular breast carcinoma compared with never users of statins[87]. Moreover, in a recent case–control study, it was found that statin use was associated with thyroid cancer in female patients[88].

Finally, mounting evidence has found that statin therapy can lead to new-onset of diabetes[89]. Interestingly, certain groups of patients are at particular increased risk for statin induced diabetes; they include both women[89,90] and the elderly[89]. Long-term observational data have indicated that diabetes is positively and significantly associated with all-cause and cancer mortality[91]. Also prediabetes has been shown to be associated with an increased risk of cancer[92]. Furthermore, statin therapy has been associated with an increase in fasting blood insulin levels[89], and chronic hyperinsulinemia can lead to increased expression of insulin-like growth factor-1 which has mitogenic effects[93]. Therefore, it is also possible that people prescribed long-term statin therapy might be at increased risk of cancer resulting from the off-target diabetogenic and hyperinsulinemic effects of these drugs.

Conclusions

We express concerns on the use of statins to prevent cardiovascular disease in certain segments of the population. They include the elderly, women and those individuals with a clinical history of cancer. Primary and secondary prevention trials largely have excluded patients with a history of cancer. In real practice situations, statins are commonly used in patients with prevalent cancer. We feel this is a leap of faith, and the shorthand long-term safety of these agents needs further prospective evaluation among patients with a history of cancer. It is unlikely that trends will be noticed as these drugs are routinely used in clinical practice, since the reporting of side effects of drugs is incomplete and the prevalence of cancer is large. Likewise, more prospective data need to be produced on the safety of statins in the elderly and immunodepressed population, who are more likely susceptible to the immunosuppressive and tumor promoting effects of statins, because of their immunosuppressive state and increased chance of harboring microscopic foci of cancer cells. Equally important, more prospective data are needed on the safety of statins in women and people at risk to develop diabetes, and high-dose statin use, in general.

Key issues

- Low cholesterol has been shown to be associated with an increased risk of cancer in numerous studies although it is difficult to prove this as well as other cause-effect relationships.

- Statins are carcinogenic in laboratory animals with blood levels similar to those seen in clinical practice.

- *In vitro* studies have shown statins to exhibit anti-proliferative properties.

- Other studies report that statins prevent risk of prostate, hepatocellular and esophageal cancer or can be effective in treating these and other malignancies.

- It has been demonstrated that these and other alleged statin benefits are due to purported pleiotropic effects rather than lipid lowering.

- Statins have other pleiotropic immunomodulatory actions that might promote existing cancer.

- Therapy guidelines have replaced lowering LDL cholesterol as a goal with an arbitrary 10-year risk assessment that would make tens of millions of additional individuals eligible for treatment.

- Statin trials have typically randomized subjects free of prevalent cancers and have been about 5 years in duration. Long-term follow-up data are limited, particularly for the development of cancer.

- More prospective data need to be produced in particular segments of the population on the safety of statins who might be more likely susceptible to the immunosuppressive and potentially tumor promoting effects of statins

Paul J. Rosch*, MD, Luca Mascitelli**, MD, Mark R. Goldstein***, MD

*Clinical Professor of Medicine and Psychiatry
New York Medical College
Chairman, The American Institute of Stress
stress124@optonline.net

**Luca Mascitelli, MD
Medical Service
Comando Brigata alpina "Julia"/Multinational Land Force
Udine, Italy
lumasci@libero.it

***Independent Investigator
markrgoldstein@comcast.net

References

1. Ukraintseva SV, Yashin AI. Individual aging and cancer risk. Dem Res 2003;9:163-96.

2. DeGregori J. Challenging the axiom: does the occurrence of oncogenic mutations truly limit cancer development with age? Oncogene 2013;32:1869-75.

3. Turner, EH, Matthews AM, Linardatos E, et al. Selective publication of antidepressant trials and its influence on apparent efficacy. N Engl J Med 2008;358:252–60.

4. Bero L, Oostvogel F, Bacchetti P, Kirby L. Factors associated with findings of published trials of drug-drug comparisons: Why some statins appear more efficacious than others. PLoS Med 2007;4:e184.

5. Ravnskov U. Rosch PJ, McCully KS. The statin-low cholesterol-cancer conundrum. QJM 2012;105:383-8.

6. Dormann H, Criegee-Rieck M, Neubert A, et al. Lack of awareness of community-acquired adverse drug reactions upon hospital admission: Dimensions and consequences of a dilemma. Drug Safety 2003;26:353–62.

7. Golomb BA, McGraw JJ, Evans MA, Dimsdale JE. Physician response to patient reports of adverse drug effects. Drug Safety 2007;30:669-75.

8. Richard Smith: Medical journals: a gaggle of golden geese BMJ July 3, 2012. http://blogs. bmj.com/bmj/2012/07/03/richard-smith-medical-journals-a-gaggle-of-golden-geese/

9. Jefferson T, Di Pietrantonj C, Debalini MG, Rivetti A, Demicheli V. Relation of study quality, concordance, take home message, funding, and impact in studies of influenza vaccines: systematic review. BMJ 2009;338:b354.

10. http://www.fda.gov/Drugs/GuidanceComplianceRegulatoryInformation/ Surveillance/AdverseDrugEffects/default.htm

11. Strom BL. How the drug safety system should be changed. JAMA. 2006;295:2072-5.

12. Williams RR, Sorlie PD, Feinleib M, McNamara PM, Kannel WB, Dawber TR. Cancer incidence by levels of cholesterol. JAMA 1981;245:247–52.

13. Salmond CE, Beaglehole R, Prior IA. Are low cholesterol values associated with excess mortality? BMJ 1985;290:422–4.

14. Schatzkin A, Hoover RN, Taylor PR, et al. Serum cholesterol and cancer in the NHANES I epidemiologic followup study. National Health and Nutrition Examination Survey. Lancet 1987;2:298–301.

15. Sherwin R, Wentworth D, Cutler J, et al. Serum cholesterol levels and cancer mortality in 361,662 men screened for the Multiple Risk Factor Intervention Trial. JAMA 1987;257:943-8.

16. Tornberg SA, Holm LE, Carstensen JM, Eklund GA. Cancer incidence and cancer mortality in relation to serum cholesterol. J Natl Cancer Inst 1989;81:1917–21.

17. Isles CG, Hole DJ, Gillis CR, Hawthorne VM, Lever AF. Plasma cholesterol, coronary heart disease, and cancer in the Renfrew and Paisley survey. BMJ 1989;298:920–4.

18. Kreger BE, Anderson KM, Schatzkin A, Splansky GL. Serum cholesterol level, body mass index, and the risk of colon cancer. The Framingham Study. Cancer 1992;70:1038–43.

19. Jacobs D, Blackburn H, Higgins M et al.: Report of the Conference on Low Blood Cholesterol: Mortality Associations. Circulation 1992; 86:1046-60.

20. Schuit AJ, Van Dijk CE, Dekker JM, Schouten EG, Kok FJ. Inverse association between serum total cholesterol and cancer mortality in Dutch civil servants. Am J Epidemiol 1993;137:966–76.

21. Chang AK, Barrett-Connor E, Edelstein S. Low plasma cholesterol predicts an increased risk of lung cancer in elderly women. Prev Med 1995;24:557–62.

22. Steenland K, Nowlin S, Palu S. Cancer incidence in the National Health and Nutrition Survey I. Follow-up data: diabetes, cholesterol, pulse and physical activity. Cancer Epidemiol Biomarkers Prev 1995;4:807–11.

23. Newman TB, Hulley SB. Carcinogenicity of lipid-lowering drugs. JAMA 1996;275:55-60.

24. Ebrahim S, Casas JP. Statins for all by the age of 50 years? Lancet 2012;380:545-7.

25. Singh PP, Singh S. Statins - the Holy Grail for cancer? Ann Transl Med 2013;1:1-3.

26. Bansal D, Undela K, D'Cruz S, et al. Statin use and risk of prostate cancer: a meta-analysis of observational studies. PLoS One 2012;7:e46691

27. Singh S, Singh PP, Singh AG, et al. Statins are associated with a reduced risk of hepatocellular cancer: A systematic review and meta-analysis. Gastroenterology 2013;144:323-32.

28. Singh S, Singh AG, Singh PP, et al. Statins and the risk of esophageal cancer: A systematic review and meta-analysis. Am J Gastroenterol 2012;107:S11-2.

29. Singh S, Singh AG, Singh PP, et al. Statins are associated with reduced risk of esophageal cancer, particularly in patients with Barrett's esophagus: A systematic review and meta-analysis. Clinical Gastroenterology and Hepatology 2013;11:620–9.

30. Demierre MF, Higgins PD, Gruber SB, et al. Statins and cancer prevention. Nat Rev Cancer 2005;5:930-42.

31. Chan KK, Oza AM, Siu LL. The statins as anticancer agents. Clin Cancer Res 2003;9:10-9.

32. Nielsen SF, Nordestgaard BG, Bojesen SE. Statin use and reduced cancer-related mortality. N Engl J Med 2012;367:1792-802.

33. Denoyelle C, Vasse M, Korner M, et al. Cerivastatin, an inhibitor of HMG-CoA reductase, inhibits the signaling pathways involved in the invasiveness and metastatic properties of highly invasive breast cancer cell lines: an in vitro study. Carcinogenesis 2001; 22:1139-48.

34. Kusama T, Mukai M, Iwasaki T, et al. Inhibition of epidermal growth factor-induced RhoA translocation and invasion of human pancreatic cancer cells by 3-hydroxy-3-methylglutaryl-coenzyme A reductase inhibitors. Cancer Res 2001;61:4885-91.

35. Jakobisiak M, Golab J. Potential antitumor effects of statins. Int J Oncol 2003;23:1055-69.

36. Platz EA, Leitzmann MF, Visvanathan K, et al. Statin drugs and risk of advanced prostate cancer. J Natl Cancer Inst 2006;98:1819-25.

37. Hamilton RJ, Banez LL, Aronson WJ, et al. Statin medication use and the risk of biochemical recurrence after radical prostatectomy: results from the Shared Equal Access Regional Cancer Hospital (SEARCH) Database. Cancer 2010;116:3389-98.

38. Ahern TP, Pedersen L, Tarp M, et al. Statin prescriptions and breast cancer recurrence risk: a Danish nationwide prospective cohort study. J Natl Cancer Inst 2011;103:1461-8.

39. Kwan ML, Habel LA, Flick ED, Quesenberry CP, Caan B. Post-diagnosis statin use and breast cancer recurrence in a prospective cohort study of early stage breast cancer survivors. Breast Cancer Res Treat 2008;109:573-9.

40. Hamilton RJ, Morilla D, Cabrera F, et al. The association between statin medication and progression after surgery for localized renal cell carcinoma. J Urol 2014;191:914-9.

41. Kaffenberger S, Lin-Tsai Stratton KL, et al. Statin use is associated with improved survival in patients undergoing surgery for renal cell carcinoma. Urologic Oncology 2015;33:21.e11-7.

42. Duncan RE, El-Sohemy A, Archer MC. Mevalonate promotes the growth of tumors derived from human cancer cells in vivo and stimulates proliferation in vitro with enhanced cyclin-dependent kinase-2 activity. J Biol Chem 2004;279:33079–84.

43. Thompson R, O'Regan C, Morant S, et al. Measurement of baseline total cholesterol: new data from The Health Improvement Network (THIN) database. Prim Care Cardiovasc J 2008;1:107–11.

44. Benn M, Tybjìrg-Hansen A, Stender S, et al. Low-density lipoprotein cholesterol and the risk of cancer: a mendelian randomization study. J Natl Cancer Inst 2011;103:508–19.

45. Panagiotakos DB, Pitsavos C, Polychronopoulos E, et al. Total cholesterol and body mass index in relation to 40-year cancer mortality (the Corfu cohort of the seven countries study). Cancer Epidemiol Biomarkers Prev 2005;14:1797–801.

46. Alsheikh-Ali AA, Trikalinos TA, Kent DM, et al. Statins, low-density lipoprotein cholesterol, and risk of cancer. J Am Coll Cardiol 2008;52:1141–7.

47. http://www.cancer.gov/cancertopics/factsheet/prevention/statins

48. Mascitelli L, Pezzetta F, Goldstein MR. The epidemic of nonmelanoma skin cancer and the widespread use of statins: Is there a connection? Dermato-endocrinology 2010;2:37-8.

49. Poynter JN, Gruber SB, Higgins PD, et al. Statins and the risk of colorectal cancer. N Engl J Med.2005;352:2184–92.

50. Bjerre LM, LeLorier J. Do statins cause cancer? A meta-analysis of large randomized clinical trials. Am J Med. 2001;110:,716–23.

51. Cholesterol Treatment Trialists' (CTT) Collaboration. Efficacy and safety of more intensive lowering of LDL cholesterol: a meta-analysis of data from 170,000 participants in 26 randomised trials. Lancet 2010;376:1670–81.

52. Emberson JR, Kearney PM, Blackwell L, et al. Lack of effect of lowering LDL cholesterol on cancer: meta-analysis of individual data from 175,000 people in 27 randomised trials of statin therapy. PLoS One 2012;7:e29849.

53. Chan KKW, Oza AM, Siu LL. The statins as anticancer agents. Clin Cancer Res 2003;9:10–9.

54. Takahashi HK, Nishibori M. The antitumour activities of statins. Curr Oncol 2007;14:246–47.

55. Kobashigawa JA, Katznelson S, Laks H, et al. Effect of pravastatin on outcomes after cardiac transplantation. N Engl J Med 1995; 333:621–7.

56. Zamai L, Ponti C, Mirandola P, Gobbi G, Papa S, Galeotti L. NK cells and cancer. J Immunol 2007;178:4011–6.

57. Vasa M, Fichtlscherer S, Adler K, Aicher A, Martin H, Zeiher AM. Increase in circulating endothelial progenitor cells by statin therapy in patients with stable coronary artery disease. Circulation 2001;103:2885–90.

58. Garmy-Susini B, Varner JA. Circulating endothelial progenitor cells. Br J Cancer 2005;93:855–8.

59. Ahn G-O, Brown JM. Role of endothelial progenitors and other bone marrow-derived cells in the development of the tumor vasculature. Angiogenesis 2009;12:159–64.

60. Naik RP, Jin D, Chuang E, et al. Circulating endothelial progenitor cells correlate to stage in patients with invasive breast cancer. Breast Cancer Res Treat 2008;107:133–8.

61. Igreja C, Courinha M, Cachaco AS, et al. Characterization and clinical relevance of circulating and biopsy-derived endothelial progenitor cells in lymphoma patients. Haematologica 2007; 92:469–77.

62. Mausner-Fainberg K, Luboshits G, Mor A, et al. The effect of HMG-CoA reductase inhibitors on naturally occurring CD4+CD25+ T cells. Atherosclerosis 2008;197:829–39.

63. Curiel TJ. Tregs and rethinking cancer immunotherapy. J Clin Invest 2007;117:1167–74.

64. Tiemessen MM, Jagger AL, Evans HG, van Herwijnen MJC, John S, Taams LS. CD4+CD25+ Foxp3þ regulatory T cells induce alternative activation of human monocytes/macrophages. Proc Natl Sci USA 2007;104:19446–51.

65. Wolf AM, Wolf D, Steurer M, Gastl G, Gunsilius E, Grubeck-Loebenstein B. Increase of regulatory T cells in the peripheral blood of cancer patients. Clin Cancer Res 2003;9:606–12.

66. Yakirevich E, Resnick MB. Regulatory T lymphocytes: pivotal components of the host antitumor response. J Clin Oncol 2007;25:2506–8.

67. Knutson KL, Dang Y, Lu H, et al. IL-2 immunotoxin therapy modulates tumor-associated regulatory T cells and leads to lasting immune-mediated rejection of breast cancers in neu-transgenic mice. J Immunol 2006;177:84-91.

68. Gruver AL, Hudson LL, Sempowski GD. Immunosenescence of ageing. J Pathol 2007;211:144–56.

69. The PROSPER Study Group. Pravastatin in elderly individuals at risk of vascular disease (PROSPER): a randomised controlled trial. Lancet 2002;360:1623–30.

70. The *LIPID* Investigators. Benefits of pravastatin on cardiovascular events and mortality in older patients with coronary heart disease are equal to or exceed those seen in younger patients: results from the *LIPID* trial. Ann Intern Med 2001;134:931–40

71. The Treating to New Targets Study Steering Committee and Investigators. Outcomes of using high- or low-dose atorvastatin in patients 65 years or older with stable coronary heart disease. Ann Intern Med 2007;147:1–9.

72. Carroll RP, Segundo DS, Hollowood K, et al. Immune phenotype predicts risk for posttransplantation squamous cell carcinoma. J Am Soc Nephrol 2010; 21:713–22.

73. Kuoppala J, Lamminpää A, Pukkala E. Statins and cancer: a systematic review and meta-analysis. Eur J Cancer 2008; 44: 2122–32.

74. Scandinavian Simvastatin Survival Study Group. Randomised trial of cholesterol lowering in 4444 patients with coronary heart disease the Scandinavian Simvastatin Survival Study (4S). Lancet 1994;344:1383–9.

75. Heart Protection Study Collaborative Group. MRC/BHF heart protection study of cholesterol lowering in 20536 high-risk individuals: a randomised placebo-controlled trial. Lancet 2002;360:7–22.

76. Sahi H, Koljonen V, Böhling T, et al. Increased incidence of Merkel cell carcinoma among young statin users. Cancer Epidemiol 2012;36:421–4.

77. Paulson KG, Iyer JG, Blom A, et al. Systemic immune suppression predicts diminished Merkel cell carcinoma-specific survival independent of stage. J Invest Dermatol 2013;133:642–6.

78. Sahi H, Kukko H, Böhling T, et al. Unusually young Merkel cell carcinoma patients are Merkel cell polyomavirus positive and frequently immunocompromised. Eur J Plast Surg 2010; 33:349–53.

79. Kaae J, Hansen AV, Biggar RJ, et al. Merkel cell carcinoma: incidence, mortality, and risk of other cancers. J Natl Cancer Inst 2010;102: 793–801.

80. Sacks FM, Pfeffer MA, Moye LA, et al.; for the Cholesterol and Recurrent Events Trial Investigators. The effect of pravastatin on coronary events after myocardial infarction in patients with average cholesterol levels. N Engl J Med 1996;335:1001–9.

81. Setoguchi S, Glynn RJ, Avorn J, Mogun H, Schneeweiss S. Statins and the risk of lung, breast, and colorectal cancer in the elderly. Circulation 2007;115:27–33.

82. Borgquist S, Djerbi S, Pontén F, et al. HMG-CoA reductase expression in breast cancer is associated with a less aggressive phenotype and influenced by anthropometric factors. Int J Cancer 2008;123:1146–53.

83. Dimmeler S, Aicher A, Vasa M, et al. HMG-CoA reductase inhibitors (statins) increase endothelial progenitor cells via the PI 3-kinase/Akt pathway. J Clin Invest 2001;108:391–7.

84. Merla R, Ye Y, Lin Y, et al. The central role of adenosine in statin induced ERK1/2, Akt, and eNOS phosphorylation. Am J Physiol Heart Circ Physiol 2007;293:H1918–28.

85. Pearson GW, Hunter T. PI-3 kinase activity is necessary for ERK1/2-induced disruption of mammary epithelial architecture. Breast Cancer Res 2009; 11:R30.

86. Naumov GN, Folkman J, Straume O. Tumor dormancy due to failure of angiogenesis: role of the microenvironment. Clin Exp Metastasis 2009;26:51–60.

87. McDougall JA, Malone KE, Daling JR, Cushing-Haugen KL, Porter PL, Li CI. Long-term statin use and risk of ductal and lobular breast cancer among women 55–74 years of age. Cancer Epidemiol Biomarkers Prev 2013;22:1529-37.

88. Hung SH, Lin HC, Chung SD. Statin use and thyroid cancer: a population-based case-control study. Clin Endocrinol (Oxf). 2015; 83:111-6.

89. Goldstein MR, Mascitelli L. Do statins cause diabetes? Curr Diab Rep 2013;13: 381-90.

90. Goodarzi MO, Li X, Krauss RM, Rotter JI, Chen Y-D I. Relationship of sex to diabetes risk in statin trials. Diabetes Care 2013;36:e100-1.

91. Campbell PT, Jacobs EJ, Newton CC, Gapstur SM, Patel AV. Diabetes and cause-specific mortality in a prospective cohort of one million U.S. adults. Diabetes Care 2012;35:1835-44.

92. Huang Y, Cai X, Qiu M, et al. Prediabetes and the risk of cancer: a meta-analysis. Diabetologia 2014;57:2261-9.

93. Gallagher EJ, LeRoith D. The proliferating role of insulin and insulin-like growth factors in cancer. Trends Endocrin Metab 2010;21:610-8.

Chapter Fourteen

Deciphering The Dilemma Of Perilous vs. Pleiotropic Effects Of Statins

Paul J. Rosch, MD

Abstract

Statins became the best selling and most profitable drugs ever because they purportedly safely lowered cholesterol, which was presumed to be the major cause of coronary atherosclerosis. Subsequent studies showed that the benefits of statins were limited to patients with a history of a heart attack and that they were not related to either cholesterol or LDL levels or their degree of lowering. The explanation for this was that statins reduced inflammation and clot formation in addition to other "pleiotropic" effects such as improved endothelial nitric oxide formation, stabilization of atherosclerotic plaque and improved immune system function. Pleiotropy refers to the observation that a gene or drug may have two or more apparently unrelated effects. These can be desirable as well as undesirable, but with respect to statins, "pleiotropic" has become a synonym for "beneficial". For example, it has been claimed that statins also reduce the risk of various malignancies, despite the fact that all statins are carcinogenic in rodents at doses similar to those used to lower cholesterol in patients. In addition, as indicated in other chapters, statin trials show an increase in breast and skin cancers, which would be the first to be detected clinically. Similarly, it has been suggested that statins may prevent or even be used to treat Alzheimer's disease since some studies show that patients on statins are much less likely to develop this disabling dementia than controls taking a placebo. The relevant literature not only contradicts this, but statin labels must now include a warning about adverse responses such as memory loss and confusion. There are no known pleiotropic effects of statins that might influence the onset or course of Alzheimer's and the best explanation for this discrepancy may be that the cohort on statins likely had high cholesterol levels for years that had a protective effect. Studies show that elderly patients with high cholesterol and LDL levels are also protected from infectious diseases and live the longest. The latest guidelines for statin therapy no longer have lowering LDL as much as possible as a goal, but target those at increased risk . This is based on arbitrary criteria of age, gender and past history that would now make an additional 12 million Americans eligible for statins. Cholesterol is not even mentioned and for some reason, family history of premature death due to coronary disease is not included. On the other hand, all type 2 diabetics over the age of 40 should be treated, despite evidence that statins cause diabetes and the warning labels also now also include this. Canada and other countries also mandate a warning that statins lower Coenzyme Q10, which "could lead to impaired cardiac function in patients with borderline congestive heart failure." This is a particular problem in the elderly that can be prevented and treated with CoQ10 supplements. Statin manufacturers are well aware of this and Merck was granted 2 patents in 1990 for a statin Q10 combination, "to help prevent the inflammation to come." Such drugs were never made or marketed since they would have called attention to adverse side effects and blemish the widespread belief that statins were extremely safe. Merck's patents also prevented any other company from marketing a statin CoQ10 combination. Such adverse effects are never included in discussions of statin pleiotropy for obvious reasons, and it is likely they will continue to be used to prevent or treat disorders in which they are more apt to do harm than good.

The Demise Of The Diet-Heart Hypothesis

The belief that fatty foods and cholesterol caused coronary atherosclerosis stemmed from experiments 100 years ago demonstrating that feeding cholesterol and saturated fat to rabbits caused their blood cholesterol to skyrocket and produced fatty deposits in arteries similar to atherosclerotic plaque in humans. Five decades later, Ancel Keys reported a close correlation between saturated fat intake, cholesterol levels, and deaths from coronary disease. As a consequence, everyone was urged to sharply restrict eggs, butter, other dairy products and fatty meats. However, these studies were flawed and the stellar success of statins is more of a tribute to promotional hype than progress in improving health. The problem is that since rabbits are herbivorous, cholesterol and saturated fat are foreign substances and these results could not be reproduced in rodents and other meat eaters. Keys had data on 21 countries but cherry-picked the six and later seven that best supported his theory.[1,2] Had he reported on all the data available, there would have been no correlation between diet, cholesterol and coronary mortality, and if he selected countries like Israel, Sweden, Germany and France, he would have concluded that the more saturated fat and cholesterol consumed, the lower the incidence of deaths from coronary heart disease.[3] And a 30-year follow-up of Framingham participants found that for each 1% drop in cholesterol, there was actually an 11 % **increase** in coronary and total mortality.[4]

The "Prudent Diet" study launched in 1957 compared two groups of healthy 49 to 59-year-old New York businessmen. One group followed a restricted diet with corn oil and margarine instead of butter, cold cereal rather than eggs, and chicken and fish to replace beef. The control group ate eggs for breakfast and meat three times per day. The results published a decade later revealed that although cholesterol levels of those on the restricted diet averaged 30 points lower than controls eating eggs and meat, they had eight deaths from heart disease compared to none in the controls. Similar trials also failed[5,6]

The World Health Organization's Monitoring of Trends and Determinants in Cardiovascular Disease (MONICA) study that began in 1971 involved thirty-two centers in twenty-one countries that monitored approximately ten million men and women aged 25-64 for ten years.[7] It found that the eight lowest saturated fat consumption countries had the highest CHD death rates and the eight highest saturated fat consumption countries had the lowest rates of CHD deaths. A Framingham follow-up study similarly showed that the more saturated fat and the more cholesterol people ate, the lower their serum cholesterol was.[8] The NIH Women's Health Initiative (WHI) study that started in 1991 was a 15-year project conducted at 40 clinical centers involving 161,808 healthy postmenopausal women.[9,10] One component of this evaluated the effect of a low-fat and high fruit, vegetable and grain diet on the prevention of CHD, compared to a control group that followed their usual eating habits. Although there was some lowering of blood lipids in the low fat intervention group, there was no reduction in CHD or stroke. In addition, over two-dozen studies have reported that coronary heart disease patients ate less or the same amount of saturated fat as healthy controls.

Cholesterol Does Not Cause Heart Disease & Statins Don't Work By Lowering Lipids

If cholesterol caused coronary atherosclerosis, then people with higher levels should have more coronary disease and lowering cholesterol should have the reverse effect. However, no association between cholesterol levels and the severity or extent of atherosclerosis has ever been found in postmortem studies of the general population. In familial hypercholesterolemia, there is no association between the very high cholesterol and LDL levels and a corresponding increased incidence or prevalence of coronary disease. Nor is LDL-cholesterol higher in those with heart disease compared to controls with no history of this.[11,12] No clinical or imaging study has found any relation between the degree of cholesterol lowering and improvement. In one angiography study in which blood cholesterol had been reduced by more than 25% in 24 patients, atherosclerosis was increased in 18 and unchanged in eight. A Mayo Clinic study similarly found that in all patients whose cholesterols had decreased by more than 60 mg., there was a significant increase in coronary atherosclerosis. High cholesterol does not increase risk for heart attacks in senior citizens, women of any age, as well as patients with diabetes or renal failure.

If statins prevented CHD by lowering cholesterol, one would expect to see a clear cardioprotective dose-response relationship but this has not been demonstrated, even in patients who have had a heart attack. Nor have statins been proven to prevent coronary events and deaths in people with no history of heart disease.[13] This is extremely important since new therapy guidelines no longer have lowering LDL as much as possible as the goal, but rather an arbitrary 10-year risk assessment of 7.5% or more.[14] This would put millions of healthy people on statins, including all diabetics 40 and older, despite the fact that statins can trigger diabetes and make it more difficult to control. A non-smoking, non-diabetic 70-year-old African American woman with fabulous numbers: total cholesterol 175, good HDL 90 and a systolic blood pressure of 115 would still require moderate to high dose statin therapy perpetually. Dutch researchers who have been following senior citizens since 1997 found that 100% of men and 65% of women would have been prescribed statins based on their risk level. Examination of the data showed that only 12.7% of men and 7.9% of women actually had a heart attack or stroke. It seems doubtful that statins would have prevented this.

Inflammation And The Beneficial Pleiotropic Side Effects Of Statins

The new statin treatment guidelines tacitly acknowledge that statins don't work via effects on lipids or lipoproteins. Cholesterol and HDL are not even mentioned and LDL is not a concern unless it is over 190 mg/dL. As a result, it is now claimed that the benefits of statins in coronary heart disease, as well as a host of unrelated disorders, are achieved by pleiotropic properties such as reducing inflammation, clot formation, platelet aggregation, angiogenesis, oxidative stress and sympathetic nervous system hyperactivity, as well as improving endothelial function and nitric oxide levels, stabilizing atherosclerotic plaque and immunomodulation.[15]

Anti-inflammatory effects seem to be the most important since inflammation is now viewed as the major cause of coronary atherosclerosis and has been implicated in Alzheimer's disease, various malignancies and other non-lipid related disorders that statins can allegedly prevent. The problem is that the Justification for the Use of Statins in Primary Prevention (JUPITER) trial, showed that statins differed in their ability to reduce inflammation, which was defined as an elevated C-Reactive Protein (CRP), and that this was not related to their effects on lowering LDL.[16] It has also been proposed that in addition to being a mere marker of inflammation, CRP is a direct cause of cardiovascular disease,[17] but how this applies to preventing Alzheimer's and cancer is not clear. To add to the confusion, there is considerable evidence that statins can cause these and other disorders they allegedly prevent, especially cancer.[18]

Why No Conclusions Can Be Drawn About Good Or Adverse Statin Side Effects

Most meta-analyses and reviews fail to find any significant adverse side effects of statins and a recent one claimed that aside from a small increase in new diabetes, there were no side effects.[19] Some of the reasons for this include the fact that over 90% of side effects are not reported because they are not recognized, and even when they are diagnosed, doctors want to avoid litigation. Most statin trials are funded by drug companies that also oversee them, raw data is not available and side effects are ignored, minimized or not reported. Trials that are stopped because of statin side effects are also not reported. This is a particular problem with cognitive side effects, especially in the elderly, since memory problems, confusion and difficulty concentrating are usually attributed to old age. Even when patients report improvement in symptoms when off the drug and a recurrence if it or another statin is resumed, physicians usually deny any possibility of a causal relationship. Statins also differ with respect to cognitive side effects depending on whether they are lipophilic or hydrophilic.[20] The FDA recently added this black box warning, "There have been rare post-marketing reports of cognitive impairment (e.g., memory loss, forgetfulness, amnesia, memory impairment, confusion) associated with statin use. These reported symptoms are generally not serious and reversible upon statin discontinuation, with variable times to symptom onset (1 day to years) and symptom resolution (median of 3 weeks)."

However, this is not an accurate assessment, since a search of the FDA Adverse Events Databases from 2004 to 2014 revealed 36,605 reports of statin related cerebral dysfunction including memory impairment, transient global amnesia, confusion, paranoia, disorientation, depression, and dementia related to statins, Since it has been estimated that less than 2.5% of statin side effects are reported, this represents well over 3.5 million people. Many of these side effects are not reversible, and an episode of global amnesia lasting 6 to 10 hours could be fatal for someone flying a plane or operating heavy machinery. Baycol was withdrawn because of a high incidence of fatal cases of rhabdomyolysis, but all statins cause this. Although rarely mentioned there have been over 1,000 rhabdomyolysis deaths in the past 7 years, but the cause of death is listed as renal failure, the reason why most rhabdomyolysis patients die.

The above is just the tip of the iceberg. All statins are carcinogenic in rodents, but it may take decades for carcinogens to surface in humans, and most statin trials or follow-ups last less than five years. Nevertheless, an increase in nonmelanoma skin and breast cancers, which would be the earliest to diagnose, has already been documented.[18] This may just be the tip of the iceberg, and with long-term follow-up and improved reporting, neuropathy, an ALS like syndrome, cataracts and especially certain cancers may be added to the warning list. Everyone, especially healthy people, should be aware of this before complying with the new guidelines, which recommend higher statin doses that are likely to increase any adverse side effects.

Paul J. Rosch

Clinical Professor of Medicine and Psychiatry
New York Medical College
Chairman, The American Institute of Stress
stress124@optonline.net

References

1. Keys A. Atherosclerosis: A problem in newer public health. J Mount Sinai Hosp NY 1953;20:118-39.

2. Keys A. Coronary heart disease in seven countries. Circulation. 1970;41 (suppl 1):1-211.

3. Yerushalmy J, Hilleboe HE. Fat in the diet and mortality from heart disease. A methodologic note. NY State J Med 1957;57:2343-54.

4. Anderson KM, Castelli WP, Levy D. Cholesterol and mortality. 30 years of follow-up from the Framingham study. JAMA 1987;257:2176-80.

5. Reiser R. Saturated fat in the diet and serum cholesterol concentration: a critical examination of the literature. Am J Clin Nutr 1973;26:524-55.

6. Ravnskov U. Cholesterol lowering trials in coronary heart disease: frequency of citation and outcome. BMJ 1992;305:15-9.

7. Stewart AW, Kuulasmaa K, Beaglehole R, for the WHO MONICA Project. Ecological analysis of the association between mortality and major risk factors of cardiovascular

disease. The World Health Organization MONICA Project. Intern J Epidemiol 1994;23:505-516.

8. Castelli WP. Concerning the possibility of a nut... Arch Intern Med. 1992; 52(7):1371-2.

9. Howard BV, Van Horn L, Hsia J, et al. Low-fat dietary pattern and risk of cardiovascular disease: the Women's Health Initiative Randomized Controlled Dietary Modification Trial. JAMA 2006;295:655–66.

10. Howard BV, Curb JD, Eaton CB, et al. Low-fat dietary pattern and lipoprotein risk factors: the Women's Health Initiative Dietary Modification Trial. Am J Clin Nutr 2010;91:860–74.

11. Neil HA, Seagroatt V, Betteridge DJ et al. Established and emerging coronary risk factors in patients with heterozygous familial hypercholesterolaemia. Heart 2004;90:1431-7.

12. Jansen AC, van Aalst-Cohen ES, Tanck MW et al. The contribution of classical risk factors to cardiovascular disease in familial hypercholesterolaemia: data in 2400 patients. J Intern Med 2004;256:482-90.

13. Redberg RF, Katz MH. Healthy Men Should Not Take Statins. *JAMA.* 2012;307(14):1491-1492. doi:10.1001/jama.2012.423.

14. Stone NJ. Lichtenstein AH, Merz CNB, *et al.* 2013 ACC/AHA Guideline on the Treatment of Blood Cholesterol to Reduce Atherosclerotic Cardiovascular Risk in Adults: A Report of the American College of Cardiology/American Heart Association Task Force on Practice Guidelines. Circulation. 2013; published online before print November 12 2013, doi:10.1161/01.cir.0000437738.63853.7a

15. Mihos CG, Salas MJ, Santana O. The pleiotropic effects of the hydroxy-methyl-glutaryl-CoA reductase inhibitors in cardiovascular disease: a comprehensive review. Cardiol Rev 2010;18:298-304.

16. Ridker PM, Danielson E, Fonseca FA, *et al.* Rosuvastatin to prevent vascular events in men and women with elevated C-reactive protein. N. Engl. J. Med. 359 (21): 2195–207. doi:10.1056/NEJMoa0807646.

17. Li JJ, Fang CH. C-reactive protein is not only an inflammatory marker but also a direct cause of cardiovascular diseases. Med Hypotheses 2004;62:499-506.

18. Ravnskov U, McCully KS, Rosch PJ. The statin-low cholesterol-cancer conundrum. QJM 2012;105:383-8.

19. Finegold JA, Manisty CH, Goldacre B, *et al.* What proportion of symptomatic side effects in patients taking statins are genuinely caused by the drug? Systematic review of randomized placebo-controlled trials to aid individual patient choice. European Journal of Preventive Cardiology. 2014; 21(4): 464-474.

20. Sahebzamani FM, Munro CL, Marroquin OC, *et al.* Examination of the FDA warning for Statins and Cognitive Dysfunction. J.Pharmacovigilance 2014; 2:4

Chapter Fifteen

Critical Review Of Recent Drug Company Sponsored Trials About Statin Efficacy And Safety

Michel de Lorgeril, MD, Mikael Rabaeus, MD

Abstract

In 2005-2006, New Regulations were introduced in the conduct and publication of randomized controlled trials (RCT). This implies that before 2005, RCTs were less reliable than afterwards. To evaluate this, we reviewed studies testing the action of the cholesterol-lowering statins and conducted before and after 2005. The four studies published after 2005 were all testing rosuvastatin. Globally they show that rosuvastatin is not effective in secondary prevention, while the results in primary prevention are highly debatable. Furthermore, studies comparing statins to each other all show that none is more effective than any other, including rosuvastatin. This implies that statins are globally not effective in cardiovascular prevention, including in diabetic patients, and that the studies published before 2005 are probably flawed.

Introduction

A careful examination of the most recent statin trials and comparing them with "ancient" trials – those conducted before the 2005 *New Regulations of clinical trials* – reveals a striking discrepancy between the two categories; indicating that collectively and for years we have been very wrong regarding the miraculous health benefits of statins. Despite recent advances in clinical research transparency, there is still need of improving independent expertise and regulation as the present ones are not sufficient and should be reinforced. Two major questions relate to the real effects of drugs (both efficacy and safety) and to trial data secrecy. A corollary question is how much transparency is enough. Full transparency means having access to the complete raw clinical data of each randomized patient. This should allow a rebuild of the original dataset, a remake of the statistical analyses from an individual patient basis, and a comparison with the data published by the investigators on one side and, on the other side, with those submitted to the Health Authorities by the industrial to obtain access to the market. Refusal to give access to these data may suggest that the industrial and/or the investigators have something to hide. Providing all the data is crucial to re-establish credibility and confidence.

To determine the clinical efficacy of a medical drug, a critical issue lies in the very quality of the randomized clinical trials (RCT) evaluating this efficacy. As drugs are commercial items, credibility of RCT data evidently depends on the credibility of the principal investigators in charge of conducting the RCTs. In particular, are they free of conflicts of interest, as for example financial links with the sponsor?

This concern is justified. As of today, the owner of the patent (very often an industrial) is usually still both sponsor and principal manager – or even investigator – of the RCT. This undermines the credibility of the overall RCT data and has led prestigious scientists to state that modern medical scientific data are generally irreproducible[1-3], often wrong,[4-8] going as far as claiming that *"an estimated 85% of research resources are wasted"*[1,2].

One could argue that national and international institutions – as for instance the US Food and Drug Administration (FDA) and the European Medicines Agency (EMA) – are supposed to ensure that industry adequately conduct RCTs and fully report drug data regarding both efficacy and safety. However, there is no rigorous control. As an example, raw clinical data are still not available.

Apart from avoiding some rather "commercial" flaws[9-11], key measures in ensuring RCT quality are concealment of patient allocation and double blinding of patients and caregivers. A lack of respect of one of these obligations may introduce unintentional bias in RCTs, in particular when clinical efficacy is based on "soft outcomes" – such as nonfatal events, revascularisation or unstable angina, when evaluating cardiovascular drugs – or composite outcomes mainly including soft outcomes[12]. A clear possibility of such an unintentional *"unblinding bias"* has been recently described[13]. The risk lies in undermining the credibility of RCT data and it is not exaggerated to say that we are facing an unprecedented wave of scepticism about medical sciences from both the public and the health professionals[14,15].

To check on this, we chose to focus on one of today's most prescribed medicines, statins to lower cholesterol.

The present study was thus initiated with the aim to examine whether the most recent statin studies provide similar results – for both efficacy and safety – as the "ancient" ones. In case of discrepancy, what would be the explanation?

It is important to remember that there are two periods in the modern history of RCTs: before and after the 2005 *New Clinical Trial Regulations*. These were instaured by the Health Authorities in Europe and USA – following in particular the Vioxx, Celebrex and other incidents – to bring the pharmaceutical industry into more transparency[16-20].

Until 2005, being the sole depositories of the data yielded by the RCTs, industrialists were tempted to publish only what they chose to.[3-5] One scenario was frequent: up to a dozen of RCTs testing a new drug was set up in different countries, but then only those providing favourable data were published. If only one RCT turned out positive but all the others negative, either only the positive one was published and not the others; or the unfavourable RCTs were just prematurely discontinued, leaving the single RCT showing that the drug treatment was effective. This is known as a publication bias[5,6]. Importantly, subsequent meta-analyses including data from various RCTs cannot correct the publication bias as the reviews are based only on the known and the not discontinued RCTs. The Legislator's parry was then to force industrialists to make public all the RCTs they were setting up with the details of their main features, notably the dates of initiation and termination, including any discontinued RCT[16-20]. These *New Regulations* were far from being perfect but they had the merit of making investigators more cautious[20]. On the other hand, by doing so, the Health Authorities implicitly admitted that previous drug assessment procedures were not satisfactory. This should prompt us to re-assess all RCTs published before 2005, and to ask: what is the scientific value of statin RCTs published before the *New Regulations*?

The logical corollary is to ask whether implementing these *New Regulations* resulted in any changes in the results provided by the statin RCTs. In other words, are those published <u>after</u> 2005-2006 different from those published <u>before</u> 2005?

The statin efficacy data

Post-2005 statin RCTs

As most statins were tested and marketed <u>before</u> the implementation of the 2005 (stricter) *New Regulations*[16-20], how can we accurately evaluate today the real effects (both safety and efficacy) of the statins?

A first step is to compare the clinical effects of the "ancient" and "young" statins. The RCTs testing the "young" statins were conducted and/or published <u>after</u> 2005-2006. If the new RCT data (efficacy and safety) testing the "young" statins are in agreement with those published <u>before</u> the implementation of the *New Regulations* (before 2005-2006), this would be extremely reassuring regarding the real effects of the "ancient" statins and the robustness of the "ancient" RCT results.

The only statin that has been tested (against placebo) <u>after</u> the implementation of the New Regulations is rosuvastatin. Whether rosuvastatin may reduce cardiovascular complications was tested in four RCTs:

- The JUPITER trial where the patients were apparently free from cardiovascular disease and carried a rather moderate risk of cardiac death[21];

- The CORONA trial where patients were all survivors of a prior acute myocardial infarction (AMI) – with various degrees of cardiac dysfunction – and at a quite high risk of AMI recurrence and cardiac death[22];

- The GISSI-HF trial where all patients had cardiac dysfunction – 50% following a previous AMI, and 50% due to other heart disease – and a high risk of cardiac death[23];

- The AURORA trial where patients presented with severe renal failure, with 50% having already suffered an AMI or other ischemic complications. Evidently they had a major risk of recurrent AMI and cardiac death[24].

Thus, a large proportion of the patients recruited in these 4 rosuvastatin RCTs were in the context of secondary prevention, thereby testing what appears as an indisputable statement, namely: "beyond any doubt, statins are effective in secondary prevention"[25-28].

A similar statement that is tested by these rosuvastatin RCT's is: "the higher the risk of AMI, the more the reduction of cholesterol levels by means of a statin will be beneficial"[25-28]. The patients in AURORA – with the highest risk – should get the greatest benefit and those in JUPITER – with the smallest risk – the least benefit.

Let us start with the patients whose risk was the lowest.

The JUPITER trial

The JUPITER trial was a primary-prevention trial[21]. About eighteen thousand participants selected on the basis of a moderately elevated CRP (C-reactive protein) were distributed randomly into two groups: one was treated with a placebo, the other with rosuvastatin[21]. The primary hypothesis was to test rosuvastatin against placebo. However, it is likely that an implicit additional objective was to test whether CRP levels could serve as indicators for the prescription of a cholesterol-lowering drug, even in patients with normal or even low blood cholesterol levels. Indeed, knowing that the main investigator of JUPITER also held part of the licence for the CRP assay kit – the other owner being one of the major Boston hospitals – indicates that very serious conflicting interests were present[21,29].

One must remember that rosuvastatin, being the last statin arriving on the market, faced a major problem: the presence of the "ancient" statins, already considered as wonder-drugs. So, how could the pharma company lay its' hands on even a small part of the market, next to or against the competitors' statins?

The pharmaceutical industry does not like to compare face-to-face one drug to another for fear that the lack of significant difference between the two treatments might lead to the rejection of the new one. JUPITER was therefore supposed to demonstrate that rosuvastatin *is* indicated in a specific "new" category of patients, i.e. those with slightly raised CRP levels. JUPITER was a potentially win-win RCT: good for the CRP assay (and licence owners) and good for rosuvastatin and its' producer[20,21,29-31].

What happened with JUPITER? The whole story has been told in several articles and book chapters[20,21,29-31]. To put it short, by the end of 2007, the investigators and the sponsor announced highly favorable results for rosuvastatin and that the trial should be discontinued[30,31]. According to them, it would have been unethical to leave millions of potential patients without treatment when they had already demonstrated the highly significant protective effect of rosuvastatin, notably on cardiovascular mortality[20,21,29-31]. Accordingly, in March 2008, a press release announced the discontinuation of the JUPITER trial, with an average follow-up of less than 2 years per patient[29-31]. The adequacy of this premature discontinuation was widely challenged[20,21,29-31]; but the investigators and the sponsor answered that the discontinuation process was scientifically validated, and ultimately decided by a committee supposedly "independent from the sponsor". However, this committee had strong ties (in general) to the pharmaceutical industry[20,21,29-31]. In November 2008, the results of JUPITER were published[21] and controversy grew further as many realised that the mortality data were not presented correctly. Criticisms abounded, and so did the answers and counter-attacks of the investigators[20,21,29-31]. As the debate progressed, new data (previously concealed) were reported by the investigators or the sponsor, accompanied by rather surprising, not to say unacceptable, modifications in the survival curves[29-31]. This definitely raised suspicion of major flaws and possibly of misconduct in the way JUPITER was conducted and reported[20,21,29-31]. For instance, at least five different versions of cardiovascular mortality data were reported[31], which obviously is unacceptable[29-31]. Cardiovascular mortality was ultimately not judged different in the placebo and rosuvastatin groups and the small difference in overall mortality was not validated by the statisticians of the FDA[29-31]. As the raw clinical data, detained by the sponsor, are not available to independent experts and have not been examined by the FDA experts, it remains however impossible to make any definite conclusion regarding the true effectiveness of rosuvastatin in JUPITER. Admittedly, the lack of effect on death rate and the existence of mortality data tampering, do not by itself call into question the effectiveness of rosuvastatin against non-lethal complications. After all, if that medicine does not lengthen survival, it could improve quality of life by reducing nonfatal cardiac complication rate. The answer was indirectly given by the three other trials testing rosuvastatin – CORONA, GISSI-HF, AURORA – which did not report any effect on non-lethal complications[22-24].

Was the premature discontinuation of JUPITER a deliberate form of tampering? Surely, the investigators must have known that they would be criticized for this, as many scientists consider that when RCTs are stopped early for benefit, they usually show implausibly large treatment effects and that their findings should therefore be seen with scepticism[32,33]. So what could have been the true reason for this methodological flaw in JUPITER? The answer might lie with the unexpected significant increase of new cases of diabetes in the rosuvastatin-treated patients. The investigators tried to minimize this finding in their first report in 2008[21] and in subsequent analyses of their data, claiming that *"the cardiovascular and mortality benefits of statin therapy exceed the diabetes hazard"*[34]. They wrongly seem to support the idea that the only consequences of diabetes are cardiovascular complications, forgetting that type-2 diabetes increases risk of many non-cardiovascular diseases such as cancers, eye and kidney diseases, dementia and cognitive decline, depression and bone damage among many others[35-40].

This statin-diabetes issue is further discussed below in the *safety* section.

Other rosuvastatin trials: CORONA and GISSI-HF

Let us start with the CORONA trial which was the first RCT to rationally test a statin in patients with chronic heart failure. It was published in 2007[22]. Over 5,000 AMI survivors aged 60 or more were randomised to receive either a placebo or rosuvastatin. Despite a striking reduction in blood cholesterol level, patients taking rosuvastatin had no clinical benefit whatsoever, particularly in terms of survival. The occurrences of cardiac death, AMI and other non-lethal ischemic complications were unambiguously similar in the two groups, indicating that in secondary prevention of AMI cholesterol-lowering with rosuvastatin does not result in any protection.

This came in complete opposition to previous post-hoc analyses of RCTs and also meta-analyses,[41-43] all claiming that statins have beneficial effects on several endpoints, including mortality and non-lethal complications, in patients with cardiac dysfunction and chronic heart failure, with or without coronary heart disease. One of the major lessons of CORONA therefore was to confirm that only RCTs testing clearly defined primary hypotheses – and only a primary hypothesis[4,7,8,20] – can provide a reliable evaluation of the efficacy of any medicine.

In other words, the well-spread theory, based on ancient RCTs, that statins are unambiguously protective in secondary prevention should be rediscussed in light of more robust data provided by more recent and more credible RCTs, such as CORONA.

But then, how can we explain the discrepancy between CORONA and "ancient" RCTs testing a statin in secondary prevention – such as 4S[44] for instance – as explaining discrepant *scientific* data is a fundamental work of independent scientists?

Some have curiously said that the failure of CORONA to show any benefit of rosuvastatin was hardly surprising since there was no reason for the statin to protect elderly heart-failure patients. According to these post-hoc claims, the statin was supposed to prevent ischemic heart attacks, certainly not to extend the life of elderly patients with ruined hearts by stopping the progression of cardiac dysfunction. The analysis of CORONA outcomes shows that this argument is not valid: most deaths occurred during a recurrent AMI, and only a minority because of progression of heart failure[22]. This is no surprise as previous studies have shown that recurrent AMI is the first cause of death following a prior AMI with cardiac dysfunction[45]; and this argument – the efficacy of statin to prevent AMI – was the true reason to conduct CORONA specifically in post-AMI patients[22]. Finally, when the authors analysed their results, there was no difference when comparing patients according to age or to degree of cardiac dysfunction at baseline: the youngest did not benefit any more than the oldest, and those who suffered from minor or no symptoms of heart dysfunction were no more protected than the most severe cases[22].

Clearly, CORONA came as an unexpected blow for the sponsor and for all those claiming that statins are effective in secondary prevention of AMI. This was reinforced when Italian investigators reported the results of the GISSI-HF trial where approximately 50% of the patients recruited had very similar characteristics to the CORONA population (except that they were younger) and where again no benefit was demonstrated in the rosuvastatin group[23].

It is pointless to discuss the GISSI-HF results in detail, although it was a remarkable piece of clinical research. All one needs to say is that, like CORONA, GISSI-HF failed to show any benefit of cholesterol-lowering with a statin in secondary prevention. Furthermore, as the results of CORONA and GISSI-HF were known by the sponsors and most statin experts before the results of JUPITER were revealed, there was no doubt as to the crucial importance for the rosuvastatin sponsor of salvaging JUPITER (and rosuvastatin) whatever the methods (including premature termination), so as to convince the sceptics.

The AURORA trial in chronic kidney disease

In the AURORA trial, rosuvastatin was tested against placebo in patients with severe chronic kidney disease, some of them with a previous AMI or other cardiac ischemic syndromes, thus again in secondary prevention[24].

Renal failure patients being at high risk of AMI, the expected benefit from lowering their cholesterol level has also been considered as very high. Indeed, for years, on the basis of meta-analyses using weak data extracted from studies not designed to primarily test the effectiveness of statins on renal failure patients[46], these patients (and their doctors) were misled into believing that their cholesterol level should be lowered as much as possible[20].

So what did AURORA show? The results were the same as in CORONA: no clinical benefit at all – for both fatal and nonfatal complications – despite a striking reduction in blood cholesterol[24].

AURORA ended the fable that cholesterol-lowering by a statin is useful in chronic renal failure. Actually, AURORA confirmed the negative results of a previous RCT named 4D,[47] discussed below in the statin-diabetes section, that had tested the effects of atorvastatin in similar kidney failure patients. Thus, AURORA and 4D again confirmed that we should not trust results of individual studies that do not respect the strict methods of RCTs based on a well-defined primary hypothesis[7,8,20]. Evidently the same goes for meta-analyses[7,8,20,25-28,32,33,41-43,4] in which such studies are included. Despite this evidence, investigators still recently published new meta-analyses mixing well-conducted RCTs (such as AURORA and 4D) with a myriad of commercial studies reporting secondary endpoints or post-hoc data[48,49], resulting in the curious claim that statins might be useful in chronic renal failure patients. The inadequacy of such methods is evidenced by the fact that the results differed. One study claimed that statins reduce the risk of cardiovascular complications in patients with chronic kidney disease, including those receiving dialysis[48] while another concluded that there was no effect in patients on dialysis[49]. One meta-analysis showed no effect of statins on stroke[48] while the other concluded that statins did reduce stroke in patients not on dialysis[49]. Such studies should be discarded.[48,49]

Curiously, in the most recent RCT testing intense cholesterol-lowering (with simvastatin plus ezetimib) in patients with chronic kidney disease, the SHARP investigators concluded that reduction of cholesterol with such a strategy *"safely reduced the incidence of major atherosclerotic events in a wide range of patients with advanced chronic disease"*, and in particular the effects were similar in patients on dialysis and those who were not[50]. In fact, in SHARP, there was no significant effect on coronary death, nonfatal AMI, any major coronary event and all-cause death. The significant effect on the composite endpoint called "total cardiovascular events" (619 events in the placebo group vs. 526 in the simvastatin plus ezetimib group) was almost totally the consequence of the between-group difference in the revascularisation procedures (352 vs. 284)[50]. As discussed earlier in that review[12,13] and elsewhere[20,30,31], revascularisation is not a complication – but a medical decision which requires unblinding – and should be considered as very soft endpoint which cannot serve to judge the efficacy of any medicine against cardiovascular disease. In addition, the trial was criticized because of some uncertainty concerning the primary endpoint and a lack of clarity in the statistical analysis plan[51].

Thus, there is no evidence behind the recommendations to lower cholesterol in chronic kidney patients. The whole story – including the "ancient" and recent RCTs – illustrates the weakness of the scientific reviewing process in medical journals and the persistence of significant links between some "experts" and commercial interests.

Summary on recent statin RCTs

A first conclusion is inevitable: taken as a whole, the 4 RCTs testing rosuvastatin – all conducted or published <u>after</u> the implementation of the 2005 *New Regulations* – show that cholesterol-lowering with that specific statin is not proven to be effective, whether in primary or in secondary prevention. This is in total contradiction with most "ancient" commercial RCTs, all published <u>before</u> the *New Regulations*.

The next question is obvious: if rosuvastatin appears ineffective, what about the "ancient" statins, allegedly remarkably effective on clinical outcomes but less effective than rosuvastatin to lower cholesterol?

Pre-2005 RCTs: are "ancient" statins better than rosuvastatin?

ATORVASTATIN

As mentioned above, statin investigators and industrials do not favour comparing two statins face-to face. Indeed, if comparative studies fail to detect any difference, it would mean that the "new" statin is no better than the old. But then, if the new statin is proven ineffective it would imply that the ancient one is also ineffective. This would be another indirect manner of demonstrating that the "ancient" commercial RCTs truly were biased.

A recent study, conducted according to the *New Regulations*, compared rosuvastatin with atorvastatin, one of the "ancient" allegedly miraculous statins. The findings are quite interesting.

The SATURN trial, published in 2011, compared the effects of rosuvastatin to those of atorvastatin, in the absence of a control (placebo) group[52]. The primary end-point was progression of atherosclerotic plaque. They claimed that plaque volume – measured with sophisticated imaging techniques – is predictive of cardiovascular complications. The number of patients was relatively small (about one thousand), as well as the duration of the follow-up (two years). The results showed no significant difference between the two statins regarding the evolution of plaque volume during follow-up, which was curiously interpreted as showing that both statins were equally effective in slowing down the plaque evolution, when there was no control group[52]. In addition, there was no difference in the number of major cardiovascular complications: 49 vs. 52[52]. This is a critical point. One could argue that the trial was rather short and the number of patients too low to expect any significant difference to emerge between both groups. However, the total lack of difference (even no trend) after two years does not raise hope that, even with many more patients, atorvastatin would suddenly recover the miraculous effects it had boasted in the publications made before the stricter New Regulations.

Thus, according to SATURN, atorvastatin is no better than rosuvastatin and, as the latter is totally ineffective[20-24,29-31], so must be atorvastatin. This leads to the consideration that what caused the change of atorvastatin, going from a wonder-drug into an ineffective one, might be the implementation of the 2005 New Regulations[16-20]. We therefore chose to reconsider the results of another RCT testing atorvastatin in secondary prevention: the MIRACL trial published in 2001 and often presented as an unambiguous demonstration that atorvastatin is effective to prevent cardiovascular complications[53,54].

Why come back on MIRACL in 2015? The MIRACL trial is quite typical of the commercial RCTs undertaken long before the 2005 New Regulations. MIRACL compared atorvastatin (80 mg) to a placebo in over 3,000 patients who had just suffered an AMI, within 24 hours to 3 days after their admission to hospital. This was a quite perfect situation to assess the effectiveness of a statin in secondary prevention. The investigators wished to demonstrate that the effect of large doses of atorvastatin was close to immediate. Importantly, the trial was totally controlled by the sponsor. Even the main statistician was a member of the sponsor staff[53].

The results were unambiguous: there were 68 deaths in the placebo group, against 64 in the atorvastatin group; 113 non-lethal AMIs in the placebo group vs. 101 in the atorvastatin group; and 10 vs. 8 cardiac arrests, respectively[53]. The hypothesis that atorvastatin may protect from recurrence in secondary prevention should therefore be rejected without any hesitation. However, MIRACL was[53,54] – and still today[55] is – presented as an unequivocal demonstration that a statin – in particular atorvastatin – should be imperatively prescribed in secondary prevention.

How did the investigators and the sponsor of MIRACL turn around the evidence? The procedure was subtle. They added a new clinical cardiac endpoint category, in place of AMI or unstable angina. In their own words, the new category was: *"recurrent symptomatic myocardial ischemia with objective evidence requiring emergency hospitalization"*[53]. These patients were not suffering AMI or unstable angina according to established criteria but of something else, i.e. *hospitalisation* – an endpoint still more soft than the *revascularisation* endpoint (discussed above) – which, in any case, can serve to judge the efficacy of a drug in scientific medicine. Moreover, the validation of that endpoint totally depended on the data collected by field investigators who belonged to the sponsor's staff. By performing this curious validation-classification of a "new" endpoint, at last something appeared to be slightly different in the two groups: they recorded 130 and 95 of these types of "events" respectively in the placebo and atorvastatin groups. One might be tempted to smile if it were not so outrageous.

The failure of statins to reduce the risk of recurrence and death in the early high-risk period following AMI or acute coronary syndromes – the worst phase in secondary prevention – has been confirmed since then in various meta-analyses[56,57] thereby also confirming that MIRACL was a flawed trial. The only conclusion then is that we do not have any evidence that rosuvastatin or atorvastatin (even at high dose) are effective in secondary prevention.

SIMVASTATIN

For years, millions of AMI survivors worldwide have been treated with simvastatin on the basis of a single trial, the 4S trial (*Scandinavian Simvastatin Survival Study*), the findings of which were published in 1994 and were showing significant effects with reduction of both cardiac death and nonfatal complications[44].

The 4S trial is the one and only published RCT assessing the effect of simvastatin in secondary prevention[44]. It is surprising that a world leader in the pharmaceutical industry set up only one trial to test such a promising drug. It is more likely that other RCTs were conducted, but that their results remained unpublished, probably because they were not as favourable as previously hoped. We would be facing again a *"publication bias"*[3-6].

The fact that the sponsor of 4S was the same company that marketed Vioxx is to be noted. And also that the trial was conducted on the field by the sponsor's staff and that, as in MIRACL, the main statistician of the trial belonged to the sponsor's staff[44] which would today be unacceptable. Nonetheless, given the ineffectiveness of atorvastatin in secondary prevention, is there any indication then that simvastatin is better that atorvastatin?

Simvastatin was compared to atorvastatin in a trial called IDEAL, published in 2005[58], at a time when investigators and sponsors began to be very prudent, 2005 being right in the middle of the transition phase between the ancient and *New Regulations*. Briefly, in IDEAL, almost 9,000 patients with coronary heart disease were treated with either atorvastatin or simvastatin. The LDL cholesterol level was a bit lower in the atorvastatin group, but the 11% reduction in the primary endpoint (nonfatal AMI + cardiac death) in this group was not statistically significant[58]. More specifically, there was no difference between groups in total death rates (374 vs. 366) nor in cardiac deaths (178 vs. 175).

In our sense, IDEAL is therefore a good source of information as it shows that atorvastatin and simvastatin are similar in terms of clinical effectiveness over a period of nearly 5 years in secondary prevention[58]. As atorvastatin is apparently ineffective, simvastatin appears to be ineffective too. The 1994 "4S miracle"[44] was not reproduced. As discussed in the Introduction section, reproducibility of scientific data is the cornerstone of their credibility[1,2].

As long as we do not have access to the raw clinical data of 4S – and because the methods used in 4S are questionable (in particular, the lack of independent statistical analyses) – it seems prudent to consider 4S as a doubtful RCT.

Is intensive lowering of cholesterol more effective?

It has been claimed that more versus less intense statin regimens is more effective to reduce cardiovascular complications[59]. Is there any difference between the "ancient" and recent RCTs?

The SHARP trial, discussed above and testing intense cholesterol-lowering (with simvastatin plus ezetimib)[50] was a first answer: no significant effect of intense cholesterol-lowering.

In fact, only one RCT investigating intensive cholesterol-lowering with a statin has been published after the 2005-2006 transition period; it is the SEARCH trial comparing 80 mg versus 20 mg of simvastatin in a huge (n=12,064) population of AMI survivors[60]. Results after a mean follow-up of almost 7 years are by no way ambiguous: there was no significant difference between groups for any cardiovascular endpoint, including the very soft composite endpoint (p=0.10). More specifically, more intense simvastatin regimen did not significantly reduce coronary death (447 vs. 439), major coronary events (1189 vs. 1225), stroke (255 vs. 279) or any death rate (964 vs. 970)[60]. The only possible conclusion is that the tested hypothesis, i.e. intensive statin therapy is more effective, must be rejected. Neither the sample size nor the duration of follow-up could explain the failure. Curiously, the investigators concluded that the SEARCH results *"were consistent with previous RCTs"* demonstrating that more intense statin therapy safely produces extra benefits[60]. This is obviously wrong and once again raises concerns about the review process in medical journals.

Summary of the studies comparing statin vs. statin

In short, rosuvastatin (which is not effective) is not different from atorvastatin which, itself, is not different from simvastatin. This leads to the conclusion – based on the comparison of statin versus statin – that the "ancient" statins (simvastatin and atorvastatin) are not different from the youngest one (rosuvastatin). Thus, cholesterol-lowering with any of these medicines yields no detectable benefit against cardiovascular disease, in particular cardiac death and nonfatal AMI, and no effect on overall survival.

This lack of difference between the "ancient" and young statins was recently, and indirectly, supported by a very large cohort study based on the huge French national health insurance database comparing the cardiac and cerebrovascular prognosis of 106,941 patients prescribed rosuvastatin with 56,860 patients prescribed simvastatin, the average follow-up being 36 months[61]. No difference between the two statins was observed in this *real-life* study, suggesting again that the lack of significant protective effect of rosuvastatin may represent the true effect of statins in general and, by extension, also of cholesterol-lowering against cardiovascular disease.

Furthermore, this is confirmed by the fact that apparently intensive statin regimen is no better than a less intensive one. Finally, the observed discrepancy between "ancient" and more recent RCTs testing the different statins implies that mixing data from these two categories of RCTs in meta-analyses should no longer be accepted.

On the contrary, to be credible, any new meta-analysis should separately analyse RCTs conducted <u>before</u> and <u>after</u> the implementation of the 2005 *New Regulations*; and should separately analyse the RCTs testing "ancient" and "young" statins.

In the same line of reasoning, *official* recommendations should be rewritten on the basis of these new systematic reviews and meta-analyses.

The noncardiovascular and safety statin data

Beyond the cardiovascular issue, statins have repeatedly been presented as medicines having "other" major health effects in relation or not with cholesterol-lowering. Some were potential benefits, others could be deleterious. There are many different aspects and all cannot be discussed in the present review. We have selected the thromboembolic and diabetes issues.

Here again, do the most recent studies, compared with the "ancient" ones, provide some new information about statins? In case of discrepancy between the "ancient" and recent noncardiovascular statin data, this would be another indication that "ancient" RCTs have been, intentionally or not, flawed.

Statins and thromboembolisms

As an example, let's return to the JUPITER trial[21]. Despite the premature termination of the trial and the fact that thromboembolism was not a primary endpoint – both considerably increasing the possibility of a chance effect and biased results – JUPITER investigators nonetheless claimed that rosuvastatin significantly reduces the occurrence of symptomatic venous thromboembolism[62]. In a subsequent meta-analysis[63] published in 2012 which analyzed published and unpublished results of statin RCTs – including JUPITER – investigators found that statins do not significantly reduce the risk of venous thromboembolism: events occurred in 0.9% of the participants who were given statins and in 1% of the participants who were given placebo. The whole issue strongly indicates (as expected) that JUPITER results about venous thromboembolism happened by chance. Until we get new and consistent data, the theory that statins may have some anticoagulant properties should be rejected. The thromboembolism/JUPITER story is another illustration that JUPITER is a flawed RCT.

Statins and new-onset diabetes

Whether statins induces new-onset diabetes is a major question because diabetes is a serious disease with many complications including indeed AMI and stroke on one side but also renal and ophthalmic diseases, cancers, depression, cognitive decline, dementia and some others[35-40]. Thus, if statins actually induce new-onset diabetes, it is clearly a relevant issue.

In fact, they do. Curiously it is only with the JUPITER trial in 2008 that the statin-diabetes issue was revealed[21] and, as discussed above, it has likely been the main reason to prematurely stop JUPITER. It took 4 additional years before the FDA sent out a warning concerning this undesirable side effect, stating that statins definitely increase the risk of de novo diabetes[64].

This means that it took at least 30 statin RCTs and 30 years – during which the statins were fully prescribed – to bring to light this toxic effect. Is it possible that during such a long period of time, investigators (and their sponsors) had seen nothing? The statin-diabetes story is a remarkable illustration of high bias in reporting of harmful outcomes within studies, including sponsored RCTs[65,66]. In fact, statins not only increase the risk of *de novo* diabetes, but even more frequently increase insulin resistance and metabolic syndrome, probably through their effect (at least in part) on skeletal muscles[67].

Nevertheless, the investigators who had seen (or reported) nothing until then, immediately reacted by claiming that we must not change anything in the way of prescribing statins[68-70]: their "reasoning" was (and still is) that as statins are highly effective in preventing AMI and stroke in diabetics, becoming a diabetic is not a problem as the patient would ultimately anyway be protected from cardiovascular problems[68-70].

Probably untrue[71,72], this reasoning does in addition not take into consideration the previously mentioned several complications of diabetes that statins cannot reduce or may even stimulate[20,30,31,35-40,73-80]. And we must remember that most patients prescribed a statin are at low risk of AMI or stroke. Even if statins were really protective – an elusive theory – only a very small proportion of the treated patients would benefit. On the other hand, among the huge number of low-risk patients treated with statins, a significant proportion (see below) can become diabetic (or insulin-resistant) and suffer complications from this – including non-cardiovascular complications – in addition to the other deleterious side-effects of statins[73-85] which have been systematically underestimated in the "ancient" statin RCTs and meta-analyses[86-89]. This is in total contradiction with fundamental medical ethics stating: *"Primum non nocere, deinde curare"* [i.e. "First do no harm, then cure"].

Risk of inducing diabetes

Because of the lack of credible information about statin safety from commercial statin RCTs –well confirmed by the fact that the diabetes-statins relation was only very recently revealed – it is difficult to know the exact prevalence of this side-effect. Taking things prudently, the pro-diabetic effect of statins could be far from negligible in clinical practice. In a real-world setting, the risk of new-onset diabetes has been reported to increase with dose regimen and as adherence with statin treatment increases; the relative risk of new-onset diabetes may reach 40 to 70% in a real-world setting[90-92]. In brief, statins could induce roughly one *de novo* diabetes for every 100 to 150 patients taking an average dose. Things would be much worse with the very large doses currently recommended. In France, for instance, this means that every year at least 47,000 *de novo* diabetes cases could result from the current treatment of roughly

7 million patients[20,30,71]. These figures are probably underestimated, considering the difficulty that exists to get reliable figures.

Do statins prevent cardiovascular complications in diabetics?

Let us first cautiously have a look at the existing data as many experts are claiming that statins do prevent cardiovascular complications in diabetics[68-70] whereas others say the opposite[71,72]. To stay in line, only robust data should be retained.

How many RCTs have tested the effects of statins in diabetics as a primary hypothesis? There are three, namely CARDS[93], ASPEN[94] and 4D[47] all three conducted and published before the 2005 *New Regulations*[16-20]. Despite the fact that these three RCTs did not show unambiguous benefits of statins in diabetics, investigators claimed the opposite. So, let us carefully examine the data.

In brief, 4D is a RCT testing atorvastatin against placebo (median follow-up 4 years) in 1255 diabetics receiving maintenance haemodialysis[47]. There was no significant difference between the 2 groups for the primary endpoint (relative risk 0.92) and for total mortality (relative risk 0.93). The risk of fatal stroke was significantly increased among patients receiving atorvastatin (relative risk 2.03). The only possible conclusion should have been that the statin did not protect diabetics[47]. The investigators actually concluded that *"initiation of statin therapy in patients with diabetes who already have end-stage renal disease may come too late to translate into consistent improvement of the cardiovascular outcome"*[47]. In a subsequent substudy of 4D however – reanalysing the dataset and making an *a posteriori* subgroup analysis, thereby drastically increasing a chance effect – they claimed that *"in patients with type 2 diabetes mellitus undergoing haemodialysis, atorvastatin significantly reduces the risk of fatal and nonfatal cardiac events and death from any cause if pre-treatment LDL-cholesterol is >145 mg/dl"*[95]. This is simply not acceptable and again raises questions about the reviewing process in some medical journals.

The failure of 4D to show a protective effect of atorvastatin is supported by the results of another RCT in patients with haemodialysis, the AURORA trial[24] discussed above, in which rosuvastatin also failed to protect against cardiovascular complications. Nonetheless, the question raised by the 4D investigators in their first original report[47] – lack of benefit because of a too late initiation of treatment – might be relevant. It has been examined in ASPEN, a RCT where diabetics with severe renal dysfunction were excluded[94].

The ASPEN trial investigated the cardiovascular effects of atorvastatin in diabetics, with or without documented coronary heart disease (CHD)[94]. The trial was originally designed as a secondary prevention trial, but updates in treatment guidelines for individuals with CHD impaired recruitment. The protocol was therefore amended to enrol subjects without prior CHD[94]. Following the new statistical calculations, the trial was powered to detect differences between the statin and placebo groups but not to detect differences in the primary or secondary prevention subgroups alone[71]. Subjects were followed up during 4 years. There was no significant difference between groups for the primary endpoint (166 and 180 events for the atorvastatin and the placebo group respectively), for cardiovascular mortality (38 and 37 deaths) and overall mortality (70 and 69 deaths). Thus, the results of ASPEN were similar to those of 4D, but in the absence of severe renal dysfunction. The extension of criteria for enrolment was likely not an important cause of bias since the statistical protocol was amended accordingly. The two trials complement each other: in 4D (diabetics with severe renal dysfunction), patients were at very high risk while in ASPEN patients were at rather low risk.

In CARDS, the third RCT testing atorvastatin against placebo, 2838 diabetic patients were included[93]. In contrast to ASPEN and 4D, significant reduction of a composite primary endpoint was reported (relative risk 0.63). However, the numbers of primary endpoints in CARDS were small (83 and 127 in the statin and placebo group) despite the fact that the investigators used a *composite* primary endpoint mixing hard and soft (such as revascularisation) events. This criticized strategy considerably increases the probability of a chance effect[12]. Indeed, there was no statistically significant difference for all-cause mortality and coronary mortality. In this context, the decision of early termination – two years before the anticipated end without a clear justification – was inadequate. Furthermore, the clinical inconsistencies seen in CARDS suggest that the validation and classification of the endpoints were questionable. In addition – because, as written by the investigators, *"site monitoring, data collection, and data entry was done by sponsor's staff*[93]" – the possibility of outcome reporting bias in CARDS must be considered. Whatsoever, it was ethically and scientifically indicated to continue the trial to definitely clarify the effect on cardiac and total mortality. The CARDS trial has to be suspected of being biased until confirmed by other trials. No such confirmation has occurred. On the contrary, both 4D and ASPEN failed to report any benefit (not even a trend toward benefit) of atorvastatin in diabetics[47,94].

Taken together, the three RCTs testing a statin in diabetics as a primary hypothesis failed to show any benefit. This was confirmed in the ACCORD trial[96] where aggressive cholesterol-lowering did also not yield any benefit in diabetics.

Summary of the statin-diabetes issue

Despite the absence of evidence, why do the "official" recommendations still state that most diabetics (if not all) should be treated with cholesterol-lowering drug[97,98]?

One explanation is that these recommendations are usually based on meta-analyses which are supposed to objectively synthetize the whole scientific knowledge about the issue. In fact, even meta-analyses examining whether statins may protect diabetics do not all show the same results. For instance, Chang et al concluded in 2013 that no significant benefit of statin is found in primary (p=0.24) as well as in secondary (p=0.26) prevention of cardiovascular complications in diabetics[72] whereas the Cholesterol Treatment Trialists' Collaborators (CTTC) concluded in 2008 that statins reduce the risk of AMI in diabetics, even stating that statin should be considered for all diabetics[99]. How can we explain such discordant conclusions?

The CTTC meta-analysis pooled the data from 14 statin RCTs but none of the statin RCTs published <u>after</u> 2005 was included thereby curiously excluding 4D[47] and ASPEN[94]. Moreover, among the 14 included RCTs, only one – CARDS[93] for which we have exposed the major methodological problems – prospectively randomized diabetic patients and thus actually tested the effect of a statin in diabetics as a primary hypothesis. Data from the other 13 trials were from nonrandomized subgroups of diabetics – representing between 1% and 35% of the total of the patients enrolled in each trial[99] – and therefore open to major bias. Even more surprisingly, 4D and ASPEN – although not included in the main analysis – were mentioned at the end of the discussion section of the CTTC report, the authors writing that "*their conclusions are not materially affected by the results of ASPEN and 4D trials*"[99]. On the contrary, true science imposes to only consider statin RCTs where diabetics were prospectively randomized – namely CARDS, 4D and ASPEN – as Chang et al did[72], rather than partial retrospective data from nonrandomized subgroups of diabetics. The CTTC meta-analysis is therefore flawed by a major selection bias[99]. Consequently, the only possible interpretation based on robust data is that statins do not protect the diabetics.

The conclusion is therefore that on the basis of the most recent statin RCTs discussed here, there is no evidence that statins reduce the risk of cardiovascular disease in diabetics while there is on the other side no question about their diabetogenic effect and other deleterious side-effects.

It is high time to re-assess the whole statins-diabetes issue.

In summary, we propose 9 key issues that put into question the scientific basis justifying the use of statins:

1. Obvious discrepancy between "ancient" – before the 2005 *New Regulations of clinical trials* – and more recent statin trials in terms of both efficacy and safety.

2. In the recent trials, rosuvastatin was not effective in secondary prevention and most probably not in primary prevention.

3. No statin has proven to be superior to rosuvastatin. Statins can therefore all be considered as ineffective.

4. Recent trials clearly indicate that intense cholesterol-lowering does not protect high-risk patients any better than less intense statin regimens, confirming that the cholesterol theory saying that "*lower is better*" is wrong.

5. More specifically, in view of the lack of evidence, cholesterol-lowering and statins are useless in chronic heart failure, chronic kidney failure and diabetic patients.

6. In primary prevention, the data showing a protective effect of statins have a high likelihood of having been tampered with.

7. Most patients prescribed a statin at present are at low risk of stroke and AMI and the expected cardiovascular benefits can at best only be very small.

8. It took 30 years to bring to light the effect of statins on new-onset diabetes. This illustrates a high level of bias in reporting harmful outcomes in commercial trials.

9. Among the dozens of millions taking a statin, a significant proportion could become diabetic and get the many complications of diabetes, in addition to the many other adverse side-effects of statins.

Because of the above, a complete reassessment of statin therapy is mandatory.

Conclusions

A careful examination of the most recent statin RCTs and comparing them with "ancient" RCTs, as done in the present review, clearly shows that collectively and for years we have been very wrong regarding the health benefits (and safety) of statins.

We are entering a new era where full access to raw data from industry-sponsored RCTs[100,101] is the only way to permit transparency and to restore the credibility of clinical research. It is time to implement completely reliable methods to conduct medical trials so as to restore mutual confidence between all participants in the patient's care[102-104].

If the 2005 *New Regulations* definitely represented a step in the right direction[16-20], it remains that investigators and industrials could still succeed in finding a way around them. Indeed, since 2006, the media in various countries report problems every week between the pharmaceutical industry (or the experts working with it) and the law courts[105-108].

So despite advances in clinical research and RCT transparency, there are still scientists and regulators – of the EMA for instance[109] – saying that the present regulations are not sufficient and should be reinforced[110]. Obviously, full access to RCT data (still not possible) would allow independent researchers to examine the risks and benefits of medicines and thereby counterbalance the industry's power to assess its own products in the "industry-sponsored" RCTs. Clearly, legitimate interests in the protection of private (industry) investments must be weighed against other legitimate interests, such as the benefit and the protection of patients. The right balance between these interests is an obvious duty for all stakeholders involved, including regulators. And truly, when industry investments have been paid back, years after publication of RCTs that justified the marketing of a new medicine, there is no reason remaining not to give free access to RCT raw data unless, of course, that there are things which are not to be shown…

We strongly call for an end to the dogmas about statin efficacy and safety, based on unrealistic clinical reports and flawed meta-analyses, leading to biased recommendations about statin use[102,103,111,112] and ultimately extravagant situations and claims[113,114].

Michel de Lorgeril, MD*, Mikael Rabaeus, MD**

* TIMC-IMAG CNRS UMR 5525, Laboratoire Coeur et Nutrition
Université Joseph Fourier
Grenoble - France
michel.delorgeril@ujf-grenoble.fr

** CIC – Groupe de Santé
1815 Clarens – Switzerland
mikael.rabaeus@bluewin.ch

It should be noted that parts of this chapter have been published January 2016 in an article signed by the two authors and entitled: "Beyond confusion and controversy, can we evaluate the real efficacy and safety of cholesterol-lowering with statins?". Journal of Controversies in Biomedical Research 2015; 1(1):67-92. Doi: http://dx.doi.org/10.15586/jcbmr.2015.11

References

1. McNutt M. Reproducibility. Science 2014;343:229

2. Collins FS, Tabak LA. Policy: NIH plans to enhance reproducibility. Nature 2014;505:612-3

3. Dwan K, Altman DG, Clarke M, et al. Evidence for the selective reporting of analyses and discrepancies in clinical trials: a systematic review of cohort studies of clinical trials. PLoS Med 2014;11:e1001666

4. Ebrahim S, Sohani ZN, Montoya L, et al. Reanalyses of randomized clinical trial data. JAMA 2014;312:1024-32

5. Landewé RB. How publication bias may harm treatment guidelines. Arthritis Rheumatol 2014;66:2661-3

6. Wieseler B, Wolfram N, McGauran N, et al. Completeness of reporting of patient-relevant clinical trial outcomes: comparison of unpublished clinical study reports with publicly available data. PLoS Med 2013;10:e1001526

7. Ioannidis JP. Why most published research findings are false. PLoS Med 2005;2: e124

8. Ioannidis JP. How to make more published research true. PLoS Med 2014;11:e1001747

A useful article (as reference 7) where the author tries to explain the unprecedented wave of scepticism about medical sciences

9. Karha J, Topol EJ. The sad story of Vioxx, and what we should learn from it. Cleve Clin J Med 2004;71:933-4, 936, 938-9

10. Alpert JS. The Vioxx debacle. Am J Med 2005;118:203-4

11. Landefeld CS, Steinman MA. The Neurontin legacy-marketing through misinformation and manipulation. N Engl J Med 2009;360:103-6

12. Cordoba G, Schwartz L, Woloshin S, Bae H, Gotzsche PC. Definition, reporting and interpretation of composite outcomes in clinical trials: systematic review. BMJ 2010;341:c3920

13. Nguyen PV. Electronic health records may threaten blinding in trials of statins. BMJ 2014;349:g5239

14. Blendon RJ, Benson JM, Hero JO. Public trust in physicians-U.S. medicine in international perspective. N Engl J Med 2014;371:1570-2

15. Duncan Moore J. U.S. Physician Leaders Suffer Loss of Public Trust. Available at: http://www.medpagetoday.com/PublicHealthPolicy/GeneralProfessionalIssues/48402 [Last accessed 30 November 2014]

16. New Clinical Trial Regulation. Available at: http://ec.europa.eu/health/files/eudralex/vol-1/dir_2005_28/dir_2005_28_en.pdf [Last accessed 30 November 2014]

17. Commission Directive 2005/28/EC of 8 April 2005 laying down principles and detailed guidelines for good clinical practice as regards investigational medicinal products for human use, as well as the requirements for authorization of the manufacturing

or importation of such products. Official Journal of the European Communities L91: 13–19. Available at: http://ec.europa.eu/enterprise/pharmaceuticals/eudralex/vol-1/ dir_2005_28/dir_2005_28_en.pdf [Last accessed 30 November 2014]

A useful document (as references 16 and 18) to understand the major changes provoked by the 2005 New Clinical Trial Regulation

18. Bollapragada SS, Norrie JD, Norman JE. Review of new regulations for the conduct of clinical trials of investigational medicinal products. BJOG 2007;114:917-21

19. Hartmann M. Impact assessment of the European Clinical Trials Directive: a longitudinal, prospective, observational study analyzing patterns and trends in clinical drug trial applications submitted since 2001 to regulatory agencies in six EU countries. Trials 2012;13:53

20. de Lorgeril M. Cholesterol and statins. Sham science and bad medicine. Thierry Souccar Publishing, Vergèze France 2014

**A longitudinal and transversal analysis of the statin story since the beginning. Useful to understand the present situation*

21. Ridker PM, Danielson E, Fonseca FA, et al; JUPITER Study Group. Rosuvastatin to prevent vascular events in men and women with elevated C-reactive protein. N Engl J Med 2008;359:2195-207

A prototype of a recent statin trial whose results were not credible because of the way of conducting it (premature termination and data manipulation)

22. Kjekshus J, Apetrei E, Barrios V, et al; CORONA Group. Rosuvastatin in older patients with systolic heart failure. N Engl J Med 2007;357:2248-61

A prototype of a recent statin trial where data interpretation does not reflect results

23. Gissi-HF Investigators, Tavazzi L, Maggioni AP, et al. Effect of rosuvastatin in patients with chronic heart failure (the GISSI-HF trial): a randomised, double-blind, placebo-controlled trial. Lancet 2008;372:1231-9

24. Fellström BC, Jardine AG, Schmieder RE, et al; AURORA Study Group. Rosuvastatin and cardiovascular events in patients undergoing hemodialysis. N Engl J Med 2009;360:1395-407

25. Baigent C, Keech A, Kearney PM, et al; Cholesterol Treatment Trialists' (CTT) Collaborators. Efficacy and safety of cholesterol-lowering treatment: prospective meta-analysis of data from 90,056 participants in 14 randomised trials of statins. Lancet 2005;366:1267-78

26. Ray KK, Seshasai SR, Erqou S, et al. Statins and all-cause mortality in high-risk primary prevention: a meta-analysis of 11 randomized controlled trials involving 65,229 participants. Arch Intern Med 2010;170:1024-31

27. Taylor F, Ward K, Moore TH, et al. Statins for the primary prevention of cardiovascular disease. Cochrane Database Syst Rev 2011;(1):CD004816

28. Abramson JD, Rosenberg HG, Jewell N, Wright JM. Should people at low risk of cardiovascular disease take a statin? BMJ 2013;347:f6123

29. de Lorgeril M, Salen P, Abramson J, et al. Cholesterol lowering, cardiovascular disease, and the rosuvastatin-JUPITER controversy: a critical reappraisal. Arch Intern Med 2010;170:1032-6

30. de Lorgeril M, Salen P, Defaye P, Rabaeus M. Recent findings on the health effects of omega-3 fatty acids and statins, and their interactions: do statins inhibit omega-3? BMC Med. 2013 Jan 4;11:5; pre-publication history available at: http://www.biomedcentral.com/imedia/5160335768195678_comment.pdf [Last accessed 30 November 2014]

31. de Lorgeril M. The JUPITER and statin controversy. American Heart Association, Los Angeles 2012. Available at: http://michel.delorgeril.info/conferences/diapositives-congres-de-l-aha-a-los-angeles [Last accessed 30 November 2014]

32. Montori VM, Devereaux PJ, Adhikari NK, et al. Randomized trials stopped early for benefit: a systematic review. JAMA 2005;294:2203-9

33. Bassler D, Briel M, Montori VM, et al. Stopping randomized trials early for benefit and estimation of treatment effects: systematic review and meta-regression analysis. JAMA 2010;303:1180-7

34. Ridker PM, Pradhan A, MacFadyen JG, Libby P, Glynn RJ. Cardiovascular benefits and diabetes risks of statin therapy in primary prevention: an analysis from the JUPITER trial. Lancet 2012;380:565-71

35. Halimi S. Do not forget that type 2 diabetes does not only expose to cardiovascular complications. Diabetes Metab 2014;40:167-8

36. Cowey S, Hardy RW. The metabolic syndrome: A high-risk state for cancer? Am J Pathol 2006;169:1505-22

37. Sieri S, Muti P, Claudia A, Berrino F, et al. Prospective study on the role of glucose metabolism in breast cancer occurrence. Int J Cancer 2012;130:921-9

38. Bordier L, Doucet J, Boudet J, Bauduceau B. Update on cognitive decline and dementia in elderly patients with diabetes. Diabetes Metab 2014;40:331-7

39. Carnevale V, Romagnoli E, D'Erasmo L, D'Erasmo E. Bone damage in type 2 diabetes mellitus. Nutr Metab Cardiovasc Dis 2014;27:1151-7

40. Pan A, Lucas M, Sun Q, et al. Bidirectional association between depression and type 2 diabetes mellitus in women. Arch Intern Med 2010;170:1884-91

41. Horwich TB, MacLellan WR, Fonarow GC. Statin therapy is associated with improved survival in ischemic and non-ischemic heart failure. J Am Coll Cardiol 2004;43:642-8

42. Mozaffarian D, Nye R, Levy WC. Statin therapy is associated with lower mortality among patients with severe heart failure. Am J Cardiol 2004;93:1124-9

43. Go AS, Lee WY, Yang J, Lo JC, Gurwitz JH. Statin therapy and risks for death and hospitalization in chronic heart failure. JAMA 2006;296:2105-11

44. [No authors listed] Randomised trial of cholesterol lowering in 4444 patients with coronary heart disease: the Scandinavian Simvastatin Survival Study (4S). Lancet 1994;344:1383-9

45. Orn S, Cleland JG, Romo M, Kjekshus J, Dickstein K. Recurrent infarction causes the most deaths following myocardial infarction with left ventricular dysfunction. Am J Med 2005;118:752-8

46. Strippoli GF, Navaneethan SD, Johnson DW, et al. Effects of statins in patients with chronic kidney disease: meta-analysis and meta-regression of randomised controlled trials. BMJ 2008;336:645-51

47. Wanner C, Krane V, März W, et al; for the German Diabetes and Dialysis Study Investigators. Atorvastatin in Patients with Type 2 Diabetes Mellitus Undergoing Hemodialysis. N Engl J Med 2005;353:238-48

48. Hou W, Lv J, Perkovic V, et al. Effect of statin therapy on cardiovascular and renal outcomes in patients with chronic kidney disease: a systematic review and meta-analysis. Eur Heart J 2013;34:1807-17

49. Palmer SC, Craig JC, Navaneethan SD, Tonelli M, Pellegrini F, Strippoli GF. Benefits and harms of statin therapy for persons with chronic kidney disease: a systematic review and meta-analysis. Ann Intern Med 2012;157:263-75

50. Baigent C, Landray MJ, Reith C, et al; SHARP Investigators. The effects of lowering LDL cholesterol with simvastatin plus ezetimibe in patients with chronic kidney disease (Study of Heart and Renal Protection): a randomised placebo-controlled trial. Lancet 2011;377:2181-92

51. TrialResults-center. SHARP trial, description and results. Available at: http://www.trialresultscenter.org/study8081-SHARP.htm [Last accessed 30 November 2014]

52. Nicholls SJ, Ballantyne CM, Barter PJ, et al. Effect of two intensive statin regimens on progression of coronary disease. N Engl J Med 2011;365:2078-87

53. Schwartz GG1, Olsson AG, Ezekowitz MD, et al; Myocardial Ischemia Reduction with Aggressive Cholesterol Lowering (MIRACL) Study Investigators. Effects of atorvastatin on early recurrent ischemic events in acute coronary syndromes: the MIRACL study: a randomized controlled trial. JAMA 2001;285:1711-8

A prototype of "ancient" flawed statin trial

54. Waters D, Schwartz GG, Olsson AG. The Myocardial Ischemia Reduction with Acute Cholesterol Lowering (MIRACL) trial: a new frontier for statins? Curr Control Trials Cardiovasc Med 2001;2:111-4

A typical misunderstanding of medical research and poor reviewing in medical journal

55. National Clinical Guideline Centre (UK). Lipid Modification: Cardiovascular Risk Assessment and the Modification of Blood Lipids for the Primary and Secondary Prevention of Cardiovascular Disease. London: National Institute for Health and Care Excellence (UK); 2014

56. Briel M, Schwartz GG, Thompson PL, et al. Effects of early treatment with statins on short-term clinical outcomes in acute coronary syndromes: a meta-analysis of randomized controlled trials. JAMA 2006;295:2046-56

57. Vale N, Nordmann AJ, Schwartz GG, et al. Statins for acute coronary syndrome. Cochrane Database Syst Rev 2014;9:CD006870

58. Pedersen TR, Faergeman O, Kastelein JJ, et al; Incremental Decrease in End Points Through Aggressive Lipid Lowering (IDEAL) Study Group. High-dose atorvastatin vs usual-dose simvastatin for secondary prevention after myocardial infarction: the IDEAL study: a randomized controlled trial. JAMA. 2005;294:2437-45

59. Cholesterol Treatment Trialists' (CTT) Collaboration, Baigent C, Blackwell L, Emberson J, et al. Efficacy and safety of more intensive lowering of LDL cholesterol: a meta-analysis of data from 170,000 participants in 26 randomized trials. Lancet 2010;376:1670-81

60. Study of the Effectiveness of Additional Reductions in Cholesterol and Homocysteine (SEARCH) Collaborative Group, Armitage J, Bowman L, Wallendszus K, et al. Intensive lowering of LDL cholesterol with 80 mg versus 20 mg simvastatin daily in 12,064 survivors of myocardial infarction: a double-blind randomised trial. Lancet 2010;376(9753):1658-69 Erratum in: Lancet 2011;377:126

A typical recent statin trial with misinterpretation of results

61. Neumann A, Maura G, Weill A, et al. Comparative effectiveness of rosuvastatin versus simvastatin in primary prevention among new users: a cohort study in the French national health insurance database. Pharmacoepidemiol Drug Saf 2014;23:240-5.

62. Glynn RJ, Danielson E, Fonseca FA, et al. A randomized trial of rosuvastatin in the prevention of venous thromboembolism. N Engl J Med 2009;360:1851-61

63. Rahimi K, Bhala N, Kamphuisen P, et al. Effect of statins on venous thromboembolic events: a meta-analysis of published and unpublished evidence from randomised controlled trials. PLoS Med 2012;9:e1001310

64. FDA announces safety changes in labeling for some cholesterol-lowering drugs. Available at: http://www.fda.gov/NewsEvents/Newsroom/PressAnnouncements/ucm293623.htm [Last accessed 30 November 2014]

65. Saini P, Loke YK, Gamble C, et al. Selective reporting bias of harm outcomes within studies: findings from a cohort of systematic reviews. BMJ 2014;349:g6501

66. Bero LA. Why the Cochrane risk of bias tool should include funding source as a standard item. Cochrane Database of System Rev 2013;(12):ED000075.

67. Muscogiuri G, Sarno G, Gastaldelli A, et al. The good and bad effects of statins on insulin sensitivity and secretion. Endocr Res 2014;39:137-43

68. Jukema JW, Cannon CP, de Craen AJ, Westendorp RG, Trompet S. The controversies of statin therapy: weighing the evidence. J Am Coll Cardiol 2012;60:875-81

69. Sattar N, Preiss D, Murray HM, et al. Statins and risk of incident diabetes: a collaborative meta-analysis of randomised statin trials. Lancet 2010;375:735-42

70. Ridker PM, Pradhan A, MacFadyen JG, Libby P, Glynn RJ. Cardiovascular benefits and diabetes risks of statin therapy in primary prevention: an analysis from the JUPITER trial. Lancet 2012;380:565-71

71. de Lorgeril M, Hamazaki T, Kostucki W, et al. Is the use of cholesterol-lowering drugs for the prevention of cardiovascular complications in type 2 diabetics evidence-based? A systematic review. Rev Recent Clin Trials 2012;7:150-7

72. Chang YH, Hsieh MC, Wang CY, Lin KC, Lee YJ. Reassessing the benefits of statins in the prevention of cardiovascular disease in diabetic patients-a systematic review and meta-analysis. Rev Diabet Stud 2013;10:157-70

A good example of correct meta-analysis

73. Hung SH, Lin HC, Chung SD. Statin use and thyroid cancer: a population-based case-control study. Clin Endocrinol (Oxf) 2014 published online 30 July 2014, doi: 10.1111/cen.12570

74. Vinogradova Y, Coupland C, Hippisley-Cox J. Exposure to statins and risk of common cancers: a series of nested case-control studies. BMC Cancer 2011;11:409

75. de Lorgeril M, Salen P. Do statins increase and Mediterranean diet decrease the risk of breast cancer? BMC Med 2014;12:94

76. Hoffman KB, Kraus C, Dimbil M, Golomb BA. A survey of the FDA's AERS database regarding muscle and tendon adverse events linked to the statin drug class. PLoS One 2012;7:e42866

77. Golomb BA, Evans MA, Dimsdale JE, White HL. Effects of statins on energy and fatigue with exertion: results from a randomized controlled trial. Arch Intern Med 2012;172:1180-2

78. Cham S, Evans MA, Denenberg JO, Golomb BA. Statin-associated muscle-related adverse effects: a case series of 354 patients. Pharmacotherapy 2010;30:541-53

79. Ravnskov U, McCully KS, Rosch PJ. The statin-low cholesterol-cancer conundrum. QJM 2012;105:383-8

An excellent comment of the cholesterol/cancer/statin issue

80. You H, Lu W, Zhao S, Hu Z, Zhang J. The relationship between statins and depression: a review of the literature. Expert Opin Pharmacother 2013;14:1467-76

81. Godlee F. Adverse effects of statins. BMJ 2014;348:g3306

82. Gøtzsche PC. Muscular adverse effects are common with statins. BMJ 2014;348:g3724

83. Redberg RF, Katz MH. Reassessing benefits and risks of statins. N Engl J Med 2012;367:776

84. Abramson JD, Rosenberg HG, Jewell N, Wright JM. Should people at low risk of cardiovascular disease take a statin? BMJ 2013;347:f6123

85. Sun GH. Statins: The Good, the Bad, and the Unknown. Available at: http://www.medscape.com/viewarticle/832841?src=wnl_int_edit_tp10&uac=78143HG [Last accessed 30 November 2014]

86. Armitage J. The safety of statins in clinical practice. Lancet 2007;370:1781-90

A prototype article (with references 87 and 88) of biased interpretation of medical knowledge

87. Armitage J, Baigent C, Collins R. Misrepresentation of statin safety evidence. Lancet 2014;384:1263-4

324

88. Collins R. Lack of adverse effect of statin therapy on common muscle-related adverse events. Eur J Prev Cardiol 2014. pii: 2047487314541732

89. Cholesterol Treatment Trialists' (CTT) Collaborators, Mihaylova B, Emberson J, Blackwell L, et al. The effects of lowering LDL cholesterol with statin therapy in people at low risk of vascular disease: meta-analysis of individual data from 27 randomised trials. Lancet 2012;380:581-90

90. Culver AL, Ockene IS, Balasubramanian R, et al. Statin use and risk of diabetes mellitus in postmenopausal women in the Women's Health Initiative. Arch Intern Med 2012;172:144-52

91. Corrao G, Ibrahim B, Nicotra F, et al. Statins and the risk of diabetes: evidence from a large population-based cohort study. Diabetes Care 2014;37:2225-32

92. Zaharan NL, Williams D, Bennett K. Statins and risk of treated incident diabetes in a primary care population. Br J Clin Pharmacol 2013;75:1118-24

93. Colhoun HM, Betteridge DJ, Durrington PN, et al; CARDS investigators.Primary prevention of cardiovascular disease with atorvastatin in type 2 diabetes in the Collaborative Atorvastatin Diabetes Study (CARDS): multicentre randomised placebo-controlled trial. Lancet 2004;364:685-96

*** A typical example of "ancient" flawed statin trial*

94. Knopp RH, d'Emden M, Smilde JG, Pocock SJ. Efficacy and safety of atorvastatin in the prevention of cardiovascular end points in subjects with type 2 diabetes: the Atorvastatin Study for Prevention of Coronary Heart Disease Endpoints in non-insulin-dependent diabetes mellitus (ASPEN). Diabetes Care 2006;29:1478-85

95. März W, Genser B, Drechsler C, et al; German Diabetes and Dialysis Study Investigators. Atorvastatin and low-density lipoprotein cholesterol in type 2 diabetes mellitus patients on hemodialysis. Clin J Am Soc Nephrol 2011;6:1316-25

96. The ACCORD Study group. Effect of combination lipid therapy in type-2 diabetes mellitus. N Engl J Med 2010;362: 1563-74

97. American Diabetes Association. Standards of medical care in diabetes 2011 Diabetes Care 2011; 34 (Suppl 1):S11-61

98. American Heart Association. Cardiovascular disease and diabetes. Available at: http://www.heart.org/HEARTORG/Conditions/Diabetes/WhyDiabetesMatters/Cardiovascular-Disease-Diabetes_UCM_313865_Article.jsp [Last accessed 30 November 2014]

99. Kearney PM, Blackwell L, Collins R, et al. Efficacy of cholesterol-lowering therapy in 18,686 people with diabetes in 14 randomised trials of statins: a meta-analysis. Lancet 2008; 371:117-25

*** A typical example of flawed meta-analysis and poor reviewing in medical journals*

100. Doshi P, Goodman SN, Ioannidis JP. Raw data from clinical trials: within reach? Trends Pharmacol Sci 2013;34:645-7

101. Strom BL, Buyse M, Hughes J, Knoppers BM. Data Sharing, Year 1 - Access to Data from Industry-Sponsored Clinical Trials. N Engl J Med 2014;371:2052-54

102. Abbasi K. The missing data that cost $20bn. BMJ 2014;348:g2695

103. Protecting citizens' health: transparency of clinical trial data on medicines in the EU. Available at: http://haieurope.org/wp-content/uploads/2013/10/HAI_Protecting-citizenshealth-transparency-of-clinical-trial-data-on-medicines-in-the-EU.pdf [Last accessed 30 November 2014]

104. Protecting citizens' health. Available at: http://english.prescrire.org/en/79/207/46302/2612/2506/SubReportDetails.aspx [Last accessed 30 November 2014]

105. Jefferson T, Jones MA, Doshi P, et al. Neuraminidase inhibitors for preventing and treating influenza in healthy adults and children. Cochrane Database Syst Rev 2012;1:CD008965

106. Heneghan CJ, Onakpoya I, Thompson M, et al. Zanamivir for influenza in adults and children: systematic review of clinical study reports and summary of regulatory comments. BMJ 2014;348:g2547

107. Nisen P, Rockhold F. Access to patient-level data from GlaxoSmithKline clinical trials. N Engl J Med 2013;369:475-8

108. Jain A, Nundy S, Abbasi K. Corruption: medicine's dirty open secret. BMJ;348:g4184

109. Eichler HG, Pétavy F, Pignatti F, Rasi G. Access to patient-level trial data-a boon to drug developers. N Engl J Med 2013;369:1577-9

110. Rabesandratana T. Europe. Drug watchdog ponders how to open clinical trial data vault. Science 2013;339:1369-70

111. Stone NJ, Robinson JG, Lichtenstein AH, et al; American College of Cardiology/American Heart Association Task Force on Practice Guidelines. 2013 ACC/AHA guideline on the treatment of blood cholesterol to reduce atherosclerotic cardiovascular risk in adults: a report of the American College of Cardiology/American Heart Association Task Force on Practice Guidelines. J Am Coll Cardiol 2014;63:2889-934

112. National Institute for Health and Care Excellence. NICE clinical guideline no. 181. Lipid modification: cardiovascular risk assessment and the modification of blood lipids for the primary and secondary prevention of cardiovascular disease. July 2014. Available at: http://www.nice.org.uk/guidance/cg181/resources/guidance-lipid-modification-cardiovascular-risk-assessment-and-the-modification-of-blood-lipids-for-the-primary-and-secondary-prevention-of-cardiovascular-disease-pdf [Last accessed 30 November 2014]

113. Gøtzsche PC. Big pharma often commits corporate crime, and this must be stopped. BMJ 2012;345:e8462

114. Ioannidis JP. More than a billion people taking statins? Potential implications of the new cardiovascular guidelines. JAMA 2014;311:463-4

Chapter Sixteen

Why Reported Statin Side Effects Are Just the Tip of a Titanic Iceberg

Duane Graveline, MD, MPH, Paul J. Rosch, MD

Editor's Note: The majority of this chapter is written in the first person since it is Dr. Graveline's compelling account of his personal experience with statins and his crusade to alert others to their sinister adverse side effects.

Abstract

I introduce the reader to an account of my two personal experiences of statin associated transient global amnesia (TGA) which led me out of retirement to a full time study of statin drug side effects. The fortuitous publication of my TGA story in the widely syndicated Peoples Pharmacy column resulted in a veritable flood of emails from statin damaged people permitting the recognition of the full scope of statin adverse effects long before Medwatch became functional in this respect. People were reporting many different forms of cognitive dysfunction, behavioral disorders, peripheral neuropathy, ALS-like disorders and rhabdomyolysis. Gradually the two faces of statins became evident. As mevalonate pathway inhibitors they block cholesterol synthesis while at the same time blocking CoQ10 and dolichols (the cause of most of our side effects) while the other face of statins inhibits nuclear factor kappa B creating both anti-inflammatory and immunomodulatory properties accounting for reduction of cardiovascular risk.

Introduction

Statins have become the most profitable and popular prescription drugs ever because of their efficacy in lowering cholesterol and LDL. The importance of this stems from the lipid hypothesis, which postulates that lowering elevated cholesterol will significantly reduce coronary morbidity and mortality. This is based on studies done 100 years ago showing that experimental animals on a high cholesterol diet developed fatty deposits similar to those found in human atherosclerotic plaque. A half-century later, epidemiologic studies in different populations showed a very close correlation between saturated fat consumption, cholesterol levels and coronary disease deaths[1,2]. The Framingham study[3] also established cholesterol as a risk factor for heart disease. However, these were observational studies with serious flaws, and only an experiment that demonstrates the benefit of an intervention can prove a cause-effect relationship. In that regard, attempts to reduce coronary disease by restricting saturated fat to lower cholesterol failed, and some reported an increase in deaths.

The NIH sponsored Coronary Primary Prevention Trial was widely hailed as proof of the lipid hypothesis since it showed that cholestyramine, a foul tasting bile binding resin, lowered LDL and cholesterol and reduced coronary events in a synchronized fashion. However, this was of little practical value because of side effects and poor adherence[4,5].

While statins subsequently seemed to avoid these drawbacks, there is no proof that they are effective in primary prevention[6]. In addition, any benefits in coronary disease patients have now been shown to be due to pleiotropic effects such as reducing inflammation and clotting tendencies rather than lipid lowering[7]. As will also be demonstrated, there are growing and serious concerns about statin safety and how it is reported[8-11].

How Were Statins Discovered And Why Do They Lower Cholesterol?

Statins were discovered in the early 1970's by Akira Endo, a Japanese biochemist, who hypothesized that penicillin and other chemicals in fungi killed bacteria by inhibiting their ability to synthesize cholesterol. After testing several thousand fungal extracts, he isolated three from a Penicillin mold, one of which, mevastatin, was the first statin[12]. Mevinolin (MK-803), the first commercial statin, was subsequently isolated from an Aspergillus mold by Alfred Alberts and co-workers at Merck[13], and received FDA approval as lovastatin in 1987. Mevastatin, also known as compactin, was never approved, but pravastatin, a derivative, was discovered by Japanese scientists in 1979 and was approved there in 1989 and by the FDA in 1991. While developing lovastatin, Merck chemists also derived MK-733; a more potent cholesterol-lowering agent that was later named simvastatin. Simvastatin was approved in Sweden in 1988 and became available in the U.S. in 1991.

Cholesterol biosynthesis is a complex process involving over 30 enzymes and coenzyme Q10. The designation statin is used to describe products that interfere with this by inhibiting the HMG-CoA reductase enzyme. As this is one of the very early steps in the creation of cholesterol in the liver, statins also block the mevalonate pathway and the production of ubiquinone (Coenzyme Q10) and dolichols, which can have dire consequences. Cholesterol is made by most mammalian cells because it is a crucial component of cell membranes, and statins can disrupt this process as well.

All Statins Are Not Created Equal

There are two subtypes of statins: those that are natural and fermentation derived, such as lovastatin (Mevacor), pravastatin (Pravachol) and simvastatin (Zocor), and others that are synthetic; atorvastatin (Lipitor), cerivastatin (Baycol), fluvastatin (Lescol), rosuvastatin (Crestor) and pitavastatin (Livalo). The chemical structures of the three natural statins are very similar since they have a common source. Synthetic statins bear no resemblance to this configuration and differ from them with respect to cholesterol lowering properties. Rosuvastatin, atorvastatin and pitavastatin appear to be the most potent, with fluvastatin being the least. However, this rating may not apply to their ability to affect low and high density lipoproteins, apolipoprotein B, or triglycerides, which are also believed to influence risk for coronary heart disease.

Statins are often classified with respect to their solubility in fat (lipophilic) and water (hydrophilic). Atorvastatin, lovastatin, and simvastatin are lipophilic, whereas pravastatin, rosuvastatin, and fluvastatin tend to be more hydrophilic. Lipophilic statins cross the blood-brain barrier more readily, which could increase the likelihood of central nervous system complaints such as cognitive disturbances, memory loss and insomnia. Statins also differ with respect to the frequency and nature of other adverse side effects that might be influenced by their lipophilic status. These include diabetes, congestive failure, neuropathy, certain cancers and rhabdomyolysis, a severe type of muscle disease. Cerivastatin (Baycol) was withdrawn because it caused rhabdomyolysis 10 to 80 times more often than other statins and was associated with over 100 deaths.

Statin interaction with other drugs can also vary considerably. Rhabdomyolysis is more frequent in patients when they are taking other drugs that increase statin blood levels. In one study, patients who took both verapamil (Calan, Verelan, Isoptin), and simvastatin (Zocor), experienced myopathy 10 times more frequently than patients who received simvastatin alone[14]. Pravastatin (Pravachol) and rosuvastatin (Crestor) levels are less likely to be elevated by other drugs because liver enzymes that eliminate them are not affected by medications that block the enzymes responsible for removing other statins.

The Reality of Statin Adverse Drug Reactions

Tens of thousands of statin users have complained to their doctors of weakness, instability, easy fatigue, muscle aches and pains, burning of their extremities, depression, personality change and faulty memory, to which their doctors generally have responded, "You have to expect this now. You are over fifty" or even, "statins do not do that."[15] Although these experienced doctors all have pointed to a reasonable presumptive diagnosis, few have been entirely comfortable with this explanation because of a curious recurring pattern in their presentation. All of these patients have been on statins of one brand or another and the transition from midlife vigor to the multiple infirmities of the elderly has been much too swift in most. In the few months since the previous office visit, an aura of senescence has evolved in these patients. Doctors deal

330

with the passage of time on a daily basis and are acutely sensitive to its telltale first traces. The complaints their patients are reporting may be common even routine in the elderly yet these people are for the most part in their sixties and seventies and sometimes even much younger!

If anything out of the ordinary can be attached to these complaints of faulty memory, weakness and various aches and pains, it is their prematurity - premature aging. Conditions are being complained about that ordinarily would not be seen until much later in life. Are these statin users being robbed of their "golden years"? Is it possible that their passage to senescence has been expedited? If so, what could be the mechanism?[16].

This series will take you on a journey where many doctors really do not want to go - not after decades of use of reductase inhibitor (statin) class of drugs. What doctor wants to admit that he or she has been wrong about the side effects of statin drugs that now appears to be much more important than originally thought?

I have been there, and I have done that, and it has not been easy. The very idea that my practice philosophy was wrong for many years is a bitter pill for me to accept and to think I was following the dictates of national leadership, marching in lockstep with everyone else to the misguided fallacy of cholesterol causation of arterial damage.

Those were the days when we doctors were delighted to have statins. After almost 40 years of treating cholesterol with ineffective medicines we finally had a drug that really worked. Cholesterol dropping 40 points in just a few weeks was a whole new world for us. And hardly a word about side effects. We were advised to look out for liver damage by doing a blood test after a few weeks and told to expect a few muscle problems in under 2% of our patients for which we needed only to drop the dose a bit.

Many physicians have doubted the hypothesis of cholesterol causation from the very beginning[17]. Gradually, very serious reports of adverse reactions started to come in along with surprising reports of studies showing benefit of statin use even when the cholesterol remained unchanged. Strangely, we observed that in almost half of the new heart attacks being reported the cholesterol levels were normal. Then reports began to accumulate of transient global amnesia, permanent myopathy, diabetes, permanent neuropathy, rhabdomyolysis, ALS and serious neuro-degenerative conditions.

Evidence of another effect of statins, independent of cholesterol, began to accumulate. The study that made a huge difference for me was a study called JUPITER[18]. This study selected men and women who ordinarily would not have been a candidate for statins with cholesterol levels all less than 130 and no significant CV risk but whose inflammatory marker, (hs)CRP, was elevated. Half of these were given a statin, the other half took a placebo. After 19 months the ethics committee forced the stopping of the study because of excess heart attacks and stroke in the placebo group. It was deemed unethical to proceed.

Naturally there was a furor of controversy about these findings and it was in anticipation of this controversy that the study had been specially crafted yet two very important things emerged from this study: one was that cholesterol level appeared to have no relationship with cardiovascular disease risk and the second was that statins did work to lower this risk level as measured by this new inflammatory marker. Doctors have been reluctant to accept this because they had accepted cholesterol causality for well over 4 decades. Drug companies had only to shift marketing gears a bit to overcome this new reality for statins had been proving to be powerful anti-inflammatory agents in addition to an inhibitor of cholesterol synthesis for which they originally were designed.

So now we have a statin drug designed to be a reductase inhibitor that suddenly turns out also to have anti-inflammatory and immuno-modulatory properties and it is this added feature of the drug that gives the benefit[19]. The reductase inhibitor function blocks the the reductase step in the mevalonate pathway which synthesizes cholesterol along with CoQ10 and dolichols. The other new function is based upon the blocking of an intracellular transcriptase known as nuclear factor kappa B (NF-kB)[20].

So where are we? Statins now block cholesterol, perhaps the most important biochemical in the body, especially vital for the cognitive function of the brain and statins also block CoQ10[21,22] and dolichols, critical to mitochondrial function and responsible for almost all of the side effects. Additionally, statins block NF-kB giving a modest anti-inflammatory benefit to high risk heart patients but decreasing our immune status, raising the specter of increasing cancer risk. The fact that this vital information was not revealed until more than a decade after statins were marketed proves that statins were marketed long before they were fully understood[23].

Cognitive Effects of Statins

With our statin drug experience of the past decade we have come to expect side effects such as liver damage, muscle pain and nerve damage. But the ever-increasing cognitive side effects from statin drugs are new and completely unexpected by both patient and physician. They strike at who we are, our very essence, for without out memory what are we?

Transient global amnesia strikes without warning[24], abruptly depriving one of the ability to formulate new memories. With no record of the past, every new face, thought, conversation or scene is a unique moment, a novel experience transiently entering a mind suddenly emptied of the past. Think of the utter horror of this instant depersonalization, the anxiety, the frustration, the constant query, "What has happened to me?"

Think of the concern of family and friends when their loved one has abruptly become a querulous being who can walk and talk but who has suddenly been transformed into a bewildered creature without memory or ability to converse, pathetically trying to cope with its strange new world.

Prior to 2000 transient global amnesia (TGA) was very rare[25], almost a medical curiosity, and deserving of only a very limited description in most neurology textbooks. My medical community knew nothing of this.

In 1999 NASA (astronaut status) had called me in for my annual physical and because of modestly elevated cholesterol (270) placed me on Lipitor 10 mg. My first TGA occurred some 6 weeks later at which time my cholesterol was 155. This episode lasted 6 hours before I came to my senses in the office of the neurologist. The neurological examination was completely normal except for the amnesia. An MRI was ordered and the neurologist made a tentative diagnosis of transient global amnesia, cause unknown. I had been on Lipitor 10 mg for six weeks at this time.

I stopped the Lipitor on my own despite my neurologist's statement that statins did not do this and had no further amnesia episodes for the next year. During that time I questioned perhaps a dozen doctors and pharmacists as to any record of Lipitor amnesia, always with a negative response.

Lipitor was again strongly recommended by my NASA doctors on my annual physical the following year, 2000. My doctors had not previously encountered any amnesia side effects from this class of drugs and it was agreed to restart at one-half the previous dose, five milligrams daily.

Six weeks went by and I experienced my second episode of transient global amnesia. During its 12-hour span, I regressed in memory back to my teens, precisely recalling details of my high school years, but with no awareness of my intervening life.

The same doctors who had treated me the year before made the same diagnosis this time: transient global amnesia, cause unknown. Again they refused to accept any possibility of a Lipitor association, although by now I was convinced that Lipitor had caused my problem. But I remained the only one convinced or even suspicious of a relationship. The prevailing opinion in the medical community was that statins do not do that[26].

Alone, I remained on a very isolated pinnacle where I became both the soapbox speaker and audience, defending my conclusion. Even my wife was ready to accept that any relationship of my amnesia episodes with Lipitor was probably coincidental, hinting that the aging process alone does terrible things to the human body. One can hardly argue with that statement but I obstinately saw it differently. These were dark days when despite my conviction, an occasional specter of doubt would reach out momentarily, almost subliminally, suggesting the unthinkable: the possibility of underlying brain disease. Statins don't do this was the stock answer of my doctors.

In desperation I had contacted Joe Graedon of the Peoples Pharmacy[27] syndicated column seeking answers to my plea for information. He told me of a new statin study in San Diego and gave me their email contact. Upon receiving my email Dr. Beatrice Golomb of the San Diego College of Medicine statin study[28] responded with a telephone call and her very first words lifted a tremendous weight from my shoulders. "I have two more amnesia cases just like yours," she said, "and both are associated with Lipitor use." I was ecstatic and was off and running with my research interest. Dr. Golomb had saved my life, so to speak, and we became close collaborators in the statin side effect study. Joe Graedon meanwhile asked me if I minded if he published my original letter to him in his Peoples Pharmacy column. I saw no problem with that. Soon my website was flooded with emails and abruptly through Peoples Pharmacy stimulation, my website became a focal point for statin damage reports. Within a few months thousands of damage reports came flooding in and, more to the point, our transient global amnesia reports jumped from 3 to 30. None of these people had any idea their problems could possibly be related to statin use. I made certain that all of my emails were forwarded to Dr. Golomb for the benefit of her studies.

Soon, Dr. Golomb recruited me and Joe Graedon as co-authors in a manuscript she was preparing on "30 cases of statin associated amnesia". Subsequently, we were appalled to learn that it was refused by one of our major medical journals, the *Annals of Internal Medicine*. I was even more appalled two months later when our manuscript was refused by the *Archives of Internal Medicine*, as well. I am not talking of shoddy, undocumented work here, for both Dr. Golomb and I were thoroughly experienced in the writing of scientific papers. Our paper was so new and counter-current to existing medical philosophy as to be indigestible to the editors and the peer review process. Dr. Golomb gave up at that point and I did not blame her.

In 2003 Wagstaff et al of Duke University submitted a paper to *Pharmacotherapy* titled "The first 60 cases of statin associated transient global amnesia"[29] upon their review of FDA's Medwatch records. From that time to the present (2014) this condition has reached seemingly epidemic proportions in emergency rooms throughout our country with over 9,000 cases of TGA or severe memory impairment being reported to FDA.

Emergency room doctors have hauled out their sometimes dusty medical books and looked with wonder from book to patient as they realize they are seeing what, for many, is their first case of transient global amnesia. These confused patients, asking over and over again, "What has happened to me?" or some similar question, are completely unable to remember the doctor's explanation offered only moments before[30].

For every case of this type of temporary amnesia, thousands of cases of lesser forms of memory disturbance such as extreme forgetfulness, disorientation and confusion have also been reported to statin drug researchers[31]. Most of these cases do not make it to the emergency rooms and are, undoubtedly, extensively under reported.

All of these cases are associated with the use of the statin drugs Lipitor, Zocor, Crestor, Lescol, Mevacor and Pravachol although Lipitor and Zocor appear to have a greater predisposition for these adverse reactions of a cognitive nature[32]. Sometimes symptoms begin within weeks of starting medication. In other cases several years might pass before the onset of symptoms. Frequently they have been associated with muscle pain and tenderness, the much more common statin drug side effects.

Although the overwhelming majority of our physicians are very aware of the association of muscle pain with statin drug use, few are aware of the possible effects of statin drugs on cognitive functions[33]. Patients, even less aware of this relationship, are reluctant to report amnesia, confusion and altered memory coming on months or even years after statin drugs are started, thinking it is just old age, an inevitable touch of senility or possibly early Alzheimer's disease. When such patients are brought to the doctor's office with these complaints, all too frequently the doctor fails to consider the very real possibility that such side effects might be due to their statin drug, the very drug he or she had placed them on for health maintenance purposes, the very drugs purported to do so much good for public health.

What is Transient Global Amnesia?

The onset of transient global amnesia is abrupt, without the slightest warning to the patient that a central nervous system catastrophe is about to strike[34]. Suddenly the patient no longer has the ability to formulate new memories, a condition known as anterograde amnesia. Any sensory input during this time will be preserved briefly, if at all, only to disappear completely and forever, as though it never happened. Although consistently aware of their own identities, patients are often perplexed as to their surroundings and the identity of those around them. Characteristically, these patients repetitively question those present about where they are and what is happening but are unable to remember any explanation. To the consternation and ultimate frustration of doctors, nurses and well-meaning companions, they ask the same question, over and over again, sometimes for hours.

In most of these cases disorientation is profound. Many, but not all, of these patients will have an extensive retrograde component to their amnesia extending back many years in their lives. Gone are memories of friends and relatives, marriages and deaths, positions held and occupations learned.

Characteristically, the neurological examination is completely normal except for the amnesia and, after periods of usually less than twelve hours, recovery spontaneously occurs. This restoration of memory takes place quite rapidly, usually within fifteen to thirty minutes after improvement begins until recovery is complete. During this time patients rapidly become aware of their emergence from amnesia and, to the profound relief of those around them, their repetitive questioning finally ceases.

The syndrome of transient global amnesia, which usually occurs in otherwise healthy middle-aged or elderly people, was first presented to the medical literature by M. B. Bender in the *Journal of the Hillside Hospital* in 1956[25]. Since that time it has become a well-described condition, although its etiology has remained an enigma until very recently.

Transient global amnesia may well be a vastly under-reported condition because of the lack of an observer. A patient recovering from such an attack has no recall for the event. For brief episodes of transient global amnesia without an observer, there might be no clue. Dozens, even hundreds, of such brief attacks, measured in durations of less than an hour, may occur undetected in some cases and lead to gross under-reporting.

Anecdotal reporting from observers indicates that routine tasks such as walking or jogging, riding a bicycle or even driving a car appear to be done as usual. One wonders what might transpire in the event there was an associated retrograde element to the amnesia, which included the time period for training for a specific non-routine task such as flying an airplane.

Precipitating factors, events occurring in the 24 hours prior to the attack that might have contributed to it, are many and varied. Moderate to severe physical exertion often precedes an episode; activities such as dragging a deer carcass out of the woods, heavy digging, felling a tree, and laying concrete. Unusual emotional stresses such as newly reported cancer, a death in the family, news of a severe accident, a lawsuit, and violent family arguments can trigger these reactions. Swimming in cold water is occasionally a factor, and some individuals appear to recognize sexual intercourse as a frequent and even consistent trigger. Occasionally, transient global amnesia is seen after routine medical procedures such as venipuncture, minor surgery or application of the Valsalva maneuver, a "grunting" expiration test commonly used to determine cardiovascular responsiveness. Another medical procedure identified as a trigger agent for a growing number of transient global amnesia cases is cerebral angiography. Whether this is due to the patient's sensitivity to the contrast agent used, or whether the perfusing fluid transiently alters brain cell metabolism has not been determined.

The advent of the statin drugs has now provided a new contributory factor, one clearly rooted in the biosynthesis of cholesterol and clearly fundamental to neurophysiologic mechanisms[35]. Reported cases of transient global amnesia associated with the stronger statins such as Lipitor do not reflect its true prevalence because so many cases go undiagnosed and misdiagnosed. Millions of patients now taking this class of drugs--particularly Lipitor, which in 2003 is expected to become the first $10 billion drug in history4--are at significant side-effect risk, and transient global amnesia is just the tip of the iceberg.

For every reported case of transient global amnesia there are hundreds of case reports of impaired memory, disorientation and confusion among an older group of patients that rarely, if ever, get mentioned. All too frequently, this group is willing to accept old age, "senior moments" or incipient senility as the cause, particularly when their physicians are also ignorant about this side effect of the statin drugs.

As to duration and frequency, most patients will have just one attack in their lifetime. The shortest attack of transient global amnesia in their group lasted 15 minutes and the longest 12 hours. All of their cases had reliable observers. Quite understandably, in the absence of an observer, short duration attacks are easily missed. Students of this condition readily appreciate this under-reporting bias by the victim during an attack of transient global amnesia is an almost universal behavior.

Lipitor and Zocor[36] seem to have more association with significant cognitive disturbances than their sister drugs Mevacor, Pravachol, Crestor and Zocor. It would seem that very subtle differences exist in this group of HMG-CoA reductase inhibitors and they contribute to variations in the incidences of certain physiological side effects. All side effects seem to be shared among the statins but to different degrees.

Recent studies have shown a strong correlation of TGA episodes with deficiency of valves within the internal jugular vein complex especially while performing the so-called Valsalva respiratory maneuver of G-protection[37].

The mechanism of action of statin drugs, that of HMG-CoA reductase inhibition with its subsequent reduction of cholesterol biosynthesis at the cellular level, brings us tantalizingly close to the 'final common pathway' of transient global amnesia, if, indeed, a single pathway exists. The recent identification of cholesterol's vital role in brain activity as described by Pfrieger[38] makes this all the more likely and opens up a fertile area for future study.

On the subject of cognitive impact of statins Medwatch data has reported 2,708 TGAs, 1,971 cases of severe memory loss, 706 cases of cognitive loss and 3,260 cases of extreme confusion from 2004 through 2012 associated with all use of all statins. Additionally for the single statin, Lipitor in the time period 1997 through 2006, 1,965 cases of TGA were reported in a separate study of Medwatch data. This figure is grossly under-reported with no attempt to estimate the brief episodes of TGAs acknowledged by Hodges and Warlow that might increase incidence estimates by ten or one hundred times. This by itself is a formidable figure for incidence of cognitive effect but it is only the very tip of the iceberg. To this must be added the lengthy list of minor effects such as confusion, disorientation, forgetfulness and dementia-like changes closely resembling Alzheimers, diagnosed only after the statin is stopped and improvement occurs.

The Broad Range of Statin Adverse Reactions

Two events occurred in 2001 that were to have an immense effect upon the course of my life. Thanks to the support of Joe and Teresa Graedon[39] and the Peoples Pharmacy[27] promotion of my statin story, thousands of emails from statin damaged people were pouring into my website. Additionally, the co-author, Dr. Paul Rosch[40] entered my life by directing me to two very important books on the subject of cholesterol and inviting me to join THINCS, The International Network of Cholesterol skeptics[41]. Those books were like seeds germinating in the fertile fields of new concepts that Dr. Rosch's referral to THINCS had placed me. Kilmer McCully's "The Homocysteine Revolution"[42] and Uffe Ravnskov's "The Cholesterol Myths"[17] had a tremendous impact on my thinking. Paul Rosch brought it all together as the enabler who wanted my material brought before the eminent scientists of THINCS.

FDA opened the shelves of Medwatch in 2006 to those of us wishing to review for ourselves the status of statin adverse drug reports (ADRs). This has been all the more imperative since FDA has been extremely reluctant to report side effect data on the statin class of drugs. I was able to access Medwatch data in 2006. The process was not easy for it meant one must tackle the immense challenge of reviewing manually some 64,000 Lipitor ADRs using the "find" mechanism on one's PC. This was necessary, I was told, since the appropriate software for reading Medwatch data was available only to FDA and drug company officials. The rest of us had to be content with the time-honored and accurate but painfully slow process of counting each case one by one using the search mechanism on our PC.

What prompted me to do this personal search of what most would agree is FDA's business were the thousands of emails from statin damaged people telling me of the almost total lack of awareness of most doctors of statin-associated cognitive dysfunction, emotional and behavioral disorders and cases of disabling neuromuscular degeneration. Clearly our doctors have not been informed about most of these reactions, yet I knew from the 30,000 emails I had received through my website (www.spacedoc.com) by 2006 that many thousands of Medwatch reports have been submitted to FDA. In many cases I have been instrumental in helping distraught victims make their FDA report. What is wrong with our ADR reporting system, I wondered? Although all statins were involved I used the Lipitor data for this report. It is important to remember that all statins are reductase inhibitors blocking a single reductase step in the synthesis of cholesterol, so what is true for one is generally true for all statins. The only real variable is strength.

Because of my personal cognitive experience with this drug[43], transient global amnesia (TGA) was the first search term I entered. Not unexpectedly, there were 1,302 case reports for TGA in the Medwatch files. Adding the search term "memory impairment" yielded me another 663 cases. This total of 1,965 reports of serious cognitive dysfunction associated with the use of Lipitor seemed to fit quite well with the total numbers of such reports I now have recorded in my repository. I have generally recommended that victims do online Medwatch reporting and had helped more than a few to do just that.

Gross under-reporting of TGA deserves to be mentioned again here. That is the nature of self-reporting systems. Additionally, only the more severe forms of cognitive dysfunction get reported - the transient global amnesia and severe memory loss. More minor forms of cognitive loss such as confusion, disorientation or unusual forgetfulness are never included, so we should not expect to find them in the database. And I must stress the category of short-term cognitive loss with durations measured in seconds and minutes. By their very nature these will rarely be recognized even by the victim, and yet they might be so critical to a pilot, the crew and passengers. As mentioned earlier their incidence may well be ten or one hundred times greater than full blown TGA attacks. We will never know for certain. The passage of time is too short for recognition, yet special studies have revealed just how common these brief lapses can be[44].

Applying additional cognitive search terms gave me 222 reports of "dementia," 523 case reports of "disorientation" and 602 reports of "confusional state."

I next searched among words that might reflect the curious effects of statin drugs on emotion and behavior now being reported. I found 347 reports using the search terms "aggressiveness," "paranoia" and "irritability" commonly reported in statin users. Use of the search term "depression" yielded 1,142 reports, of which 118 expressed "suicidal ideation."

The next search term I entered was rhabdomyolysis, an especially serious form of muscle damage with a fatality rate of 10%[45]. You may recall that it was rhabdomyolysis that led to the Baycol withdrawal from the market. Some 60 deaths in the year 2004 made it untenable for Bayer to continue selling Baycol. Death in these cases is due to the blockage of renal tubules by the muscle cell fragments from ruptured muscle cell membranes and been carried to the kidney by the circulation.

I counted 2,731 Medwatch reports of rhabdomyolysis presumably resulting in 273 kidney failure deaths up to 2006. Applying additional search terms bearing on the muscular system, I found 1325 reports of "myalgia" and 494 reports of "musculoskeletal stiffness". It should be mentioned here that just recently I have received upgraded Medwatch data on rhabdomyolysis deaths. A recent study involving Dr. Golomb on the total muscle impact of all statin drugs reported from 2006 to 6 months beyond 2012[46] found 8,111 rhabdomyolysis hospitalizations for a presumed death toll (from kidney failure) of 811. Somehow the media did not pick up on this. We all recall the media uproar in 2004 resulting in Bayer's removal of Baycol from marketing. I must assume that their being labelled kidney failure deaths prevented the media uprising that almost certainly would have resulted from 811 rhabdomyolysis deaths, had they known.

My response to use of the search term "neuropathy" in 2006 was 1,294 reports to Medwatch. It should be mentioned that almost all of these peripheral neuropathy reports have proven to be very resistant to traditional treatment and now deserve to be called permanent. Using the term "Guillain-Barre syndrome" gave 98 reports, and prompted by hundreds of case reports I have received complaining of leg and arm pain, the search term "pain in extremity" gave 3,498 reports. This figure better reflects the statin neuropathy load.

Next I put in the search term, "hepatitis." Before I tell you the number, I first must qualify it by warning you that there are many different kinds of hepatitis. There is hepatitis A, B, C, cholestatic, autoimmune, fulminating, acute, chronic and viral, including cytomegalovirus. All of these terms are used in this compilation of Lipitor damage reports. However, the overwhelming majority of these reports said simply, "hepatitis" with no qualifier. Since hepatitis always has been a concern from statin use, you must make up your own mind in interpreting the 2,102 total cases that resulted. When I realized that "liver function abnormalities" also was being used in the Medwatch diagnosis list, I used it as a search term, reporting 842 liver function abnormalities in addition to my 2,102 hepatitis cases for a grand total of 2,944.

Since Ralph Edwards[47] of the World Health Organization reported excessive numbers of peripheral neuropathy and atypical ALS cases associated with the use of Lipitor world wide using their Vigibase data, my next investigation of Lipitor Medwatch data was for search terms that might give a measure of ALS occurrence. "Unusual weakness" turned up 2,516 case reports, "balance disorders" gave 596 responses and "coordination abnormalities" gave 195 responses. Since I have this condition, I can speak with authority on the subject of balance disorders. A kindly neighbor lady was so concerned on seeing me walk by her home she offered to drive me the rest of the way. Until that moment I was unaware of the effect of my walking on the public eye. Clearly this good Samaritan sensed me as disabled. My transition to walker took place the following day.

The Peoples Pharmacy website carries an unexpected gold mine of ALS incidence data in the following link: http://www.peoplespharmacy. com/2009/07/31/statins-and-als/ [48] Please check out this resource. Joe Graedon started this link in 2007. In it he has invited anyone struck down by statins with symptoms suggestive of ALS (Lou Gehrig's Disease) to comment on their status for the benefit of others. The last time I dug for gold here I was quite certain I had found at least 300 solid cases of ALS with hundreds of others who still might go in that direction since, as many of you understand, it sometimes takes years for ALS to unmask itself. There is no single definitive test. Seven years later (2014) this link remains very active with many hundreds of reports of ALS-like and neuromuscular degeneration cases associated with statin use.

Relevant to diabetes, it is now generally accepted that the incidence rate of new diabetes in statin users is close to 12% - an amazing user penalty for a medicine that is supposed to diminish the risk of cardiovascular disease! I used the search term "pancreatitis" to see how much of this diabetes might reflect organ damage. I found 604 reports of pancreatitis.

I next tried the search term "cardiac failure" and turned up 720 reports. CoQ10 inhibition is felt to be the major contributor to this condition. My next search was "myocardial infarction" out of curiosity as to how many might there be in a group already on Lipitor. The figure was 2,520 - another attention getter - especially when I got 610 additional reports using the search term "coronary artery occlusion." With a total of 3,030 cardiac events in a group already on statins, I wonder just how much protection is being offered. Use of the search term "cerebrovascular accident" (stroke) yielded 1,562 reports, with another 159 inferred by the use of the search term "aphasia."

FDA has a first rate monitoring system but it is grossly deficient for reporting findings back to the medical community. The average primary care physician in our country today, knowing that only a minority of patient problems get reported to FDA, would be startled to see these figures, especially the ones for cognitive dysfunction, neuropathy, rhabdomyolysis, depression and hepatitis. These are the people who write prescriptions for statin use.

From my 23 years of experience as a primary care doctor, I would say that any doctor attempting to practice medicine without full information on adverse reactions is liable for malpractice. Only with this information can proper, informed judgments for treatment plans be made. It pains me to see my colleagues being maneuvered into this position.

Mechanisms of Action of the Statin Drugs

Ubiquinone and dolichol inhibition is well known to the pharmaceutical industry, which has toyed with the idea of recommending that supplementaloenzyme Q10 be used by patients on statins. Although in 1990 the drug company Merck obtained a patent for the combination of CoQ10 with statins in one prescribed dose[49], no further action was ever taken on this matter nor did Merck share with the medical community their concerns on the matter. Of interest are the words of their patent justification: to help prevent the inflammation to come."

This oversight by Merck laid the groundwork for Dr. Sidney Wolfe's Public Citizen petition of 20 August 2001[50] and Dr. Julian Whitaker's 23 May 2002 petition with the Food and Drug Administration (FDA)[51]. Dr. Wolfe's petition called for special "black box" warnings to doctors and patients about the life threatening muscle damage of statin drugs, calling attention to the fact that 81 people had died from statin-related rhabdomyolysis since the time the drugs were first marketed in 1987. Dr. Whitaker's petition called on the commissioner of the FDA to change the package insert on all statin drugs and to issue a "black box" warning to consumers of the need to take Coenzyme Q10 (CoQ10)[21,22] whenever they take a statin drug however no action was taken on this petition. Of relevance here is the fact that in Canada the Lipitor warning label is strengthened to include warnings not only about CoQ10 depletion but also includes warnings on the closely related L-carnitine deficiencies.

For those statin victims desiring background information on their statin associated myopathy, neuropathy, ALS-like condition and even cognitive dysfunction, this section should suffice, for this condition can occur in any tissue: muscle, nerve, or brain.

The diminished bioavailability of intracellular CoQ10 and dolichols associated with the use of statins has the potential for seriously increasing oxidative damage and mitochondrial DNA mutations[52]. The anti-inflammatory benefits of statins are mediated by their special effect on the NF-kB cellular transcriptases and aggravated by inhibition of such anti-oxidants as Co-enzyme Q10[53]. The logical consequence of this is premature aging and the progressive development of such chronic conditions of aging as muscle weakness, burning pain and in-coordination and faulty memory - exactly the clinical picture we are seeing in tens of thousands of statin users.

The clinical responses we are seeing from this process of progressive mitochondrial damage is highly variable, more of a spectrum than any predictable, precise display of symptoms. We first have to accept that most statin users appear to do quite well on statins. This tells me that in some people our mevalonate pathway must take several different forms, by-pass channels if you will, that allow sufficient CoQ10, dolichols, selenoproteins etc to be available despite blockade of the basic mevalonate pathway.

We also find that some persons are completely unresponsive to statins, strongly supporting this possible presence of alternative pathways. In my 23 years of clinical medicine I soon discovered that doctors are fortunate if six out of every ten patients gave the expected response to a given medicine. We soon learn that "That's the way we are made!" There are many ways we biologic organisms evolve to get from A to B.

We also can say that premature aging and the earliest forms of neuropathy and myopathy may not yet be clinically apparent. Dull aches, slight numbness, senior moments and personality change all can be so minor as to escape recognition as possibly significant, so at least some of those who appear to be tolerant may actually have sub-clinical decrement. Just as we have to accept the fact that many, even most patients appear tolerant to statins, many thousands of people have been disabled by statins and for them, their prescribing doctor directly contributed to their problem and, in their eyes, no longer wears a completely white jacket[52].

I have generally categorized the symptoms as cognitive, emotional, neuropathic, myopathic and neurodegenerative but in reality there is much overlap. Hovering above all of these categories is the frequent presentation of tiredness and easy fatigability, pointing directly at deficient energy. Fatigue is the end result of ATP lack, so with sufficient mitochondrial DNA damage fatigue becomes inevitable[52].

The cognitive manifestations of statins may be just episodes of transient global amnesia, or increasing confusion, disorientation and forgetfulness or progressive dementia, which could be called Alzheimers-like, differing only in underlying pathology. Only when one stops the statins and sees regression of symptoms can the true cause be inferred.

So an individual can present with any one or all of these symptoms. It all depends upon what kind of body tissue is the most involved with mitochondrial deterioration. Every cell comes equipped with mitochondria, the energy producers of the cell[52].

Ubiquinone is also vital to the formation of elastin and collagen formation. Tendon and ligament inflammation and rupture have frequently been reported by statin drug users and it is likely that the mechanism of this predisposition to damage is related to some yet unknown compromise of ubiquonine's role in connective tissue formation.

The cells of slowly metabolizing tissue may be composed of only a few mitochondria because its energy needs are minimal. Muscle, heart and brain cells come equipped with hundreds and thousands of mitochondria because of the urgency of their metabolic demand.

There is no way to predict how any one person will respond to this progressive mitochondrial deterioration triggered by statins. Therefore, a cognitively impaired victim may also present with emotional symptoms, painful neuropathy, disabling myopathy or an ALS-like manifestation or with just cognitive dysfunction alone. It all depends on the roll of the dice[10]. Since the year 2000 I have devoted my full time to a study of the adverse reactions of statin drugs and the mechanisms by which they influence human physiology. My website at www.spacedoc.com with its busy forum is based upon my receipt of some 30,000 emails from statin damaged people and contains some 250 articles on the subject of statin side effects. In the year 2000 statin associated transient global amnesia was unknown. Fours years would pass before excess rhabdomyolysis deaths would take Baycol off the market. Despite the apparent benefits claimed in many of the clinical trials, men like Drs. Uffe Ravnskov and Kilmer McCully strongly doubted cholesterol causation and by 2002 Dr. Ora Shovman already had written his review of the "Anti-inflammatory and Immuno-modulatory Properties of Statins, exposing the truth about reductase inhibitors. Yes they lowered cholesterol but it was their anti-inflammatory effects mediated by nuclear factor kappa B (NF-kB) that lowered coronary risk. Cholesterol lowering by mevalonate blockade had nothing to do with it. After four decades of hype by Big Pharma and the drug companies acceptance was to come slowly. Even now doubters remain but the evidence can no longer be denied. Statin doses of the future must be those that enhance the NF-kB mechanism without adversely influencing our vital mevalonate pathway..

Conclusion and Key Issues

I have every reason to believe that statins will continue to sell but expect some falloff in sales figures as the medical community increasingly accepts inflammation rather than cholesterol causality and begins to accept much lower statin dosing levels. Since cholesterol no longer is the accepted cause of atherosclerosis and it is now back to whole milk, eggs and real butter, it makes no sense to continue to dose statins at 20, 40 and 60 mg levels to lower cholesterol. Cholesterol is not the problem. All we are doing at those dosage levels is creating more adverse reactions from mevalonate pathway blockade.

Dosing statins at cholesterol lowering doses does nothing but increase adverse reactions by the inevitable blockade of the mevalonate pathway decreasing the synthesis not only of cholesterol but also of CoQ10, dolichols selenoproteins and other biochemicals vital to cellular function.

We have learned that stains have two primary actions. They were designed to inhibit the reductase step in the mevalonate pathway thereby reducing the synthesis of cholesterol but more recently we have learned that there is a different side of statins one that affects the intracellular transcriptase nuclear factor kappa B mechanism leading to suppression of inflammation and immune functions. This is the mechanism that reduces coronary risk but also leads to increased susceptibility to cancer.

Lack of sufficient CoQ10 leads to diminished energy production and increased tendency for congestive heart failure. Diminished dolichols lead directly to diabetes. We who study these reactions knew that diabetes was inevitable years before the first cases appeared. The greater the statin dose the greater these side effects.

The only meaningful screening test for coronary artery dsease is (hs) CRP, a test for inflammation that correlate well for predisposition to heart disease. The JUPITER study proved the validity of this test as well as the irrelevance of cholesterol in screening for coronary proneness.

If your present statin dose lowers cholesterol you are giving too much statin.

Duane Graveline*, MD, MPH, Paul J. Rosch, MD**

*Duane Graveline MD MPH
Former NASA Astronaut and family physician
spacedoc@cfl.rr.com
www.spacedoc.com

**Clinical Professor of Medicine and Psychiatry
New York Medical College
Chairman, The American Institute of Stress
stress124@optonline.net

References

1. Keys A, Anderson JT, Grande F. Prediction of serum cholesterol responses ofmen to changes in fats in the diet. *Lancet.*1957;2:959-966.

2. Keys A. Coronary heart disease in seven countries. *Circulation.* 1970;41 (suppl 1):1-211.

3. Anderson KM, Castelli WP, Levy D. Cholesterol and mortality. 30 years of followup from the Framingham study. *JAMA.* 1987;257[16]:2176-80.

4. Lipid Research Clinics Program. The Lipid Research Clinics Coronary Primary Prevention Trial results, I: reduction in the incidence of coronary heart disease. *JAMA.* 1984;251:351-364.

5. Lipid Research Clinics Program. The Lipid Research Clinics Coronary Primary Prevention Trial results, II: the relationship of reduction in incidence of coronary heart disease to cholesterol lowering. *JAMA.* 1984;251:365-374.

6. Heneghan C. Considerable uncertainty remains in the evidence for primary prevention of cardiovascular disease [editorial]. *Cochrane Database Syst Rev.* 2011 Jan14;[8]:ED000017.

7. Shovman O. and others. Anti-inflammatory and immunomodulatory properties of statins.*ImmunoRes.*2002;25[3]: 272-85.

8. Graveline D *Lipitor, Thief of Memory, entire book,* 2002

9. Graveline D *Statin Drugs Side Effects,* entire book, 2004

10. Graveline D *Statin Damage Crisis,* entire book, 2006.

11. Graveline D *The Dark Side of Statins,* entire book, 2008

12. Endo A, Kuroda M, Tsujita Y. ML-236A, ML-236B, and ML-236C, new inhibitors of cholesterogenesis produced by Penicillium citrinium". *Journal of Antibiotics* (Tokyo) 29^{12}: 1346–8. (December 1976).

13. Alberts, A. W. et al. Mevinolin: a highly potent competitive inhibitor of hydroxymethylglutaryl-coenzyme A reductase and a cholesterol- lowering agent. *Proc. Natl. Acad. Sci.* 77, 3957–3961 (1980)

14. Graham DJ, Staffa JA, Shatin D, Andrade SE, Schech SD, La Grenade L. Incidence of hospitalized rhabdomyolysis in patients treated with lipid- lowering drugs. *JAMA.* 2004;292:2585-90.

15. Graveline D. *Lipitor Thief of Memory*, pages 8-10, 2002.

16. Graveline D. *Statin Damage Crisis*, page 18, 2006

17. Ravnskov U, *The Cholesterol Myths*, New Trends Publishing, entire book, 2000.

18. Ridker P, Justification for the Use of Statin in Prevention: An Intervention Trial -Evaluating Rosuvastatin (JUPITER): Rationale and Prespecified Analyses. *Circulation: Cardiovascular Quality and Outcomes.* 2009; 2: 279-285.

19. Shovman O. et al. Anti-inflammatory and immunomodulatory properties of statins. *ImmunoRes.*2002;25^3: 272-85.

20. Hilgendorff A and others. Statins differ in their ability to block NF-kB activation in human blood monocytes. International Journal of clinical pharmacology and therapeutics; 41^9: 397- 401, 2003.

21. Ely JTA, Krone CA. A brief update on ubiquinone (Coenzyme Q10). *JOrthomol Med* 15^2: 63-8, 2000.

22. Ely JTA, Krone CA. Urgent update on ubiquinone (Coenzyme Q10). (www.faculty.washington.edu/ely/turnover.html), 2000.

23. Masato E and others. Statin prevents tissue factor expression in human endothelial cells. *Circulation* 105:1756, 2002.

24. Hodges J and Warlow C. Syndrome of transient amnesia – towards a classification. A study of 153 cases. *J Neurol Neurosurgery Psychiatry.* Oct 1990; 53^{10}: 834-843.

25. Bender MB, Syndrome of isolated episode of confusion with amnesia. *Journal of the Hillside Hospital.* 1956; 5: 212-215.

26. Personal communication with many MDs and pharmacists

27. http://www.peoplespharmacy.com/

28. http://www.statineffects.com/info/

29. Wagstaff. LR and others. Statin-associated memory loss: analysis of 60 case reports and review of the literature. *Pharmacotherapy.* 2003;23^7: 871-8887.

30. Graveline D. *Lipitor, Thief of Memory. Page 27,* 2002

31. Graveline D. *Statin Drugs Side Effects*. Page 127, 2004

32. Sander K and Sander D. New insights into transient global amnesia: recent imaging and clinical findings. *The Lancet Neurology*. July 2005; 4[7]: 437-442.

33. Graveline D. *Statin Damage Crisis. Page 61,* 2006.

34. Hodges J and Warlow C. Syndrome of transient amnesia – towards a classification. A study of 153 cases. *J Neurol Neurosurgery Psychiatry*. Oct 1990; 53[10]: 834-843.

35. Pfrieger F. Brain researcher discovers bright side of ill-famed molecule. *Science*, 9 November, 2001.

36. Graveline D. *Lipitor, Thief of Memory*, page 47, 2002.

37. Akkawi N. Transient Global Amnesia and venous flow patterns. *The Lancet*, 24 February 2001; 357(9256): 639-643.

38. Pfrieger F. Role of cholesterol in synapse formation. *Biochimica et Biophysica Acta (BBA) – Biomembranes.* 10 Mar 2003;1610[2]:271-280.

39. http://www. spharmacy.com/about/

40. http://www.stress.org/about/founder/

41. http://www.thincs.org/

42. McCully KS. *The Homocysteine Revolution*. Keats, entire book, 1997.

43. Graveline D. *Lipitor, Thief of Memory*, page 4, 2002.

44. Hodges J and Warlow C. Syndrome of transient amnesia – towards a classification. A study of 153 cases. *J Neurol Neurosurgery Psychiatry.* Oct 1990; 53[10]: 834-843.

45. http://www.citizen.org/pressroom/pressroomredirect.cfm?ID=1657.

46. Keith B. Hoffman et al. Survey of the FDA's AERS Database Regarding Muscle and Tendon Adverse Events Linked to the Statin Drug Class. *PLOS one.* Published: August 2012 DOI: 10.1371/journal.pone.0042866.

47. Edwards R, Star K and Kiuru A. Statins, Neuromuscular Degenerative Disease and an Amyotrophic Lateral Sclerosis-Like Syndrome: An Analysis of Individual Case Safety Reports. *Drug Safety* 2007; 30[6]:515-525.

48. http://www.peoplespharmacy.com/2009/07/31/statins-and-als/

49. Merck Patent No. 4,929,437 and Patent No. 4,933,165. 29 May 1990.

50. http://www.fda.gov/ohrms/dockets/ac/03/slides/3968OPH1_01_Wolfe.pdf

51. Whitaker J. *Life Extension Magazine.* May 23, 2002.

52. Golomb BA, Evans, MA 2008. "Statin Adverse Effects: A Review of the Literature & Evidence for a Mitochondrial Mechanism." *American Journal of Cardiovascular Drugs.* 8[6]: 373-418.

53. Masato E et al. Statins prevent tissue factor expression in human endothelial cells. *Circ* 103: 1736, 2002

Chapter Seventeen

Systemic Evaluation of Statin Therapy Side Effects.
Do the Accrued Adverse Effects Outweigh the
Benefits?

*Sherif Sultan, MCh, MD, FRCS, EBQS/VASC, FACS, PhD, Edel P.
Kavanagh, BSc, PhD, Niamh Hynes, MD*

Abstract

Statin studies have shown that the rate of adverse side effects that
surface in post-marketing studies is very much greater compared
to those reported in company sponsored clinical trials designed to
obtain approval. This may be due to the highly selective nature of such
trials that are conducted in populations not representative of those
who ultimately receive statins. As a consequence, the overall adverse
effects on the population have not been adequately determined.

A comprehensive objective review of articles pertaining to statin
therapy was conducted to clarify their role within contemporary
clinical practices. These showed that statin therapy leads to both
beneficial and detrimental effects. Statin side effects included an
increased risk of diabetes, myopathy, cognitive deficiencies, amnesia,
peripheral neuritis, premature cataract development, erectile
dysfunction, chronic fatigue syndrome, intra-cerebral bleeding,
interstitial pneumonitis, and rhabdomyolysis. Some recent studies
have also documented that statin therapy increases the risks of
atherosclerosis, Parkinson's disease, cancer and congestive heart
failure (CHF). These results are clearly alarming and provoke the
possibility of not only the lack of primary cardiovascular protection
by statin therapy but highlight the very real possibility of augmented
cardiovascular risk in women, patients with diabetes, octogenarians
as well as the young.

Introduction

The endovascular revolution has brought about unprecedented changes in our cardiovascular practice over the last twenty-five years. In the course of this insurgence, we contemplated that gene and stem cell therapy would supplant all technologies. However, after phase three human trials and more than 7 billion euro squandered globally on research and development, all that we have attained is the realization that we are remote from any ground breaking clinical outcome.

Cholesterol is established in every human cell body, and plays significant roles as part of cell walls or membranes, in the manufacture of hormones, and helps promote the absorption of fat from our diet. Cholesterol and fat is insoluble in the blood and binds with apoproteins in order to keep them soluble. Low-density lipoproteins (LDL) are the main types involved in transporting cholesterol in the blood. It is the vehicle that mobilises cholesterol, but not a marker as wrongly labelled.

Recently statins have gotten bad press in relation to causing adverse side affects such as muscle pain and inflammation, increased risk of development of diabetes mellitus, and neurological side effects. Studies show that the rate of adverse side effects in post-marketing studies is greater than that found in the pre-marketing studies. This is due to the highly selective nature of clinical trial populations. The populations may therefore not represent those who ultimately receive statin therapy. Consequently, the overall adverse effects are not determined.

Cholesterol is crucial for energy, immunity, fat metabolism, leptin, thyroid hormone activity, liver related synthesis, stress intolerance, adrenal function, sex hormone syntheses and brain function. We must keep in mind before prescribing a statin therapy that the body has increased its cholesterol level as a defensive mechanism. For example seasonal level adjustments and the effects on metabolism must be considered, especially in northern countries that lack sunshine in winter.

Statin Induced Side effects

Diabetes Mellitus

Diabetes is a life-long medical condition, which inhibits the body's natural process of effectively using energy from the intake of food. Those with diabetes tend to have a higher disposition towards cardiovascular related events. Patients diagnosed with diabetes are often concomitantly prescribed a statin therapy, which is thought to combat the rising levels of cholesterol, thereby reducing cardiovascular risk.

Conversely, a study by the US veterans affair healthcare system conducted on 15 million veterans in 10 hospital centres in the US established that statins affect both fasting and postprandial glucose levels by inducing a state of hyperglycemia in diabetic as well as non diabetic patients.[1] A sub-analysis of the JUPITER study showed that statin therapy can in fact induce full blown type 2 diabetes in women.[2]

This was shown in the sub-study of PROVE-IT TIMI 22, which assessed intensive lipid lowering in diabetics. Results showed there was a significantly increased risk (6 %) of developing an elevated glycated hemoglobin (HBA1c) level in both diabetics and non diabetics.[3] Furthermore, Huptas et al. demonstrated that daily atorvastatin (10 mg/day) statin therapy actually encouraged insulin resistance in patients with a metabolic syndrome.[4]

Culver et al. investigated statin use and its risk of developing diabetes in 153,840 post-menopausal women without Diabetes Mellitus.[5] Results documented 10,242 incidences of diabetes over 1,004,466 person-years of follow-up. Statin use at baseline was associated with an increased risk of diabetes and this association remained after adjusting for other potential confounders and was observed for all types of statin medications. The authors concluded that the increased risk for diabetes in post-menopausal women is a medication class effect of statins. These results confirmed that of the JUPITER sub-analysis.

A critical appraisal of the JUPITER trial by de Lorgeril et al. elucidated that the results of statin therapy trials do not support the use of statin treatment for primary prevention of cardiovascular diseases.[6] Prescribing a statin in old age has a 9 % increase in the risk of developing diabetes.[7] It is another iatrogenic risk factor that must be avoided and it is mandatory to add glucose level testing to the list required for monitoring patients on statin therapy, and is equally as important as liver function and creatine kinase (CK) tests.

Preiss et al. conducted a meta-analysis of data from 5 major statin trials. There was an increased incidence of new onset diabetes with statin therapy, and evidence of a dose dependent association by assessing intensive versus moderate dose therapy.[8] As well as a dose dependent association, large scale randomized controlled trials demonstrated differences in risk between individual statin medications. Pravastatin tends to reduce risk of new onset of diabetes, while atorvastatin, rosuvastatin and simvastatin together significantly increase risk of new onset of diabetes.[9]

A meta-analysis of individual data from 27 randomised trials published in the Lancet revealed an excess incidence of diabetes of 0.1 % per year in patients at low risk of developing vascular disease.[10] The Cholesterol Treatment Trialists' (CTT) Collaboration authors reported a 10 % increase in the relative risk of developing diabetes while taking statins, yielding an estimated excess of 5 new diagnoses per 1000 people over 5 years.[11] Data from the JUPITER trial by Mora et al, showed a 25 % increase in frequency of physician reported incidence of diabetes, and a 50 % increase in women alone, corresponding to an estimated 11 new diagnoses per 1000 women over 1.9 years.[12]

In 14 primary prevention trials that involved 46,262 participants, treatment with statins was associated with an increase in the absolute risk of diabetes of 0.5 %.[13] The study found that only the risk of developing new onset diabetes mellitus was significantly higher in patients taking statins than in those taking a placebo.[13]

A meta-analysis of 6 statin trials that included 57,593 participants revealed a 13 % increase in the relative risk of new-onset diabetes.[14] Similarly, a meta-analysis of 13 randomized statin trials with 91,140 participants showed an odds ratio of 1.09 for a new diagnosis of diabetes.[7]

With increasing incidence of new diagnosis, costs may spiral. A study by Briggs et al. predicted that prescribing statins to everyone over the age of 50 years will lead to 12,300 diagnoses of diabetes.[15] The total extra cost of statin treatment from the drug alone is estimated at £180m.[15] Prescribing statins to everybody over 30 years old is estimated to produce 24,400 excess diabetes diagnoses at a cost of £360m.[15]

Statins may increase the risk of new-onset diabetes, particularly in patients already at risk of developing the disease by disrupting a number of regulatory pathways including insulin signalling, which may affect insulin sensitivity, pancreatic β-cell function, and adipokine secretion.[16,8] A study by Cederberg et al. showed that statin treatment increased the risk of type 2 diabetes and was attributable to decreases in insulin sensitivity and insulin secretion in a study of 8,749 non-diabetic participants.[17]

From the literature we can see there is overwhelming evidence to suggest that prescribing statins to non-diabetics can lead to disastrous effects such as full-blown development of type 2 diabetes. Statins manipulate glucose metabolism as a consequence of inhibitory effects on adipocytes. They induce insulin resistance through reduction in insulin-stimulated glucose uptake with a strong impact on glycemic control in non-obese patients. Patient metabolic conditions as well as whether statins can amend or impair insulin resistance, and ultimately type 2 diabetes mellitus impairs the poise of utilizing statins and its clear outcomes.

Myopathy and Incapacitation

Myopathy is a disease of the muscle fibres, which leads to dysfunction and muscle weakness as a result. There is an increasing amount of evidence to suggest that statin therapy induces myopathy as an adverse effect in those prescribed statins. In fact, myopathy is the most common adverse effect of statin treatment, manifested by muscle aches and pains, weakness, instability, and easy fatigue.[18,19] It is seen most often in women and elderly people.[20-23] In one randomized trial of 1,016 healthy men and women given statins or a placebo, 40 % of the women taking statins suffered exertional fatigue or decreased energy.[20] Other studies demonstrated increased muscle fatigability of 30 %.[24,25]

Statin therapy induces inflammatory myopathy, including necrotizing autoimmune myopathy with immunosuppression. Statin-related myopathy can last for 12 months. Myalgia or myopathy were the most common category of statin-related events, affecting 27 % of patients who had any statin-related event documented and 4.71 % of all patients.[26] Among the 3,858 patients who had a statin-related event, had the original statin discontinued, and were then re-challenged with another statin, a second statin-related event was subsequently documented for 510 (13.2 %) patients. Only 381 (9.9 %) of these patients had myalgia or myopathy that was severe enough to warrant discontinuation of the re-challenge statin.[26] Prescribing statins to everyone over the age of 50 years is predicted to lead to 1,200 excess cases of myopathy, with a total extra cost of statin treatment from the drug alone estimated at £180m.[15]

A cross sectional analysis of data from the National Health and Nutrition Examination Survey database by Buetter et al. similarly showed that the occurrence of muscle pain in patients prescribed with a statin therapy was 50 % greater when compared to patients with no prescription.[27] A retrospective cohort study that included 13,626 participants taking statins and 32,623 controls found a greater incidence of musculoskeletal disorders overall, and injuries in those taking statins.[28] Sinzinger et al.[22] has reported that muscular weakness and pain occur in 1 out of 4 statin treated patients who exercise regularly. They also noted that 17 out of 22 professional athletes with familial hypercholesterolemia (FH) treated with statins stopped because of that particular side effect.[36,23] Golomb et al.[20] performed a randomized controlled trial that included 1,016 healthy men and women with high LDL-C. Participants were divided into 3 groups that were given 20 mg simvastatin, 40 mg pravastatin or placebo. After 6 months treatment, 40 % of the women on statin treatment experienced adverse effects to energy or exertional fatigue.[20]

All statins have been reported to cause myopathy, with the severity ranging from asymptomatic increases in creatine kinase to myalgia and myositis to fatal rhabdomyolysis, commonly characterized by massive muscle necrosis, myoglobinuria and acute renal failure.[29-31] People on statins may have muscular problems although their CK is normal,[32] and even people on statins without any symptoms may have microscopic evidence of muscular damage.[33] Myopathy is dose dependent and may occur after therapy has been tolerated for up to 1 year.[29]

It is our experience that patient's who present with statin therapy-induced myopathy, have complete resolution of symptoms relatively quickly, or upon cessation of therapy. Some patients can take between

9 and 12 months to feel near normal again, or may present with more severe side effects such as muscle damage, rhabdomyolysis or in some cases complete incapacitation as a result. Reviewing the literature demonstrates a definitive link between statin therapy and myopathy. This should be tentatively taken into account when making the decision to prescribe a statin therapy.

Amnesia and Incapacitation

Statin therapy has been directly associated with memory loss.[20,34,35] Most reports were from individuals older than 50 years of age. Time to onset of the impairment was highly variable, ranging from 1 day to years after statin exposure. An association between cognitive impairment and a specific statin, a specific age group, a particular statin dose, or concomitant medication use was not observed. Furthermore, the cognitive impairment did not appear to be associated with fixed or progressive dementia, such as Alzheimer's disease, and was not detectable in controlled clinical trials measuring longer-term cognition.[36-38]

A large-scale study by Strom et al. including almost a million subjects compared a statin user to a non-statin user group. The authors observed a strong association between first exposure to statins and acute memory loss, which was diagnosed within 30 days immediately following exposure. The increase in memory loss was 4.4 times compared with non-statin users. The non-statin lipid lowering drugs increased memory loss 3.6 times compared with people not on lipid lowering medicines. Both statin and non-statin drugs substantially dented acute memory to a similar degree. They concluded that either all lipid-lowering drugs cause acute memory loss regardless of drug class or the association is the result of detection bias rather than a causal association.[39]

Memory problems were reported for 0.06 % (n = 70 / 107035) of patients in a study by Zhang et al.[26] In a study of 143 patients with memory loss or other cognitive problems associated with statin therapy, they reported that 90 % of them improved, sometimes within days of statin discontinuation.[40]

In a study by Padala et al., older statin-treated patients with Alzheimer's disease were asked to stop their statin treatment.

Twelve weeks later, their performance on several cognition tests had improved significantly and after having started the treatment again, their performance on the tests worsened significantly.[41] There is a strong argument for the view that statin treatment may cause adverse central nervous system effects. In a study by Sahebzamani et al. of adverse events from statin treatment reported to the FDA, there was a disproportionately greater incidence of adverse cognitive events reported by patients who were treated with lipophilic statins.[42]

Reports of memory loss, or cognitive deficiencies are difficult to cultivate from patients on a statin therapy. This risk factor is difficult to measure since it is not a quantitative measure, but nonetheless, evidence from the literature has shown a strong link between statin therapy and amnesia.

Peripheral Neuritis

Peripheral neuritis occurs as a result of damage to the peripheral nerves. This in turn causes pain, weakness, and numbness. There is a dearth of published studies that examine statin induced peripheral neuritis. Although, statin therapy has been associated with a wide range of adverse events including neuropathy.[19,43] Gaist et al. conducted a study on 465,000 people in Denmark. They asked all patients who had polyneuropathy of unknown cause, how many were on statin treatment. This was then compared with the general population in the county. They calculated that the risk for definite polyneuropathy was 16-times higher for current statin users than for non-users, and even higher for those who had used statins for more than 2 years.[44]

Arterial Calcification and Sclerosis

Arterial calcification and sclerosis is a silent disease, which can remain asymptomatic throughout the life of an individual, and may ultimately lead to a life-threatening vascular event. It is associated with accumulation of LDL, macrophages, T cells, smooth muscle cells, proteoglycans, collagen, calcium and necrotic debris in the vessel wall.[45] Arterial calcification can result from an initial injury to the

358

vascular wall, where the endothelial cells have been disturbed, or a change in velocity of the blood on the intra arterial wall. This leads to endothelial dysfunction and inflammation.

Reducing carbohydrates, as opposed to fat, seems to have more favourable effects on atherogenic dyslipidemia, inflammation, thrombogenic and atherosclerotic surrogate markers, hence the development of atherosclerosis, heart disease, diabetes, obesity and the metabolic syndromes.[46-54] Couse et al. assessed whether statin therapy could slow progression and/or cause regression of carotid intima-media thickness (CIMT) over 2 years, and found that Rosuvastatin did not induce disease regression.[55]

The Ezetimibe and Simvastatin in Hypercholesterolemia Enhances Atherosclerosis Regression (ENHANCE) trial reported no difference in carotid intima-media thickness in patients with heterozygous familial hypercholesterolemia who were treated with simvastatin and ezetimibe or with simvastatin and placebo, despite significantly greater LDL-C lowering with the combination.[56] In the Simvastatin and Ezetimibe in Aortic Stenosis (SEAS) study,[57] 1,873 subjects with mild to moderate aortic stenosis were randomized to ezetimibe 10 mg/day and simvastatin or to placebo. After 4 years, combination therapy with ezetimibe reduced LDL-C by 61% as compared with the effect of placebo administration. Although there was no effect on requirement for aortic valve surgery.

In 2 randomized double blind trials, the effect of statin therapy on progression of coronary artery calcification (CAC) was studied. Over a period of 12 months, intensive atorvastatin therapy was unable to attenuate CAC progression compared with standard atorvastatin therapy.[58]

Literature shows that statin therapy has reduced the incidences of cardiovascular related events however, no definitive link has been made between statins and reduction in atherosclerosis. This absence of association between cholesterol levels and the degree of atherosclerosis in unselected people was originally described in 1936.[59] Similarly, over 50 years ago, heart surgeon Michael DeBakey and his team found no correlation between blood cholesterol levels and severity of atherosclerosis in patients undergoing surgical treatment of atherosclerotic cardiovascular disease.[60] The fact is that older adults with low levels of cholesterol are just as atherosclerotic as those with high levels.[61] Despite the many contradictory findings, the advocates have praised statins as 'miracle drugs' which are 'the best anti-atherosclerotic insurance'.[62]

Premature Cataract

Cataract is a clouding of the lens in the eye, leading to impaired vision. It is caused by coagulation of protein within the lens in a small area, which is the clouded area. Statin therapy has been associated with a wide range of adverse events including cataracts.[5,19,34,63,64,65] For normal healthy individuals who are using statins as a method of primary prevention, it was discovered that for every 10,000 people taking a statin, there were 307 extra patients with cataracts.[63,66,67] There is in fact a 50 % probability of cataract development in statin users at an earlier age then non-statin users, who develop them at a significantly later age.[64] These published findings,[65-73] although not in a large number may represent a further clinical side effect which is theoretically linked to statin therapy.

Cancer

Cancer is the notorious silent killer. As well as the life-threatening genetic link, there is strong evidence that low cholesterol and statin use, in particular, are both associated with an increased risk of cancer. The carcinogenicity of lipid lower drugs has been demonstrated in animal studies.[74] Hypo-cholesteremic patients have a higher incidence of intra-cerebral bleeds, depression and cancer.[75] One systematic review found evidence that statin therapy increased risk of non-melanoma skin cancers.[76]

Vinogradova et al. documented that long-term statin use was associated with an increased risk of colorectal cancer, bladder cancer and lung cancer.[67] The ILLUMINATE trial was undertaken to investigate a drug that increases HDL but the investigators found that the drug actually resulted in an increased risk of mortality and morbidity, with high cancer rates.[77] A study on statin use and thyroid cancer showed that statin use was indeed associated with thyroid cancer in female patients.[78]

The West of Scotland Coronary Prevention Study (WOSCOPS) trial evaluated 40 mg/day pravastatin in men with hyper-cholesterolemia reported an increase in the overall incidence of cancer.[79] A study of long-term statin use and the risk of invasive ductal carcinoma (IDC) and invasive lobular carcinoma (ILC) demonstrated that current users of statins for 10 years or longer had a 1.83-fold increased risk of IDC and a 1.97-fold increased risk of ILC, compared to never users of statins. Among women diagnosed with hyper-cholesterolemia, current users of statins for 10 years or longer had more than double the risk of both IDC and ILC compared to never users.[80]

The CARE trial was a secondary-preventive trial of pravastatin and included 4,159 patients with MI and average cholesterol levels. Half of the patients were administered 40 mg pravastatin, half of them placebo. After 5 years treatment, the most serious adverse event was breast cancer, which occurred in 12 of the women (4.2 %) in the pravastatin group but in only 1 of the women (0.34 %) in the placebo group.[81] Moreover, at least 9 cohort studies have shown that low cholesterol measured 10-30 years previously is a risk factor for cancer later in life.[82]

The PROSPER trial examined pravastatin in elderly individuals with a history of, or risk factors for, vascular disease. Half of them were given pravastatin, the other half a placebo. At follow-up 3.2 years later, a substantial number of patients had died from cancer. Furthermore, the cancer difference between the two groups increased year over year.[36]

In the two first simvastatin trials, 4S and Heart Protection Study (HPS), more patients in the treatment groups were diagnosed with non-melanoma skin cancer.[83,84] Another statin trial where cancer occurred more often in the treatment group is SEAS. In this trial, 1,873 patients with various degrees of aortic stenosis and elevated total cholesterol were included. Half of them were treated with simvastatin and ezetimibe, the other half with a placebo. After 4.3 years treatment, cancer appeared in 105 patients (11.1 %) in the treatment group, but only in 70 patients (7.5 %) in the control group.[57]

The literature shows that evidence linking statin therapy use to cancer development in general, let alone a specific cancer type is mostly heterogeneous. There has been to date no cell based analysis data that evaluates the specific causative effects of statins within the body that lead to the development of cancers. It is hypothesized that in women, the lowering levels of oestrogen and progesterone have a direct effect on cholesterol levels, especially in women over the ages of 50. The body begins to produce more cholesterol to balance decreasing levels of oestrogen and progesterone due to menopause. Women then receive statins, which in turn may increase the risk of cancer development.

Erectile Dysfunction

Case reports and clinical trial evidence supported the suggestion that statins can cause erectile dysfunction (ED). Some information on possible mechanisms was obtained, but the mechanism remains uncertain.[85] A recent study of 150,000 patients who were taking statins showed unacceptable side effects, including erectile dysfunction in 20 % of participants, resulting in discontinuation of the drug.[26]

ED in association with statins was first reported by Halkin et al. where both lovastatin and pravastatin separately caused ED in a 57-year-old man.[86] Jackson reported 5 cases of ED with simvastatin at doses of 10 mg and 20 mg.[87] Sexual function was restored within 1 week of stopping the drug. Two patients were further re-challenged only to find that impotence recurred.

In the 4S study, a prospective randomized trial, 37 patients of 1,814 on simvastatin developed ED, as did 28 of 1,803 on a placebo.[84] The Australian Adverse Drug Reaction Advisory Committee (ADRAC) reported 42 cases of ED in association with simvastatin.[88] Details of cases of ED on lipid-lowering therapy reported to the UK Committee on Safety of Medicines (Yellow Card Scheme) identified 170 cases of ED.[85]

Erectile dysfunction (ED) is not mentioned in most statin trials, however, when specifically examined, around 20 % of men appear to be affected.[89] It is hypothesized that statin therapy may reduce levels of testosterone thereby exacerbating the symptoms of ED.[90]

Chronic Fatigue Syndrome

Statin therapy has been associated with decreased energy and exertional fatigue.[20] Myopathy, which is the most common adverse effect of statin treatment, is manifested by muscle aches and pains, weakness, instability, and easy fatigue.[18,19]

A double blind randomised controlled trial that compared 1,016 low risk patients receiving simvastatin 20 mg or pravastatin 40 mg with placebo showed that both drugs had a significant adverse effect on energy/fatigue exercise score with 40 % of women reporting reduced energy or fatigue with exertion.[20]

Benign Essential Tremor & Parkinson Plus Syndromes

Benign essential tremor also known as essential or familial tremor is a neurological disorder marked by recurrent shaking. Parkinson plus syndromes are a group of neurological disorders, which mimic Parkinson's disease and are difficult to distinguish and diagnose as a result. Cholesterol levels are the main determinant of coenzyme Q10, an important antioxidant and mitochondrial electron receptor.[91] Coenzyme Q10 is neuroprotective and there is evidence that it may slow the progression of Parkinson's disease.[92] Parkinson's disease and ataxia like syndrome are increasing in nature in a subcategory of old patients. Cholesterol is a critical component of neuronal cell membranes and synapses, and plays an important role in their proper functioning. A strong association between lower cholesterol and Parkinson's disease risk has been reported, such that each mmol/L increase in total cholesterol was accompanied by a 23 % decrease in the risk of developing Parkinson's disease. The risk reduction was significant in women but not in men.[93]

With this positive effect however, one should consider, is prescribing a patient with a tremor syndrome unethical due to the known adverse side effects that the patient may experience? This should be tentatively considered when prescribing statins in particular patients.

Intra-Cerebral Bleeds

High cholesterol levels have been found to be protective in the elderly against intra-cerebral bleeds and Hypo-cholesteremic patients had higher incidence of intra-cerebral bleeds.[75] Therefore, avoiding statins should be considered for patients with a history of intra-cerebral haemorrhage (ICH).[94]

Meier et al. analysed 311 consecutive patients who received intra-arterial thrombolysis. Statin pre-treatment was present in 18 %. The authors demonstrated that prior statin use is associated with a higher frequency of any ICH after intra-arterial thrombolysis.[95] Long-term treatment with lovastatin was associated with a significant reduction of fibrinogen levels and platelet aggregation induced by ADP in type-IIa hyper-cholesterolemic patients.[96]

Eichel et al. recruited 399 patients with ICH, of which 101 (25 %) were using statins. Treatment with statins prior to ICH failed to show a significant impact on outcome in this analysis despite lower haematoma volumes.[97]

The literature predominantly shows that statin therapy is in face associated with a higher risk of intra-cerebral haemorrhage. Simvastatin treatment depresses blood clotting, which leads to reduced rates of prothrombin activation, factor Va generation, fibrinogen cleavage, factor XIII activation, and an increased rate of factor Va inactivation.[98]

Interstitial Pneumonitis

Statin-induced ILD (interstitial lung disease) has been reported with most statins, suggesting that statin-induced ILD is a class effect and not a specific statin effect.[99] Kim et al. outlined a case study of statin-induced interstitial pneumonitis caused by rosuvastatin.[100] Another case study by Lantuejoul et al. described an incident of statin-induced fibrotic nonspecific interstitial pneumonia. The authors proposed that because statins are increasingly prescribed, statin-induced interstitial lung disorders might be more frequently observed.[101]

A large-scale cohort study of over 1.4 million patients from the Quebec health administrative databases was carried out between 1990-2005. 6,665 possible or probable cases of ILD were identified during follow-up.[102]

Congestive Heart Failure

Congestive Heart Failure (CHF) is characterized by a build up of fluid in the body, which emanates from a progressive decrease in pumping power of the heart. Briggs et al. examined 136,936 patients for side effects of statins. Of those prescribed higher potency statins, 16.3 % were diagnosed with CHF. Of those prescribed lower potency statins, 17.5 % were diagnosed with CHF. In total, there were 3,629 cases of new onset diabetes in the first 2 years of follow-up study population. New cases demonstrated a slightly greater prevalence of congestive heart failure.[103]

Overall, statins have been linked with CHF but studies are mixed in their conclusions.

Rhabdomyolysis

Rhabdomyolysis is the breakdown of muscle tissue resulting in the release of muscle fibre contents i.e. myoglobin into the blood. This protein and its determinants are harmful to the kidneys, which are responsible for filtrating it out of the blood. Preiss et al. predicted in an analysis of data from 5 major statin trials, an 11.3 % enhanced risk of rhabdomyolysis with utilization of high-dose statin therapy,[8] while prescribing statins to everyone over the age of 50 years is predicted to lead to 200 excess cases of rhabdomyolysis.

In a systematic review of statins with about 35,000 people and 158,000 person years in both treated and placebo groups, rhabdomyolysis was diagnosed in 8 treated and 5 placebo patients, none with serious illness or death.[104] Taylor et al. found that 0.03 % of patients experienced rhabdomyolysis, in a total of 17.3 % participants that experienced an adverse event.[105]

Rhabdomyolysis represents the least frequent side effect of statins. Although it is a potentially fatal complication caused by skeletal muscle breakdown, which is released into the blood. The rates of rhabdomyolysis have been estimated from clinical trial and cohort data as 3 per 100,000 person-years during statin treatment.[106]

When taking the previously discussed factors into account, there is a need for definitive long-term arduous data to support the use of statins, which begin in childhood. We can see that there has been a plethora of studies investigating the effects of statins in adults, however this has not been shown to any extent in children. Therefore estimating the risks in relation to statin use for children and young adults is difficult. But one can see that the risks would probably not be zero in comparison. From the literature discussed, statins do lead to increased risk of development of a number of serious side effects such as diabetes, peripheral neuritis, ICH, interstitial pneumonitis, and rhabdomyolysis.

Young adults often suffer from a genetic form of high cholesterol known as Familial hypercholesterolemia (FH). The principal treatment for FH in young adults is lifestyle modification. The recommended dietary approach for lowering LDL-C is a low saturated fat diet, devoid of trans-fat and high in fruits and vegetables, with an emphasis on fibre. Dietary advice trials have shown both the safety and the benefits of this approach in the general paediatric population,[107-109] and a meta-analysis of nutrition and physical activity trials shows that lifestyle modification can lower LDL-C and improve other cardiovascular disease risk factors in obese children.[110]

Various supplements have been used to lower LDL-C and total cholesterol.[111,112] Stanol esters have been evaluated in several studies of children with hyper-cholesterolemia, and regular intake in the form of prepared muffins, margarine spreads, or chews shows reasonable but small decreases in LDL-C of 5 % to 7 %.[113] Red rice yeast extract has to date the strongest LDL-C reducing effect described in the adult literature. One paediatric trial tested a combination of red yeast rice extract and policosanols, and produced an 18 % lowering of LDL-C in hyper-cholesterolemic children over the course of 8 weeks.[114]

Fibre is recommended as a supplement that produces a satisfactory improvement in LDL-C, depending on the baseline diet.[115,116] Bile acid binding resins have been shown in several paediatric trials to lower LDL-C by as much as 15 %.[117,118] Their use has been hampered by difficulties with adherence due to unpalatability and adverse effects such as bloating and constipation.[119] Fibrates have been used extensively in children and adolescents and again show similar efficacy to adults, with better tolerability than bile acid sequestrants but lesser efficacy in reducing LDL-C levels.[120,121] Niacin has previously been used extensively in adolescents and has similar lipid-lowering efficacy to bile acid sequestrants and fibrates.[122] Ezetimibe has been shown to reduce LDL-C levels by 20 % in children with homozygous FH.[123]

In adolescents, statins should not be used as a principal method of lowering cholesterol; rather lifestyle changes and supplements should be utilized where possible. Where adolescents are concerned, compliance to lifestyle changes such as diet change is often an issue. But examining the possible side effects that can occur with prolonged use, statins in adolescents may need to be avoided at all costs, or at least only as a final resort.

Conclusion

From the literature discussed, there is an increased risk of diabetes, myopathy, cognitive deficiencies, peripheral neuritis, cataract development, erectile dysfunction, fatigue, intra-cerebral bleeding, interstitial pneumonitis, and rhabdomyolysis. Evidence shows that statin therapy failed in primary prevention but helps patients through secondary prevention with reduction of non-cardiovascular death over 10 years. The unexpected increase of cancer and congestive cardiac failure in statin users must be scrutinised.

The majority of company funded drugs trials in the past have overestimated the benefits of statin therapy, while grossly underestimating their harms. Results provoke the possibility of not only the lack of primary cardiovascular protection by statin therapy but highlight the very real possibility of augmented cardiovascular risk in women, octogenarians, patients with diabetes and the young.

Sherif Sultan, MCh, MD, FRCS, EBQS/VASC, FACS, PhD,***, Edel P. Kavanagh, BSc, PhD**, Niamh Hynes, MD***

* Western Vascular Institute, Department of Vascular and Endovascular Surgery, University College Hospital Galway, National University of Ireland sherif.sultan@hse.ie

** Department of Vascular and Endovascular Surgery, Galway Clinic

References

1. Sukhija R, Prayaga S, Marashdeh M, et al. Effect of statins on fasting plasma glucose in diabetic and nondiabetic patients. *J Investig Med.* 2009; 57: 495-9.

2. Jupiter subanalysis Rosuvastatin for cardiovascular prevention: too many uncertainties. *Prescrire Int.* 2009; 18: 176.

3. Ahmed S, Cannon CP Murohy SA, Braunwald E. Acute coronary syndromes and diabetes: Is intensive lipid lowering beneficial? Results of the PROVE IT-TIMI 22 trial. *Eur Heart J.* 2006; 27: 2323-9

4. Huptas S, Geiss HC, Otto C, Parhofer KG. Effect of atorvastatin (10 mg/day) on glucose metabolism in patients with the metabolic syndrome. *Am J Cardiol.* 2006; 98: 66-9.

5. Culver AL, Ockene IS, Balasubramanian R, et al. Statin Use and Risk of Diabetes Mellitus in Postmenopausal Women in the Women's Health Initiative. *Arch Intern Med.* 2012; 172: 144-52.

6. de Lorgeril M, Salen P, Abramson J, et al. Cholesterol lowering, cardiovascular diseases, and the rosuvastatin-JUPITER controversy: a critical reappraisal. *Arch Intern Med.* 2010; 170: 1032-6.

7. Sattar N, Preiss D, Murray HM, et al. Statins and risk of incident diabetes: a collaborative meta-analysis of randomised statin trials. *Lancet.* 2010; 375: 735-42.

8. Preiss D, Seshasai SR, Welsh P, et al. Risk of Incident Diabetes with Intensive-Dose Compared With Moderate-Dose Statin Therapy A Meta-analysis. *JAMA.* 2011; 305: 2556-64.

9. Koh KK, Sakuma I, Quon MJ. Differential metabolic effects of distinct statins. *Atherosclerosis.* 2011; 215: 1-8.

10. Cholesterol Treatment Trialists' (CTT) Collaborators. The effects of lowering LDL cholesterol with statin therapy in people at low risk of vascular disease: meta-analysis of individual data from 27 randomised trials. *Lancet.* 2012; 380: 581-90.

11. CTT (Cholesterol Treatment Trialists' Collaboration). www.ctsu.ox.ac.uk/ research/meta-trials/ctt/ctt-website. Accessed November 19, 2015

12. Mora S, Glynn RJ, Hsia J, et al. Statins for the primary prevention of cardiovascular events in women with elevated high-sensitivity C-reactive protein or dyslipidemia. *Circulation.* 2010; 121: 1069-77.

13. Finegold J, Manisty C, Goldacre B, Barron A, Francis D. What proportion of symptomatic side effects in patients taking statins are genuinely caused by the drug? Systematic review of randomized placebo-controlled trials to aid patient choice. *Eur J Preventive Cardiol.* 2014; 21: 464-74.

14. Rajpathak SN, Kumbhani DJ, Crandall J, Barzilai N, Alderman M, Ridker PM. Statin therapy and risk of developing type 2 diabetes: a meta-analysis. *Diabetes Care.* 2009; 32: 1924-9.

15. Briggs ADM, Mizdrak A, Scarborough P. A statin a day keeps the doctor away: comparative proverb assessment modelling study. *BMJ.* 2013; 347: f7267.

16. Goldfine, A.B. Statins: is it really time to reassess benefits and risks? *N Engl J Med.* 2012; 366: 1752-5.

17. Cederberg H, Stančáková A, Yaluri N, Modi S, Kuusisto J, Laakso M. Increased risk of diabetes with statin treatment is associated with impaired insulin sensitivity and insulin secretion: a 6 year follow-up study of the METSIM cohort. *Diabetologia*, 2015; 58: 1109-17.

18. Diamond DM, Ravnskov U. How statistical deception created the appearance that statins are safe and effective in primary and secondary prevention of cardiovascular disease. *Expert Rev Clin Pharmacol.* 2015; 8: 189-99.

19. Golomb BA, Evans MA. Statin adverse effects: a review of the literature and evidence for a mitochondrial mechanism. *Am J Cardiovasc Drugs.* 2008; 8: 373-418.

20. Golomb BA, Evans MA, Dimsdale JE, White, HL. Effects of statins on energy and fatigue with exertion: results from a randomized controlled trial. *Arch Intern Med.* 2012; 172: 1180-2.

21. Golomb BA. Statins and activity: proceed with caution. *JAMA Intern Med.* 2014; 174: 1270-2.

22. Sinzinger H, Wolfram R, Peskar BA. Muscular side effects of statins. *J Cardiovasc Pharmacol.* 2002; 40: 163-71.

23. Sinzinger H, O'Grady J. Professional athletes suffering from familial hypercholesterolaemia rarely tolerate statin treatment because of muscular problems. *Br J Clin Pharmacol.* 2004; 57: 525-8.

24. Parker BA, Augeri AL, Capizzi JA, Ballard KD, Troyanos C, Baggish AL, et al. Effect of Statins on Creatine Kinase Levels Before and After a Marathon Run. *Am J Cardiol.* 2012; 109: 282-7.

25. Fernandez G, Spatz ES, Jablecki C, Phillips PS. Statin myopathy: A common dilemma not reflected in clinical trials. *Cleve Clin J Med.* 2011; 78: 393-403.

26. Zhang H, Plutzky J, Turchin A. Discontinuation of statins in routine care settings: a cohort study. *Ann Intern Med.* 2013; 158: 526-34.

27. Buettner CA, Davis RB, Leveille SG, Mittleman MA, Mukamal KJ. Prevalence of musculoskeletal pain and statin use. *J Gen Intern Med.* 2008; 23: 1182-6.

28. Mansi I, Frei CR, Pugh MJ, Makris U, Mortensen EM. Statins and musculoskeletal conditions, arthropathies, and injuries. *JAMA Intern Med.* 2013; 73: 1-10.

29. Graham, D.J. Staffa JA, Shatin D, et al. Incidence of hospitalized rhabdomyolysis in patients treated with lipid-lowering drugs. *JAMA.* 2014; 292: 2585-90.

30. Joy TR, Hegele RA. Narrative review: statin-related myopathy. *Ann Intern Med.* 2009; 150: 858-68..

31. Bellosta S, Paoletti R, Corsini A. Safety of statins: focus on clinical pharmacokinetics and drug interactions. *Circulation.* 2004; 109: III50-7.

32. Phillips PS, Haas RH, Bannykh S, et al. Statin-associated myopathy with normal creatine kinase levels. *Ann Intern Med.* 2002; 137: 581-5.

33. Draeger A, Monastyrskaya K, Mohaupt M, et al. Statin therapy induces ultrastructural damage in skeletal muscle in patients without myalgia. *J Pathol.* 2006; 210: 94-102.

34. Graveline D. Adverse effects of statin drugs: a physician patient's perspective. *J Am Phys Surg.* 2015; 20: 7-11.

35. Tatley M, Savage R. Psychiatric adverse reactions with statins, fibrates and ezetimibe implications for the use of lipid-lowering agents. *Drug Safety.* 2007; 30: 195-201.

36. Shepherd J, Blauw GJ, Murphy MB, et al. Pravastatin in elderly individuals at risk of vascular disease (PROSPER): a randomised controlled trial. *Lancet.* 2002; 360: 1623-30.

37. McGuinness B, O'Hare J, Craig D, Bullock R, Malouf R, Passmore P. Cochrane review on 'Statins for the treatment of dementia'. *Int J Geriatr Psychiatry.* 2013; 28: 119-26.

38. Pandey RD, Gupta PP, Jha D, Kumar S. Role of statins in Alzheimer's disease: a retrospective meta-analysis for commonly investigated clinical parameters in RCTs. *Int J Neurosci.* 2013; 123: 521-5.

39. Strom BL, Schinnar R, Karlawish J, Hennessy S, Teal V, Bilker WB. Statin Therapy and Risk of Acute Memory Impairment. *JAMA Intern Med.* 2015;175:1399-1405.

40. Evans MA, Golomb BA. Statin-associated adverse cognitive effects: survey results from 171 patients. *Pharmacotherapy.* 2009; 29: 800-11.

41. Padala KP, Padala PR, McNeilly DP, Geske JA, Sullivan DH, Potter JF. The effect of HMG-CoA reductase inhibitors on cognition in patients with Alzheimer's dementia: a prospective withdrawal and rechallenge pilot study. *Am J Geriatr Pharmacother.* 2012; 10: 296-302.

42. Sahebzamani FM, Munro CL, Marroquin OC, .Diamond DM, Keller E, Kip, KE. Examination of the FDA warning for statins and cognitive dysfunction. *J Pharmacovigil.* 2014; 2: 141.

43. Tierney EF, Thurman DJ, Beckles GL, Cadwell BL. Association of statin use with peripheral neuropathy in the U.S. population 40 years of age or older. *J Diabetes.* 2013; 5: 207-15.

44. Gaist D, Jeppesen U, Andersen M, García Rodríguez LA, Hallas J, Sindrup SH.. Statins and risk of polyneuropathy: a case-control study. *Neurology.* 2002; 58: 1333-7.

45. Flavahan NA. Atherosclerosis or lipoprotein-induced endothelial dysfunction. Potential mechanisms underlying reduction in EDRF/nitric oxide activity. *Circulation* 1992; 85: 1927-38.

46. Volek JS, Fernandez ML, Feinman RD, Phinney SD. Dietary carbohydrate restriction induces a unique metabolic state positively affecting atherogenic dyslipidemia, fatty acid partitioning, and metabolic syndrome. *Prog Lipid Res.* 2008; 47: 307-18.

47. Forsythe CE, Phinney SD, Fernandez ML, Quann EE, Wood RJ, Bibus DM, Kraemer WJ, Feinman RD, Volek JS. Comparison of low fat and low carbohydrate diets on circulating fatty acid composition and markers of inflammation. Lipids. 2008; 43: 65-77.

48. Tribble DL, Holl LG, Wood PD, Krauss RM. Variations in oxidative susceptibility among six low density lipoprotein subfractions of differing density and particle size. Atherosclerosis. 1992; 93: 189-99.

49. Dreon DM, Fernstrom HA, Campos H, Blanche P, Williams PT, Krauss RM. Change in dietary saturated fat intake is correlated with change in mass of large low-density-lipoprotein particles in men. Am J Clin Nutr. 1998; 67: 828-36.

50. Foster GD, Wyatt HR, Hill JO, et al. A randomized trial of a low-carbohydrate diet for obesity. N Engl J Med. 2003; 348: 2082-90.

51. Stern L, Iqbal N, Seshadri P, et al. The effects of low-carbohydrate versus conventional weight loss diets in severely obese adults: one-year follow-up of a randomized trial. Ann Intern Med. 2004; 140: 778-85.

52. Gardner C, Kiazand A, Alhassan S, et al. Comparison of the Atkins, Zone, Ornish, and LEARN diets for change in weight and related risk factors among overweight premenopausal women. JAMA. 2007; 297: 969-77.

53. Yancy WS Jr, Olsen MK, Guyton JR, Bakst RP, Westman EC. A low-carbohydrate, ketogenic diet versus a low-fat diet to treat obesity and hyperlipidemia: a randomized, controlled trial. Ann Intern Med. 2004; 140: 769-77.

54. Shai I, Schwarzfuchs D, Henkin Y, et al. Weight loss with a low-carbohydrate, Mediterranean, or low-fat diet. N Engl J Med. 2008; 359: 229-41.

55. Crouse JR, Raichlen JS, Riley WA, et al. Effect of Rosuvastatin on Progression of Carotid Intima-Media Thickness in Low-Risk Individuals With Subclinical Atherosclerosis: The METEOR Trial. JAMA. 2007; 297: 1344-53.

56. Kastelein JJ, Akdim F, Stroes ES, et al. Simvastatin with or without ezetimibe in familial hypercholesterolemia. N Engl J Med. 2008; 358: 1431-43.

57. Rosseb AB, Pedersen TR, Boman K, et al. Intensive lipid lowering with simvastatin and ezetimibe in aortic stenosis. N Engl J Med. 2008; 359: 1343-56.

58. Schmermund A, Achenbach S, Budde T, et al. Effect of intensive versus standard lipid-lowering treatment with atorvastatin on the progression of calcified coronary atherosclerosis over 12 months: a multicenter, randomized, double-blind trial. Circulation. 2006; 113: 427-37.

59. Lande KE, Sperry WM. Human atherosclerosis in relation to cholesterol content of blood serum. Arch Pathol. 1936; 22: 301-13.

60. Garret HE, Horning EC, Creech RG, DeBakey M. Serum cholesterol values in patients treated surgically for atherosclerosis. JAMA. 1964; 189: 655-9.

61. Ravnskov U. Is atherosclerosis caused by high cholesterol? QJM. 2002; 95: 397-403.

62. Roberts WC. The underused miracle drugs: the statin drugs are to atherosclerosis what penicillin was to infectious disease. Am J Cardiol. 1996; 78: 377-8.

63. Hippisley-Cox J, Coupland C. Unintended Effects of Statins in Men and Women in England and Wales: Population Based Cohort Study Using the Q Research Database. *BMJ.* 2010; 340: c2197.

64. Machan CM, Hrynchak PK, Irving EL. Age- Related Cataract Is Associated with Type 2 Diabetes and Statin Use. *Optom Vis Sci.* 2012; 89: 1165-71.

65. Foody J. Statin use associated with increased risk of cataract, myopathy, liver dysfunction and acute renal failure with varying numbers needed to harm. *Evid Based Med.* 2010; 15: 187-8.

66. El-Salem, K Ababneh B, Rudnicki S. Prevalence and Risk Factors of Muscle Complications Secondary to Statins. *Muscle Nerve.* 2011; 44: 877-81.

67. Vinogradova Y, Coupland C, Hippisley-Cox J. Exposure to Statins and Risk of Common Cancers: A Series of Nested Case-Control Studies. *BMC Cancer.* 2011; 11: 409.

68. Bates TR, Connaughton VM, Watts GF. Non-adherence to statin therapy: a major challenge for preventive cardiology. *Expert Opin Pharmacother.* 2009; 10: 2973-85.

69. Bouchard MH, Dragomir A, Blais L, Berard A, Pilon D, Perreault S. Impact of adherence to statins on coronary artery disease in primary prevention. *Br J Clin Pharmacol.* 2007; 63:698-708.

70. Leuschen J, Mortensen EM, Frei CR, Mansi EA, Panday V, Mansi I. Association of statin use with cataracts: a propensity score-matched analysis. *JAMA Ophthalmol.* 2013; 131: 1427-34.

71. Perreault S, Blais L, Dragomir A, et al. Persistence and determinants of statin therapy among middle-aged patients free of cardiovascular disease. *Eur J Clin Pharmacol.* 2005; 61: 667-74.

72. Perreault S, Blais L, Lamarre D, et al. Persistence and determinants of statin therapy among middle-aged patients for primary and secondary prevention. *Br J Clin Pharmacol.* 2005; 59: 564-73.

73. Poluzzi E, Strahinja P, Lanzoni M, et al. Adherence to statin therapy and patients' cardiovascular risk: a pharmacoepidemiological study in Italy. *Eur J Clin Pharmacol.* 2008; 64: 425-32.

74. Newman TB, Hulley SB. Carcinogenicity of lipid-lowering drugs. *JAMA.* 1996; 275: 55-60.

75. S. Sultan, N. Hynes, Cardiovascular Disease: Primary Prevention, Disease Modulation and Regenerative Therapy. *Vascular.* 2012; 20: 243-50.

76. Kuoppala J, Lamminpää A, Pukkala E. Statins and Cancer: A Systematic Review and Meta-Analysis. *Euro J Cancer.* 2008; 44: 2122-32.

77. Barter PJ, Caulfield M, Eriksson M. For the Illuminate Investigators. Effects of Torcetrapib in Patients at High Risk for Coronary Events. *New Eng J Med.* 2007; 357: 2109-22.

78. Hung SH, Lin HC, Chung SD. Statin use and thyroid cancer: a population-based case–control study. *Clin Endocrinol (Oxf).* 2015; 83: 111-6.

79. Shepherd, J. Cobbe SM, Ford I, et al. Prevention of coronary heart disease with pravastatin in men with hypercholesterolemia. West of Scotland Coronary Prevention Study Group. *N Engl J Med.* 1995; 333: 1301-7.

80. McDougall JA, Malone KE, Daling JR, Cushing-Haugen KL, Porter PL, Li CI. Long-term statin use and risk of ductal and lobular breast cancer among women 55 to 74 years of age. *Cancer Epidemiol Biomarkers Prev.* 2013; 22: 1529-37.

81. Sacks FM, Pfeffer MA, Moye LA, et al. The effect of pravastatin on coronary events after myocardial infarction in patients with average cholesterol levels. Cholesterol and recurrent events trial investigators. *N Engl J Med.* 1996; 335: 1001-9.

82. Ravnskov U, Rosch PJ, McCully KS. The statin-low cholesterol-cancer conundrum. *QJM.* 2012; 105: 383-8.

83. Heart Protection Study Collaborative Group. MRC/BHF Heart Protection Study of cholesterol lowering with simvastatin in 20,536 high-risk individuals: a randomized placebo-controlled trial. *Lancet.* 2002; 360: 7-22.

84. Scandinavian Simvastatin Survival Study Group. Randomised trial of cholesterol lowering in 4444 patients with coronary heart disease: the Scandinavian simvastatin survival study (4S). *Lancet.* 1994; 344: 1383-9.

85. Rizvi K, Hampson JP, Harvey J N. Do lipid-lowering drugs cause erectile dysfunction? A systematic review. *Fam Prac.* 2002; 19: 95-98.

86. Halkin A, Lossos IS, Mevaorach D. HMG-CoA reductase inhibitor-induced impotence (letter). *Ann Pharmacother.* 1996; 30: 192.

87. Jackson G. Simvastatin and impotence. *Br Med J.* 1997; 315: 31.

88. Adverse Drug Reactions Advisory Committee. Simvastatin and adverse endocrine effects in men. *Aust Adverse Drug React Bull.* 1995; 14: 10.

89. Solomon H, Samarasinghe YP, Feher MD, et al. Erectile dysfunction and statin treatment in high cardiovascular risk patients. *Int J Clin Pract.* 2006; 60: 141-5.

90. Cai X, Tian Y, Wu T, Cao CX, Bu SY, Wang KJ. The role of statins in erectile dysfunction: a systematic review and meta-analysis. *Asian J Androl.* 2014; 16: 461-6.

91. Shults CW, Oakes D, Kieburtz K, et al. Effects of Coenzyme Q10 in Early Parkinson Disease: Evidence of Slowing of the Functional Decline. *Arch Neurol.* 2002; 59: 1541-50.

92. Lieberman A, Lyons K, Levine J. Myerburg R. Statins, Cholesterol, Co-Enzyme Q10, and Parkinson's Disease. *Parkinsonism Relat Disord.* 2005; 11: 81-4.

93. Huang X, Chen H, Miller WC, et al. Lower Low-Density Lipoprotein Cholesterol Levels Are Associated with Parkinson's Disease. *Mov Disord.* 2007; 22: 377-81.

94. Westover MB, Bianchi MT, Eckman MH, Greenberg SM. Statin Use Following Intracerebral Hemorrhage: A Decision Analysis. *Arch Neurol.* 2011; 68: 573-9.

95. Meier N, Nedeltchev K, Brekenfeld, C, et al. Prior statin use, intracranial hemorrhage, and outcome after intra-arterial thrombolysis for acute ischemic stroke. *Stroke.* 2009; 40: 1729-37.

96. Mayer J, Eller T, Brauer P, et al. Effects of long-term treatment with lovastatin on the clotting system and blood platelets. *Annals Hematol.* 1992; 64: 196-201.

97. Eichel R, Khoury ST, Ben-Hur T, Keidar M, Paniri R, Leker RR. Prior use of statins and outcome in patients with intracerebral haemorrhage. *Euro J Neurol.* 2010; 17: 78-83.

98. Undas A, Brummel KE, Musial J, Mann KG, Szczeklik A. Simvastatin depresses blood clotting by inhibiting activation of prothrombin, factor V, and factor XIII and by enhancing factor Va inactivation. *Circulation.* 2001; 103: 2248-53.

99. Fernández A, Karas R, Alsheikh-Ali A, Thompson P. Statins and interstitial lung disease: a systematic review of the literature and of food and drug administration adverse event reports. *Chest.* 2008; 134: 824-30.

100. Kim SY, Kim SJ, Yoon D, Hong SW, Park S, Ock CY. A Case of Statin-Induced Interstitial Pneumonitis due to Rosuvastatin. *Tuberc Respir Dis (Seoul).* 2015; 78: 281-5.

101. Lantuejoul S, Brambilla E, Brambilla C, Devouassoux G. Statin-induced fibrotic nonspecific interstitial pneumonia. *Eur Respir J.* 2002; 19: 577-80.

102. Saad N, Camus P, Suissa S, Ernst P. Statins and the risk of interstitial lung disease: a cohort study. *Thorax.* 2013; 68: 361-4.

103. Dormuth CR, Filion KB, Paterson JM, et al. Higher potency statins and the risk of new diabetes: multicentre, observational study of administrative databases. *BMJ.* 2014; 348: g3244.

104. Law MR, Wald NJ, Rudnicka AR. Quantifying effect of statins on low density lipoprotein cholesterol, ischaemic heart disease, and stroke: systematic review and meta-analysis. *BMJ.* 2003; 326: 1-7.

105. Taylor F, Huffman MD, Macedo AF, et al. Statins for the primary prevention of cardiovascular disease. *Cochrane Database Syst Rev.* 2013; 1:CD004816.

106. Law M, Rudnicka AR. Statin safety: a systematic review. *Am J Cardiol.* 2006; 97: 52C-60C.

107. Expert panel on integrated guidelines for cardiovascular health and risk reduction in children and adolescents: summary report. *Pediatrics.* 2011; 128: S213-56.

108. Efficacy and safety of lowering dietary intake of fat and cholesterol in children with elevated low-density lipoprotein cholesterol. The Dietary Intervention Study in Children (DISC). The Writing Group for the DISC Collaborative Research Group. *JAMA.* 1995; 273: 1429-35.

109. Niinikoski H, Lagstrom H, Jokinen E, et al. Impact of repeated dietary counseling between infancy and 14 years of age on dietary intakes and serum lipids and lipoproteins. The STRIP Study. *Circulation.* 2007; 116: 1032-40.

110. Ho M, Garnett SP, Baur L, et al. Effectiveness of lifestyle interventions in child obesity: systematic review with meta-analysis. *Pediatrics.* 2012; 130: e1647-71.

111. Musa-Veloso K, Poon TH, Elliot JA, Chung C. A comparison of the LDL-cholesterol lowering efficacy of plant stanols and plant sterols over a continuous dose range: results of a meta-analysis of randomized, placebo-controlled trials. *Prostaglandins Leukot Essent Fatty Acids.* 2011; 85: 9-28.

112. Li Y, Jiang L, Jia Z, et al. A meta-analysis of red yeast rice: an effective and relatively safe alternative approach for dyslipidemia. *PLoS One.* 2014; 9 :e98611.

113. Tammi A, Ronnemaa T, Gylling H, et al. Plant stanol ester margarine lowers serum total and low-density lipoprotein cholesterol concentrations of healthy children: the STRIP project. Special Turku Coronary Risk Factors Intervention Project. *J Pediatr.* 2000; 136: 503-10.

114. Guardamagna O, Abello F, Baracco V, Stasiowska B, Martino F. The treatment of hypercholesterolemic children: efficacy and safety of a combination of red yeast rice extract and policosanols. *Nutr Metab Cardiovasc Dis.* 2011; 21: 424-9.

115. Kwiterovich PO Jr. The role of fibre in the treatment of hypercholesterolemia in children and adolescents. *Pediatrics.* 1995; 96: 1005-9.

116. Dennison BA, Levine DM. Randomized, double-blind, placebocontrolled, two-period crossover clinical trial of psyllium fibre in children with hypercholesterolemia. *J Pediatr.* 1993; 123: 24-9.

117. Tonstad S, Knudtzon J, Sivertsen M, Refsum H, Ose L. Efficacy and safety of cholestyramine therapy in peripubertal and prepubertal children with familial hypercholesterolemia. *J Pediatr.* 1996; 129: 42-9.

118. Liacouras CA, Coates PM, Gallagher PR, Cortner JA. Use of cholestyramine in the treatment of children with familial combined hyperlipidemia. *J Pediatr.* 1993; 122: 477-82.

119. McCrindle BW, O'Neill MB, Cullen-Dean G, Helden E. Acceptability and compliance with two forms of cholestyramine in the treatment of hypercholesterolemia in children: a randomized, crossover trial. *J Pediatr.* 1997; 130: 266-73.

120. Becker M, Staab D, Von BK. Long-term treatment of severe familial hypercholesterolemia in children: effect of sitosterol and bezafibrate. *Pediatrics.* 1992; 89: 138-42.

121. Wheeler KA, West RJ, Lloyd JK, Barley J. Double blind trial of bezafibrate in familial hypercholesterolaemia. *Arch Dis Child.* 1985; 60: 34-7.

122. Stein EA. Treatment of familial hypercholesterolemia with drugs in children. *Arteriosclerosis.* 1989; 9: I145-51.

123. Gagne C, Gaudet D, Bruckert E. Efficacy and safety of ezetimibe coadministered with atorvastatin or simvastatin in patients with homozygous familial hypercholesterolemia. *Circulation.* 2002; 105: 2469-75.